# Register Now for Online Access to Your Book!

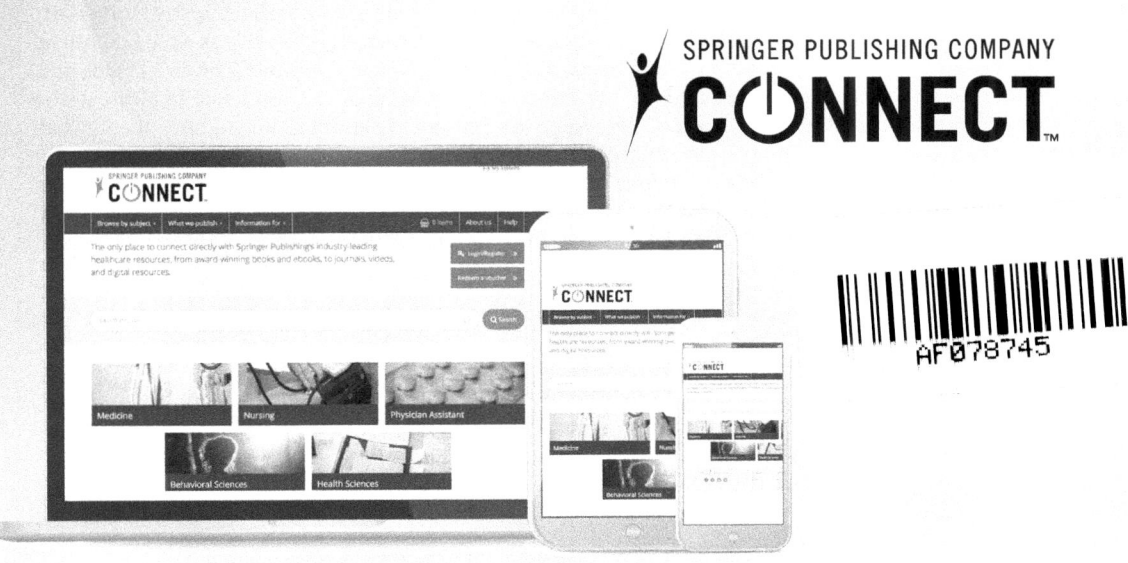

Your print purchase of *Neuroscience Certification Review for Nurses* **includes online access to the contents of your book**—increasing accessibility, portability, and searchability!

**Access today at:**

http://connect.springerpub.com/content/book/978-0-8261-8822-9
or scan the QR code at the right with your smartphone
and enter the access code below.

**2KL0XE1L**

*Scan here for quick access.*

If you are experiencing problems accessing the digital component of this product, please contact our customer service department at cs@springerpub.com

The online access with your print purchase is available at the publisher's discretion and may be removed at any time without notice.

**Publisher's Note:** New and used products purchased from third-party sellers are not guaranteed for quality, authenticity, or access to any included digital components.

**SPRINGER PUBLISHING COMPANY**
View all our products at springerpub.com

**Kendra Menzies Kent, MS, RN, CENP, CCRN, CNRN, SCRN, TCRN,** graduated from the University of Texas in Arlington in 1985 with her BSN. She successfully completed and graduated from Parkland Memorial Hospital's Critical Care and Trauma Internship. She has worked in the Surgery/Trauma, Thoracic and Neurosurgical ICU at Parkland Memorial Hospital as a staff nurse and nurse educator. Ms. Kent has been a manager on a trauma floor and the director of critical care at Zale Lipshy University Hospital in Dallas. She has her master's of nursing from Texas Women's University as a clinical nurse specialist (CNS) and has worked as a CNS in the surgical trauma ICU at Parkland Memorial Hospital. Ms. Kent moved to Florida and is currently the director of the Marcus Neuroscience Institute associated with Boca Raton Regional Hospital. Ms. Kent has presented seminars throughout the United States, Canada, and Oman. She has also published multiple chapters and books, including the books *Adult CCRN® Certification Review* and *Trauma Certified Registered Nurse (TCRN®) Examination Review*, published by Springer Publishing Company. Ms. Kent has been known to be engaging and supportive to nurses desiring certification. She receives emails from nurses who are excited that they have successfully passed their examinations.

# Neuroscience Certification Review for Nurses

## Think in Questions, Learn by Rationales

Kendra Menzies Kent, MS, RN, CENP, CCRN, CNRN, SCRN, TCRN

SPRINGER PUBLISHING COMPANY

Copyright © 2020 Springer Publishing Company, LLC

All rights reserved.

No part of this publication may be reproduced, stored in a retrieval system, or transmitted in any form or by any means, electronic, mechanical, photocopying, recording, or otherwise, without the prior permission of Springer Publishing Company, LLC, or authorization through payment of the appropriate fees to the Copyright Clearance Center, Inc., 222 Rosewood Drive, Danvers, MA 01923, 978-750-8400, fax 978-646-8600, info@copyright.com or on the Web at www.copyright.com.

Springer Publishing Company, LLC
11 West 42nd Street
New York, NY 10036
www.springerpub.com
http://connect.springerpub.com

*Acquisitions Editor*: Elizabeth Nieginski
*Compositor*: Amnet Systems

ISBN: 978-0-8261-8818-2
ebook ISBN: 978-0-8261-8822-9
DOI: 10.1891/9780826188229

19 20 21 22 23 / 5 4 3 2 1

The author and the publisher of this Work have made every effort to use sources believed to be reliable to provide information that is accurate and compatible with the standards generally accepted at the time of publication. Because medical science is continually advancing, our knowledge base continues to expand. Therefore, as new information becomes available, changes in procedures become necessary. We recommend that the reader always consult current research and specific institutional policies before performing any clinical procedure. The author and publisher shall not be liable for any special, consequential, or exemplary damages resulting, in whole or in part, from the readers' use of, or reliance on, the information contained in this book. The publisher has no responsibility for the persistence or accuracy of URLs for external or third-party Internet websites referred to in this publication and does not guarantee that any content on such websites is, or will remain, accurate or appropriate.

Springer Publishing Company recognizes that the Certified Neuroscience Registered Nurse (CNRN®) exam is a registered service mark of the American Board of Neuroscience Nursing (ABNN). The American Board of Neuroscience Nursing neither sponsors nor endorses this product.

**Library of Congress Cataloging-in-Publication Data**

Names: Menzies Kent, Kendra, author.
Title: Neuroscience certification review for nurses : think in questions, learn by rationales / Kendra Menzies Kent.
Description: New York, NY : Springer Publishing Company, [2020] | Includes bibliographical references and index.
Identifiers: LCCN 2019028574 (print) | ISBN 9780826188182 (paperback) | ISBN 9780826188229 (ebook)
Subjects: MESH: Neuroscience Nursing | Central Nervous System Diseases—nursing | Examination Question
Classification: LCC RT55 (print) | LCC RT55 (ebook) | NLM WY 18.2 | DDC 610.73076—dc23
LC record available at https://lccn.loc.gov/2019028574
LC ebook record available at https://lccn.loc.gov/2019028575

Contact us to receive discount rates on bulk purchases.
We can also customize our books to meet your needs.
For more information, please contact: sales@springerpub.com

Kendra Menzies Kent: https://orcid.org/0000-0003-3978-3324

**Publisher's Note:** New and used products purchased from third-party sellers are not guaranteed for quality, authenticity, or access to any included digital components.

Printed in the United States of America.

*To my wonderful husband, Robby, and to my parents,
Sid and Judy, for all of the love and support they have given me.*

# Contents

*Preface*   ix

*Introduction: Think in Questions*   xi

1. Chronic Neurological Disorders   *1*
2. Cerebrovascular Disorders   *29*
3. Tumors of the Brain and Spinal Cord   *49*
4. Immune Infections, Part 1   *69*
5. Immune Infections, Part 2   *83*
6. Seizures   *105*
7. Pediatric and Developmental Disorders   *123*
8. Neurological Trauma: Traumatic Brain Injury   *141*
9. Neurological Trauma: Spinal Cord Injury   *161*
10. Practice Exam   *177*
11. Chapter Review Answers and Rationales   *213*
12. Answers and Rationales for the Practice Exam   *223*
13. Bonus Exam Questions   *257*
14. Answers and Rationales for the Bonus Exam Questions   *285*

*Index*   313

# Preface

Welcome to the first edition of *Neuroscience Certification Review for Nurses*. This book was created specifically for neuroscience nurses as a comprehensive review book to prepare for successful completion of the national certification examination. It presents question styles and content material used by the American Board of Neuroscience Nursing.

This book can be used to enhance study habits, hone test-taking skills, prepare for the Certified Neuroscience Registered Nurse exam, reinforce knowledge, and avoid test-taking errors. This book can also be used for continuing education for all neuroscience nurses, even if they are not planning on taking the examination.

The book provides an overview of the certification exams written specifically by the certification organizations themselves. Distinctive to this book is a format of asking a question and thinking through a response with rationales. This review book is unique in its "think in questions" format, which helps readers to anticipate the kinds of questions that might be asked and to promote critical thinking throughout the exam. The content review comprises bite-sized sections for easier learning and memorization that includes thousands of unfolding questions, answers, and hints.

The book contains practice questions in content areas that are tested on the exams. To reinforce your knowledge, each question is associated with a rationale explaining why it is correct. A practice exam that is representative in length, variety, and complexity of the board exam questions is provided and can be taken in a timed format to assess your abilities under pressure.

I am eager to receive feedback on this book regarding the questions and rationales and offering suggestions for additions so that we can make the next edition even more superior. Please send any comments, suggestions, feedback, or criticisms to Kendra Kent at kendrakentcr@aol.com.

*Kendra Menzies Kent*

# Introduction
## Think in Questions

## INTRODUCTION

Welcome to the journey toward certification. This book was written to help guide you on the journey. It is written in a question/answer format to encourage you to think in questions when studying for the examination. I encourage you, when you study, to ask yourself, "What can they ask about this particular topic? What would be a good question?" This prepares you for questions rather than just attempting to memorize content for the certification examination.

The book provides multiple-choice questions similar to the questions that are found on the Certified Neuroscience Registered Nurse examination. These questions allow the nurse to practice taking an exam and will assist the nurse in determining areas that require further study prior to taking the Certified Neuroscience Registered Nurse examination. The answers and rationales, including some test-taking skills, are provided for each question, further preparing the nurse for the real examination.

## WHY CERTIFICATION?

The most important reason for certification is to do it for yourself (Box I.1). Certification is viewed as a mark of excellence in an area of specialty. It is an achievement and qualification that can be seen by peers, physicians, healthcare institutes, and patients/families. Becoming certified takes a dedication to neuroscience nursing and demonstrates a level of competency. The Certified Neuroscience Registered Nurse examination is developed to verify knowledge in trauma nursing.

**Box I.1** Reasons to Become Certified

| |
|---|
| Validate your knowledge of neuroscience to your hospital and peers |
| Validate your knowledge of neuroscience to the patients |
| Validate your knowledge of neuroscience to the physician |
| Promote continuing excellence in the nursing profession |
| Demonstrate competency |
| Promote self-confidence |
| Encourage continuing education |
| Hospital credentialing |
| Monetary benefit (from some hospitals) |

## CERTIFIED NEUROSCIENCE REGISTERED NURSE EXAMINATION INFORMATION

The Certified Neuroscience Registered Nurse examination was developed by the American Board of Neuroscience Nursing (ABNN) and incorporates care of neuroscience patients from prevention to rehabilitation. The exam covers all ages, pediatrics through geriatrics. The examination follows the test plan developed by the ABNN, and the test is developed and reviewed by experts in neuroscience nursing. Access www.abnncertification.org for the *Certified Neuroscience Registered Nurse Application Handbook*. The exam application can be completed online. The Certified Neuroscience Registered Nurse is a 5-year certification for neuroscience nurses.

## EXAMINATION

The Certified Neuroscience Registered Nurse examination has 220 scored multiple-choice questions, and 20 of the questions are not scored and will not count for or against you. Those 20 questions are being tested for use in future examinations. You will not know which questions count, so complete all 220 questions as if they do count. The test is not arranged per system but is randomized. You may have one question on chest trauma and the next on spinal cord injury. The time allowed to complete the examination is 4 hours.

Eligibility to take the Certified Neuroscience Registered Nurse examination requires a registered nurse (RN) licensure and at least 1-year of full-time (2,080 hours) direct or indirect neuroscience nursing practice as an RN during the past 3 years at the time of application.

The Certified Neuroscience Registered Nurse examination is offered as a computer-based test (CBT). Once ABNN receives the application, applicants may schedule an appointment to sit for the examination through PSI Services at the www.goAMP.com website. Immediate test results with score breakdowns are available. Following successful completion of the exam (which I know everyone will have), a certificate will be sent in the mail within 4 to 6 weeks.

Renewal of your Certified Neuroscience Registered Nurse certification can be done through continuing education (CE) or retaking the examination. Applications to recertify by CE are due in October of the year that certification expires and involve two options depending on the neuroscience practice hours.

- Option A: 4,160 neuroscience nursing practice hours in the past 5 years (equivalent to 2 years' full-time work) and 75 CE hours
- Option B: 2,500 neuroscience nursing practice hours in the past 5 years (equivalent to 2 years' part-time work) and 100 CE hours

For more details on renewal, use the ABNN's website for recertification and for understanding the CE.

## TEST PLAN

The Certified Neuroscience Registered Nurse test plan is a blueprint for the exam content. Each major system is divided into subheadings and topics (Box I.2).

**Box I.2** Certified Neuroscience Registered Nurse Test Plan

| Major System | Percentage of Test | Topics |
|---|---|---|
| Trauma | 18% | Traumatic brain injuries<br>  1. Blast<br>  2. Blunt<br>  3. Penetrating<br>  4. Hematoma/hemorrhage (SDH, EDH, ICH, SAH)<br>  5. Diffuse axonal injury<br>  6. Contusions<br>  7. Concussions<br>Spinal injuries |
| Cerebrovascular | 26% | Transient ischemic attack<br>Aneurysm<br>Arteriovenous malformation<br>Arteriovenous fistula<br>Carotid stenosis<br>Cavernous angiomas<br>Carotid dissection<br>Vertebral dissection<br>Ischemic stroke<br>  1. Thrombotic<br>  2. Embolic<br>  3. Lacunar<br>Hemorrhagic stroke<br>  1. Intracerebral hemorrhage<br>  2. Subarachnoid hemorrhage<br>  3. Intraventricular hemorrhage<br>  4. Hemorrhagic conversion<br>Anoxic injury |
| Tumors | 13% | Brain tumors<br>  1. Neuroepithelial tissue<br>  2. Cranial and spinal nerves<br>  3. Meningeal and related tissues<br>  4. Hematopoietic<br>  5. Endocrine<br>  6. Metastatic<br>Spinal cord tumors<br>  1. Primary<br>  2. Metastatic<br>  3. Neurofibroma |
| Immune/infections | 11% | Abscesses<br>Amyotrophic lateral sclerosis<br>AIDS<br>Bell's palsy<br>Encephalitis<br>Demyelinating polyneuropathy<br>  1. GB syndrome<br>  2. ADEM |

*(continued)*

**Box I.2** Certified Neuroscience Registered Nurse Test Plan (*continued*)

| Major System | Percentage of Test | Topics |
|---|---|---|
| | | 3. CIDP<br>4. Meningitis<br>5. Multiple sclerosis<br>6. Myasthenia gravis<br>7. Prion disease<br>8. Encephalopathies |
| Seizures | 9% | Partial<br>Generalized<br>Status epilepticus<br>Nonepileptic seizures |
| Pediatric and developmental | 8% | Chiari malformation<br>Cerebral palsy<br>Spina bifida |
| Chronic neurological | 15% | Headache<br>  1. Acute<br>  2. Chronic<br>Pain<br>  1. Acute<br>  2. Chronic<br>  3. Neuropathic<br>Dementia<br>  1. Alzheimer's disease<br>  2. Vascular<br>Movement disorders<br>  1. Parkinson's disease<br>  2. Dystonia<br>  3. Benign essential tremor<br>  4. Tourette's syndrome<br>  5. Huntington's syndrome<br>  6. Restless leg syndrome<br>Sleep disorders<br>Chemical dependency<br>Degenerative spine disease<br>  1. Degenerative disc disease<br>  2. Vertebral compression fractures<br>  3. Lumbar spondylolisthesis<br>  4. Spinal stenosis<br>  5. Herniated nucleus pulposus<br>Balance and dizziness disorders<br>Peripheral nerve injury<br>Repetitive stress injury<br>Hydrocephalus<br>  1. Communicating<br>  2. Noncommunicating<br>  3. Normal pressure |

ADEM, acute disseminating encephalomyelitis; CIDP, chronic inflammatory demyelinating polyneuropathy; EDH, extradural hematoma; GB, Guillain–Barré syndrome; ICH, intracerebral hemorrhage; SAH, subarachnoid hemorrhage; SDH, subdural hematoma.

For clinical practice categories, the nursing process will be distributed as shown in Box I.3.

**Box I.3** Nursing Process Distributions in Clinical Practice Categories of the Certified Neuroscience Registered Nurse Test

| Clinical Practice Category | Nursing Process Distribution |
|---|---|
| Basic physiology | 20% |
| Complex physiology | 36% |
| Behavior | 15% |
| Family and culture | 9% |
| Safety | 11% |
| Health system | 9% |

## PREPARATION

Be positive! Avoid any negative thoughts about passing the examination. These can be self-fulfilling. Set the test date and then establish a realistic schedule for preparing for the examination. Set your priorities: Study the areas you are less familiar with first. Look at the percentage of each body system and establish timelines based on the largest to smallest percentage of questions. Know how you study the best: by yourself or in study groups. Study in the manner that works best for you. There are flash cards, practice questions, review courses, study books in outline format, and study books in narrative format available for studying. Practice your test questions within a set time limit to become accustomed to the time limitations. Allow 2 minutes or less per question (remember the 50-questions-per-hour rule).

When using the practice test questions to study, determine several things when the answers and rationales are being reviewed. Analyze why you missed the question: Did you just not know the content? Go back and restudy this section. Did you misread the question? Did you misread the answers? Did you miss an important element in the question or scenario? Was there a clue based on age, timeline, or symptoms?

## DAY OF THE TEST

Eat healthfully and limit the amount of liquids (to avoid the need for breaks during the exam) before the examination. Remember, restroom breaks are allowed, but the test time does not stop!

Do not try to cram immediately before this test; this will increase your anxiety level. After the exam, make plans to do something special for yourself.

Know where you are going before the actual day of the test. Know how long it will take to get there at the time of day you are scheduled to take the examination. Running late and feeling hurried will increase your anxiety and can poorly affect your test-taking skills. Plus, if you are more than 15 minutes late, they will not let you in to take the examination.

Bring your letter of approval and two forms of identification (one picture ID). You cannot bring anything into the test room, so leave everything in the car or at home (they will usually have a locker in which you can put personal items during the exam).

You are allowed to do a tutorial on the computer before you start your exam if you need some assistance with CBT. The test time begins once you start the first question of the actual exam. Leaving the test site without authorization results in an automatic voiding of the test. You can take a bathroom break during the test, but know that the test time does not stop. You will be allowed only 4 hours from the time the test is started.

Results of the examination will be presented on site at the completion of your exam following a test evaluation.

## TEST-TAKING SKILLS

Frequently, the difference between passing and failing has to do with test-taking skills. An important reminder: Do not read into the question; take the question and information provided at face value. Answer all questions; do not leave any questions blank. A blank answer will be counted against you. Answering the question, even if it is an "educated" guess, will give you a one-out-of-four chance of being correct.

Keywords are important phrases or words used to focus attention on what the question is specifically asking. Examples include *always, earliest, first, on admission, best, least, immediately,* and *initial.*

> ▶ **HINT:** If the question asks for the "best" response, that indicates all answers are probably correct but you need to determine the best answer for that particular scenario.

Eliminate incorrect options first. Sometimes you will immediately see an answer that is incorrect. Mark through it to narrow down your answers and improve your odds. Frequently, you can get the choices down to two answers that are more correct.

> ▶ **HINT:** This gives a 50/50 chance for an educated guess of the correct answer.

Avoid those answers with words such as *always* or *never.* There is rarely a time in the medical field that you will always or never do a particular action. If three of the four answers are similar, choose the answer that does not sound similar.

Do not change answers unless you are absolutely sure. You can "bookmark" a question that you are not sure about to return to it at the end of the test. Sometimes you will feel more comfortable with the answer after you come back to it.

> ▶ **HINT:** First impressions are usually good! Do not use too much time on any one question.

Do not let it worry you if you do not know all the answers. Take a deep breath and keep going. Rejoice in those you know and find easy!

> ▶ **HINT:** You really are not supposed to know all the answers.

Do not try to establish patterns, such as using "two As in a row" for answers.

If there is a long scenario with large amounts of data, read the question first, then read the scenario, and then reread the question. Sometimes there will be erroneous data that are not required to answer the question. Too much time may be spent in trying to comprehend the whole scenario.

> ▶ **HINT:** Do not forget to reread the question to make sure you read it correctly the first time.

Read all answers before you make a choice; there may be more than one correct answer, but one will be the better answer for the question.

▶ **HINT:** Do not answer the first one that appears to be correct. Use the most correct answer.

Read the question closely, and answer only the question asked. Do not read into the question or want more information/data to answer the question.

▶ **HINT:** The question will provide you with all the information needed to correctly answer the question.

Timing questions are frequently used in the test. Use the timing to assist with making the correct choice. Example: Which complication of subarachnoid hemorrhage is seen 7 to 10 days after the bleed?

▶ **HINT:** All answers may be correct, but only one will occur more commonly during the time frame provided in the question.

Questions may be worded using the lead-in "What is the gold standard?" This is not asking "What is the most common routine?" but "What is the most reliable and accurate?"

Scenarios: Read the patient's description, word for word. Read the question and then formulate an answer. Read answers and choose one closest to your formulated answer. Reread the question after answering to ensure you understand the question.

▶ **HINT:** Once the question is answered, it is done. Move on to the next question. Do not second-guess yourself.

Look for answers that facilitate the patient. Facilitative words include *nurture, aid, support, reinforce, encourage,* and *assist*.

This review book will guide you in your studies toward being certified in the amazing field of neuroscience nursing. Read the chapters and take the sample tests. Always refer back to the ABNN test plan to review all of the topics listed on the plan. Congratulations and good luck!

# 1

# Chronic Neurological Disorders

## INTRODUCTION

■ **What type of pain is frequently described as shooting pain or burning pain?**
■ **Neuropathic pain**

Neuropathic pain is often described as pain that is *tingling, shooting, "burning, aching," throbbing,* and *sharp*. It is often described as an "odd" sensation in an old surgical site.

> ▶ **HINT:** The affected area can be sensitive to light touch, such as clothing rubbing against the skin.

■ **What type of patient is at risk for thalamic pain syndrome?**
■ **A poststroke patient**

Thalamic pain syndrome occurs when a stroke damages the thalamus or parietal lobe. The ischemic injury causes neurons in the affected areas to misfire, leading to chronic disabling pain. It can occur immediately, or weeks, months, to years after the stroke. The pain typically increases in severity over time.

> ▶ **HINT:** The thalamus is the primary pain center of the brain.

■ **What is peripheral neuropathy pain involving multiple nerves called?**
■ **Polyneuropathy**

Peripheral pain is initiated or caused by a primary lesion or dysfunction in the peripheral nervous system. A polyneuropathy involves multiple nerves and a mononeuropathy involves a single nerve. *Radiculalgia* is pain distributed along one or more sensory nerve roots. Potential causes of neuropathy include ischemia, vasculitis, diabetes, and musculoskeletal injury (Box 1.1).

> ▶ **HINT:** The lesion can affect the nerve root, plexus, or peripheral nerve itself.

**Box 1.1** Causes of Neuropathic Pain

| | |
|---|---|
| Infections | Postherpetic neuralgia/shingles (herpes zoster) |
| Trauma | Diabetes mellitus, diabetic sensory motor polyneuropathy |
| Metabolic abnormalities | Thyroid dysfunction |
| Chemotherapy | Vinca alkaloid derivatives |
| Surgery | Amputations |
| Inherited neurodegenerative | Tooth extractions |
| Nerve compression | Multiple sclerosis |
| Irradiation | Spinal stenosis |
| Inflammation | Trigeminal neuralgia |
| Tumor infiltration | Complex regional pain syndrome |
| Spinal cord injury | Autoimmune disorder |

■ *What is a chronic pain condition that causes extreme, sporadic, sudden burning, or shock-like pain to the face?*
■ **Trigeminal neuralgia (TN)**

TN, also called *tic douloureux*, is a chronic pain condition that causes extreme, sporadic, sudden burning, or shock-like facial pain. The disorder is characterized by recurrences and remissions.

> ▶ **HINT:** TN is not fatal, but due to the intensity of the pain, even the fear of an impending attack may prevent normal activities of daily living, and successive recurrences may incapacitate the patient.

■ *What is the most common cause of trigeminal neuralgia (TN), which presents at a younger age?*
■ **Multiple sclerosis (MS)**

TN is commonly found to be the initial presentation of MS. The demyelination of the trigeminal nerve in MS patients commonly presents with facial pain. Development of TN in a young person (<45 years) raises the possibility of MS, which should be investigated.

> ▶ **HINT:** Although TN typically is caused by a dysfunction in the trigeminal nerve itself, a lesion within the central nervous system (CNS) may also cause similar problems (Box 1.2).

**Box 1.2** Etiology of Trigeminal Neuralgia

| |
|---|
| Blood vessel pressing on the trigeminal nerve |
| Demyelination of trigeminal nerve |
| Compression by brain tumor |
| Chronic meningitis |
| Aneurysm or AVM compressing trigeminal nerve |

AVM, arteriovenous malformation.

# 1. CHRONIC NEUROLOGICAL DISORDERS

■ *What is the most common chronic benign headache?*
■ **Migraine**

Migraine headaches are classified as benign recurrent headaches and are one of the more common causes of benign headaches. Benign headaches can be severe and affect quality of life, but are not considered life-threatening (Box 1.3).

▶ **HINT:** Life-threatening causes of headache should be ruled out before the diagnosis of a benign headache is made.

**Box 1.3** Types of Benign Recurrent Headaches

| |
|---|
| Migraine |
| Tension |
| Cluster |
| Chronic daily |

■ *Which of the benign headaches is more common in the male population?*
■ **Cluster headaches**

Cluster headaches are more common in males. Migraines and other benign headaches tend to be more common in females. Cluster headaches occur frequently but last for shorter periods of time than migraines (Box 1.4).

▶ **HINT:** Cluster headaches more commonly occur in middle age, whereas migraines tend to occur at younger ages.

**Box 1.4** Benign Headache Types and Variables

|  | Migraine | Tension | Cluster | Chronic Daily |
|---|---|---|---|---|
| Age of onset | 10–30 years | All ages | Middle age | 30–40 years |
| Gender | Female > Male | Female > Male | Male > Female | Female > Male |
| Duration | 4–72 hours | 30 minutes to 7 days | 15–180 minutes | Constant to near constant |
| Frequency | Variable | Occasional to daily | Daily for weeks | Daily or constant |
| Time of day | Any time | Later in day | Nocturnal | Constant |

■ *What is the neurological disease process that is characterized by severe episodes of vertigo?*
■ **Ménière's disease**

Ménière's disease is a neurological disorder affecting the acoustic nerve (cranial nerve VIII). It is characterized by severe intermittent attacks of vertigo. It is more common in women than men and commonly occurs between the ages of 30 to 40 years.

▶ **HINT:** Sporadic episodes are followed by spontaneous recovery hours to days after onset.

# 4 NEUROSCIENCE CERTIFICATION REVIEW FOR NURSES

■ *Is Alzheimer's disease (AD) a cortical or subcortical dementia?*
■ **Cortical dementia**

Dementia can be classified as cortical or subcortical depending on the area of the brain affected. Cortical dementia, such as AD, involves the degeneration of the cortical area of the brain and affects memory. This is demonstrated by significant neuronal loss and brain atrophy.

▶ **HINT:** An example of a subcortical dementia is Parkinson's disease. The subcortical area of the brain controls motor skills.

■ *What are the two known risk factors for AD?*
■ **Age and genetic predisposition**

There are two known risk factors for the development of AD. Age is one known risk that doubles every 10 years over the age of 65 years. The second known risk is genetic predisposition. There are other potential risk factors for AD.

▶ **HINT:** Dementia likely results from multiple factors, not just one (Box 1.5).

**Box 1.5** Known and Potential Risks of Dementia

| | |
|---|---|
| Environmental factors | Exposure to aluminum |
| | Excessive zinc |
| | Toxins in the food |
| | Viral infections |
| Traumatic brain injury | |
| Gender | Greater incidence in women |
| Lower educational levels | More formal education lowers risk of developing AD |
| Cardiovascular risks | Hypercholesterolemia |
| | Hypertension |
| | Diabetes mellitus |
| | Smoking |
| Other known dementia risks | Tumors |
| | Strokes |
| | Diseases (e.g., Parkinson's disease) |
| | Long-term alcohol dependence |
| | Encephalitis |

AD, Alzheimer's disease.

■ *What is the neurological disease process that is a progressive, degenerative CNS) disorder characterized by resting tremor and cogwheel rigidity?*
■ **Parkinson's disease (PD)**

PD is a progressive, degenerative, neurological disorder of the CNS characterized by resting tremor, cogwheel rigidity, and bradykinesia. There are recognized various forms of Parkinson's, which are collectively called *parkinsonism*. PD is the most common of all forms.

# 1. CHRONIC NEUROLOGICAL DISORDERS

▶ **HINT:** One of the more common forms of parkinsonism is medication induced; neuroleptic agents included.

■ *What is the most common cause of PD?*

■ **Idiopathy**

Etiology of PD may be primary or secondary. The most common cause of primary is idiopathic and suggests no definitive cause. Familial history and genetic mutation account for the other primary causes of PD.

▶ **HINT:** There are several theories about causes of PD, including viral infection or an environmental toxin (Box 1.6).

**Box 1.6** Potential Secondary Causes of Parkinson's Disease

| |
|---|
| Medication induced: Neuroleptics |
| Toxin induced: Carbon monoxide<br>      Cyanide<br>      Manganese<br>      MPTP (illicit drug—synthetic type of heroin)<br>      Insecticides<br>      Agent orange |
| Infectious sources |
| Other neurological disorders: Brain trauma<br>           Brain tumors<br>           Vascular anomalies<br>           Metabolic disorders |

MPTP, 1-methyl-4-phenyl-1,2,3,6-tetrahydropyridine.

■ *What is the neurological disorder that is a result of an imbalance between the production and reabsorption of cerebrospinal fluid (CSF)?*

■ **Hydrocephalus**

Hydrocephalus is a result of the imbalance between the production of CSF and the reabsorption of CSF, resulting in excessive CSF in the CNS.

▶ **HINT:** CSF is absorbed through arachnoid villi into the venous sinuses. A blockage of the arachnoid villi can decrease reabsorption of CSF.

■ *An obstruction of CSF between the third and fourth ventricle is classified as which type of hydrocephalus: communicating or noncommunicating?*

■ **Noncommunicating**

Noncommunicating hydrocephalus is the obstruction to flow of CSF and is often caused by brain tumors, cysts, scarring, or infections. The obstruction commonly occurs in the ventricles, but can occur anywhere in the ventricular/CSF system.

▶ **HINT:** The most common site for obstruction is the Aquaduct of Sylvius (narrowest portion of ventricular system) located between the third and fourth ventricle.

■ **What is the most common cause of communicating hydrocephalus?**
■ **Decreased reabsorption**

The decreased reabsorption of CSF is a result of a thickening or blockage of the arachnoid villi. This is where CSF is reabsorbed into the venous sinuses. Potential causes of communicating hydrocephalus include subarachnoid hemorrhage (SAH) and meningitis (Box 1.7).

> ▶ **HINT:** In communicating hydrocephalus, there is no obstruction to flow in the ventricles, but there is an excessive volume of CSF usually due to an inability to reabsorb it.

**Box 1.7** Etiology of Hydrocephalus

| Congenital | Chiari malformations<br>Spina bifida<br>Aqueductal stenosis |
|---|---|
| Acquired | Meningitis<br>Intraventricular hemorrhage<br>Tumors<br>Encephalitis<br>Traumatic brain injury<br>Subarachnoid hemorrhage<br>Cysts |
| Idiopathic | |

■ **What is the general name of the group of spine disorders caused by the aging process?**
■ **Degenerative spine disorders**

In degenerative spine disorders, normal tissue structure and function of the spine are lost as a result of the aging process (Box 1.8). Changes are gradual unless an acute traumatic event accelerates the degenerative process.

> ▶ **HINT:** When degenerative changes cause symptoms, this is referred to as *osteoarthritis*.

**Box 1.8** Terminology of Degenerative Spine Disorders

| Osteoarthritis | Inflammation of bones and cartilage of a joint |
|---|---|
| Spondylosis | Symptomatic, degenerative changes of osteoarthritis, which include degenerative disc disease and spinal stenosis |
| Myelopathy | Involves compression of the spinal cord and tends to be the result of central stenosis |
| Radiculopathy | Involves compression of nerve roots and is associated with lateral recesses or foraminal stenosis |

■ **Disc protrusion into the spinal canal can cause what type of stenosis?**
■ **Central stenosis**

Disc protrusion can narrow the central cord canal, causing a central stenosis (Box 1.9). Hypertrophy of the facet joints can result in compression of nerve tracts. Osteophytes can impinge either laterally or centrally, causing cord or nerve involvement.

▶ **HINT:** With most common causes, the stenosis can be either developmental or acquired.

**Box 1.9** Locations of Stenosis

| Central stenosis | Narrowing of the spinal canal or cauda equina area |
|---|---|
| Lateral recess stenosis | Narrowing of the tract where the nerve root exits the central canal |
| Foraminal stenosis | Narrowing of the individual nerve roots as the nerves exit out of the body |

# PATHOPHYSIOLOGY

■ *Which portion of the spinal cord do the sensory impulses enter from the peripheral nerves?*

■ **Dorsal horn**

The dorsal horn receives the sensory impulses from the peripheral nerves, and the ventral horn contains the cells that send out the motor impulses. In neuropathic pain, sympathetic nerve fibers sprout in the dorsal horn. This is called *deafferentation of pain*. It results in increased nociceptive neurons and responsiveness in the CNS.

▶ **HINT:** Neuropathic pain arises as a direct consequence of a lesion or disease affecting the central somatosensory system.

■ *What portion of the inner ear is involved in the symptoms of Ménière's disease?*

■ **Labyrinth**

The symptoms of Ménière's disease are associated with a change in fluid volume within a portion of the inner ear known as the *labyrinth*. The labyrinth has two parts: bony labyrinth and membranous labyrinth. The membranous labyrinth, which is encased by bone, is necessary for hearing and balance and is filled with a fluid called *endolymph*. An increase in endolymph, however, can cause the membranous labyrinth to balloon or dilate, a condition known as *endolymphatic hydrops*.

▶ **HINT:** When the head moves, endolymph moves, causing nerve receptors in the membranous labyrinth to send signals to the brain about the body's motion. This controls equilibrium.

■ *What area of the brain is critical for memory?*

■ **Hippocampus**

The entire brain is involved in memory (Box 1.10). Short-term memory is located in the cortex, primarily the prefrontal cortex and frontal and parietal lobes. But the area of the brain most critical to memory is the hippocampus. It is responsible for acquiring and temporarily storing memory, playing a big role in consolidation of short-term memory into long-term memory.

▶ **HINT:** In Alzheimer's disease (AD), the hippocampus undergoes significant neuronal loss.

**Box 1.10** Types of Memory

| Declarative memory (conscious recall) | Semantic memory<br>  Involves the conscious thoughts<br>  Involves episodic memory<br>  Memory of experiences or events |
|---|---|
| Implicit memory (procedural memory) | Information learned without the conscious involvement of the person |
| Motor memory | Memory of tasks involving motor skills |
| Affective memory | Memory that is triggered by feelings or emotions |

- *What is produced in the brain that results in the main pathological change in AD?*
- **Amyloid plaque**

Amyloid plaque and neurofibrillary fibers are produced in the brain and can be found primarily on autopsy. The symptoms seen in AD are the result of the death of many neurons in the hippocampus and cerebral cortex.

▶ **HINT:** Definitive diagnosis of AD is on autopsy.

- *What is the primary role of the extrapyramidal tracts in the the basal ganglia?*
- **Inhibits muscle tone**

The extrapyramidal tract in the basal ganglia inhibit muscle tone. The portions of the brain involved in Parkinson's disease (PD) are the basal ganglia, subthalamic nucleus, and the substantia nigra (part of the midbrain). These areas in the brain and the motor neurons of the cord form the extrapyramidal system (Box 1.11).

▶ **HINT:** The symptoms of PD are the result of abnormal extrapyramidal tracts.

**Box 1.11** Roles of Extrapyramidal Tracts

| |
|---|
| Control upright position |
| Regulate muscle tone and coordination |
| Regulate initiation of automatic movements |
| Control facial expressions |
| Arm swing when walking |
| Control opposing movements to maintain balance during activity |

- *What is the neurotransmitter responsible for inhibition of muscle tone?*
- **Dopamine**

The neurotransmitter responsible for inhibiting muscle tone is dopamine. The neurons in the substantia nigra are responsible for producing and projecting dopamine to the striatum in the basal ganglia. The excitatory neurotransmitter (in opposition) is acetylcholine. In PD, the nigra–striatal pathway degenerates, resulting in an imbalance between dopamine and acetylcholine. Acetylcholine then has a greater effect, resulting in increased muscle tone.

▶ **HINT:** When approximately 80% of the dopamine-producing cells are lost, symptoms of PD begin to occur.

## 1. CHRONIC NEUROLOGICAL DISORDERS    9

▪ *Where does the CSF get reabsorbed in the brain?*
▪ **Arachnoid villi**

CSF is produced in the choroid plexus, circulates through the ventricles and in the subarachnoid space, and is then reabsorbed through the arachnoid villi into the venous sinuses. CSF is continually produced and reabsorbed to maintain the circulating volume.

> ▶ **HINT:** The brain produces about 500 mL of CSF a day, but only circulates 150 to 200 mL.

▪ *As one ages, what typically happens to the discs in the spinal column?*
▪ **Compression**

The intervertebral discs will lose height and volume during the aging process. This compression causes narrowing of the disc spaces. The disc becomes less resistant and resilient to loading forces.

> ▶ **HINT:** Loss of disc volume occurs most frequently in the cervical and lumbar areas.

▪ *What are the bony projections that occur in the vertebral bodies called?*
▪ **Osteophytes**

Osteophytes are bony projections, also known as *bone spurs*, that develop in an attempt to stabilize excessive motion. They may cause compression on neurological structures. Sclerosis is the increased bone formation of the subchondral bone adjacent to the endplate of the bone.

> ▶ **HINT:** Degeneration can also occur within the facet joints.

▪ *What is the largest avascular structure in the spinal column?*
▪ **The disc**

Discs are present between the vertebral bodies and provide cushioning. Degenerative changes and injury can cause disc injury. The disc, being avascular, is unable to heal, therefore internal disruption and damage to discs is permanent (Box 1.12).

> ▶ **HINT:** Degenerative change in the intervertebral spine is a part of the normal aging process.

**Box 1.12** Degrees of Disc Herniation

| | |
|---|---|
| Nuclear herniation | Occurs when nucleus ruptures through innermost fibers of the annulus fibrosis<br>No disruption of outer annular fiber |
| Disc protrusion (or prolapse) | Ruptured nucleus distorts the outermost fibers of the annulus<br>Causes bulge outward |
| Nuclear extension | Complete split of annulus<br>Allows nuclear material to leak out of surrounding spaces<br>Protruded material remains attached to the nucleus remaining inside the disc |
| Sequestered nucleus | Extruded nuclear substance is no longer attached to material remaining within disc<br>Sequestered fragments may float around the spinal canal<br>May become totally remote from the site |

## ASSESSMENT/SYMPTOMS

▪ *What is it called when a patient experiences pain in a nonexistent limb following an amputation?*
▪ **Phantom limb pain**

Phantom limb pain is a sensation that the deafferented body part is still present (Box 1.13). Residual limb pain is also known as *stump pain* or *phantom leg pain*. Pain also can occur in the area adjacent to an amputated body part.

> ▶ **HINT:** Neuropathic pain will almost never be completely eliminated, even with the most advanced treatment.

**Box 1.13** Symptoms of Phantom Leg Pain

| |
|---|
| Pain |
| Itching |
| Tingling |
| Cramping |
| Involuntary movement |
| Electric sensations |

▪ *What chronic pain syndrome is a complication triggered by nerve or tissue injury?*
▪ **Complex regional pain syndrome (CRPS)**

CRPS is a chronic pain syndrome that results from injury to tissue or nerve. It is classified as CRPS I and CRPS II. CRPS I is frequently triggered by tissue injury; those with CRPS II experience similar symptoms, but is clearly associated with nerve injury. CRPS results in dramatic changes in the color and temperature of the skin over the affected limb or body part (Box 1.14).

> ▶ **HINT:** The key is continuous, intense pain out of proportion to the severity of the injury.

**Box 1.14** Symptoms of Complex Regional Pain Syndrome

| |
|---|
| Intense burning pain |
| Skin sensitivity |
| Changes in skin texture |
| Excessive sweating |
| Swelling and stiffness in joints |
| Motor disability |

▪ *What term is used to describe a painful stimulus that is more painful than normal in neuropathic pain?*
▪ **Hyperalgesia**

*Hyperalgesia* is a term used to describe a stimulus that is perceived as more painful than normal in a patient with neuropathic pain. Assessment for hyperalgesia is testing with a bilateral pinprick that compares one site with the other.

> ▶ HINT: *Allodyne* is a term used to describe a normally nonpainful sensation that is experienced as painful.

■ **In TN, the pain is typically intermittent. Where is it most commonly located?**
■ **Unilateral face**

The pain typically involves one side of the face (unilateral) and is commonly described as *shooting* or *electric-like* pain. Rarely does the pain occur simultaneously bilaterally on the face. The pain follows the unilateral sensory distribution of the trigeminal nerve (cranial nerve V), radiating to the maxillary (V2) or mandibular (V3) area. Ophthalmic division (V1) pain alone occurs infrequently.

> ▶ HINT: Episodes can last for days, weeks, or months at a time and then disappear for months or years.

■ **Which of the benign headaches can commonly be associated with an aura?**
■ **Migraines**

Migraines can be associated with an aura or a hallucinatory associated sign (Box 1.15). Focal neurological signs can be associated with migraines, including visual disturbances, unilateral numbness or paresthesia, aphasia, and speech disturbances.

> ▶ HINT: Migraine headaches can be a stroke mimic.

**Box 1.15 Characteristics of Benign Headaches**

|  | Migraine | Tension | Cluster | Chronic Daily |
|---|---|---|---|---|
| Severity | Moderate to severe | Mild to severe | Severe | Variable |
| Quality |  | Dull, aching | Sharp | Variable |
| Location | Temporal and retro-orbital lobes | Bilateral temporal lobe | Unilateral retro-orbital lobe | Variable |
| Associated symptoms | Nausea and vomiting, photophobia, aura | Rarely associated with other symptoms | Ipsilateral autonomic symptoms | None |

■ **Which of the benign headaches can have associated symptoms involving the autonomic system?**
■ **Cluster headaches**

Ipsilateral autonomic signs can be associated with cluster headaches. These signs include lacrimation; nasal congestion, or rhinorrhea; facial sweating; miosis; and eyelid swelling.

> ▶ HINT: Chronic daily headaches are commonly associated with a history of migraines or substance abuse.

### What is the most predominant sign of Ménière's disease?
### Vertigo

Vertigo is the primary presenting symptom of Ménière's disease. It is characterized by attacks of severe vertigo, vomiting, tinnitus, and aural fullness or pressure. The vertigo can cause injuries and falls due to its severity and rapid onset.

> ▶ HINT: Hearing loss can be a complication of Ménière's disease.

### What is the most prominent cognitive change that occurs with AD?
### Memory loss

There are eight cognitive impairments that occur with AD (Box 1.16). Memory loss is the most prominent cognitive change that occurs. Memory deficits are the early signs of AD and affect all of the other cognitive functions.

> ▶ HINT: Memory and learning are two different processes. Memory is required for learning to occur.

**Box 1.16** Cognitive Impairments of Alzheimer's Disease

| |
|---|
| Memory |
| Language |
| Perceptual skills |
| Attention |
| Constructive abilities |
| Orientation |
| Problem solving |
| Functional abilities |

### Which of the findings found in stage I is most predictive of AD?
### Word substitution

Stage I AD presents insidiously and may not be recognized as AD (Box 1.17). Memory loss is the first sign, and at first, these memory deficits are erratic and inconsistent and may appear to be a result of age. Sporadic loss of words or word substitution of inappropriate words is the most predictive sign of the development of AD. This stage can last up to 2 years.

> ▶ HINT: The person may also realize something is wrong but cannot do anything about it.

**Box 1.17** Symptoms of Stage I Alzheimer's Disease

| |
|---|
| Short-term memory loss |
| Loss of spontaneity |
| Sporadic loss of words or word substitution |
| Easy to anger |
| Less discrimination with choices |

■ *In stage II of AD, patients may begin to hoard or stockpile items excessively or pick items up that do not belong to them. What is this called?*
■ **Rummaging and pillaging**

*Rummaging and pillaging* refers to AD patients hoarding or stockpiling items excessively and picking up items up that do not belong to them and then putting these things somewhere they cannot remember. Symptoms will begin to worsen at this stage, and the memory deficits may begin to interfere with activities of daily living (Box 1.18). This stage may last 2 to 5 years.

▶ **HINT:** Stage II AD is characterized by increased disorientation.

**Box 1.18** Symptoms of Stage II Alzheimer's Disease

| |
|---|
| Disorientation to time and place |
| Impaired communication (unable to express thought) |
| Difficulty in making decisions or plans |
| Loss of impulse control |
| Mistakes in judgment |
| Decreased concentration |
| Increased self-absorption |
| Avoidance of new situations |
| Delusions |
| Rummaging and pillaging |
| Wandering and pacing |

■ *Can AD eventually result in death?*
■ **Yes**

Stage IV is the terminal stage of AD. This stage may last for 5 to 10 years. Physically, the patient may not have medical complications, but eventually the disease overpowers the person, resulting in death (Box 1.19).

▶ **HINT:** During stage III, short-term memory is almost nonexistent and long-term memory may begin to be lost.

**Box 1.19** Symptoms of Stages III and IV Alzheimer's Disease

| Stage III | Stage IV |
|---|---|
| Sundowning | Inability to communicate |
| Catastrophic reactions | No recognition of others |
| Failure to recognize family and friends | Total dependence |
| Hyperorality (unexplained movements of mouth and tongue) | |
| Preservation (continual activity after the stimulus is removed, i.e., continue to chew even though the food is ready to be swallowed) | |
| Latency (inability to begin an activity) | |
| Agnosia (inability to recognize commonly used tools, e.g., toothbrush) | |
| Apraxia (inability to perform a task with an item, e.g., unable to brush teeth with toothbrush) | |

■ **What triad of symptoms occur in PD?**
■ **Tremors, rigidity, bradykinesia**

The triad of signs characteristic of PD includes tremors, rigidity, and bradykinesia (Box 1.20). The loss of dopamine results in motor difficulties associated with the increased muscle tone in intentional movement and posture.

> ▶ **HINT:** An infarction or hemorrhage within the basal ganglia results in paresis or paralysis.

**Box 1.20** Signs of Parkinson's Disease

| |
|---|
| Tremor |
| Cogwheel rigidity |
| Bradykinesia |
| Postural instability |
| Autonomic dysfunction |
| Dementia |
| Depression |
| Dysphagia |
| Sialorrhea (drooling) |
| Seborrhea |

■ **What is the characteristic tremor in PD called?**
■ **"Pill rolling"**

PD patients exhibit tremors, which occur at rest and will stop during a purposeful movement. Tremor is due to the imbalance between dopamine and acetylcholine. The tremor has been described as a "pill rolling" type movement especially of the hands, jaw, and lower extremities.

> ▶ **HINT:** The tremors are not present while sleeping and will worsen with emotional stress.

■ **In PD, passive range of motion (PROM) involves stiffness and difficulty bending the extremity; what is this frequently called?**
■ **"Lead pipe" rigidity**

*Rigidity* refers to an increase in muscle tone and occurs either unilaterally or bilaterally. PROM will demonstrate as a stiffness and difficulty to bend the extremity. It is frequently described as "lead pipe" rigidity. Cogwheel rigidity is another motor symptom in which a flexion or extension movement is jerky, like a cogwheel.

> ▶ **HINT:** PD patients lose the smoothness of normal movement in both passive and active range of motion.

■ **What is an inability to initiate movement or change a movement in PD called?**
■ **Bradykinesia**

Bradykinesia is the inability to initiate movement or change a movement. This results in a slowing of movement. Patients with PD lose the ability to move automatically and require greater time to react. They may even require visual or auditory cues to initiate or complete a movement. This is caused by the decreased ability to coordinate opposing muscles to initiate movement. When walking they show hesitation in initiating a step and have a shuffling gait due to rigidity, and their arms do not swing as they walk but rather stay at their sides.

> ▶ **HINT:** The combination of "slowness" of movement and rigidity causes the altered posture and walk commonly seen in PD.

- **What is an assessment technique for hydrocephalus unique to children under 2 years of age?**
- **Measurement of head circumference**

Under the age of 2 years, the skull is pliable and will increase in size to compensate for CSF volume. This is called *decompensated congenital hydrocephalus*. The hydrocephalus may have been asymptomatic for years prior due to the expandability of the cranial vault.

> ▶ **HINT:** If the measurement of the head circumference is significantly larger than normal, hydrocephalus was probably present since birth.

- **A presentation of nausea and vomiting, headache, and papilledema would indicate which of the following hydrocephalus etiologies: decompensated congenital hydrocephalus, normal-pressure hydrocephalus (NPH), or acute hydrocephalus?**
- **Acute hydrocephalus**

Acute hydrocephalus commonly presents with signs of increased intracranial pressure (Box 1.21). This includes vomiting, headache, and papilledema. Decompensated congenital hydrocephalus presents with symptoms similar to NPH.

> ▶ **HINT:** Symptoms of NPH can be remembered by the terms *wet*, *wacky*, and *wobbly*. *Wet* refers to urinary incontinence, *wacky* to cognitive abnormalities, and *wobbly* to gait abnormalities.

**Box 1.21** Symptoms of Hydrocephalus

| Decompensated Congenital Hydrocephalus | Normal-Pressure Hydrocephalus | Acute Hydrocephalus |
|---|---|---|
| Gait disturbances | Gait disturbances | Nausea and vomiting |
| Bladder-control issues | Bladder-control issues | Headache |
| Cognitive abnormalities | Cognitive abnormalities | Papilledema |
| | | Altered mentation |

- **What is it called when pain in the legs increases with walking due to spinal degeneration?**
- **Neurogenic claudication**

Lumbar spinal stenosis may be associated with spondylolisthesis and can present with neurogenic claudication. The initial pain is in the back followed by pain descending to legs when standing upright that intensifies with walking. Relief of symptoms is commonly seen by flexing forward, sitting, or lying in a fetal position.

▶ **HINT:** Patients with neurogenic claudication are comfortable leaning over a shopping cart or mowing the lawn due to the leaning-over position.

- *A cervical stenosis usually presents with altered sensations in what part of the body?*
- Hand

Cervical stenosis usually presents with unilateral radiculopathy of the C5, C6, and C7 nerve roots. These nerve roots innervate the arm and hands. The overall symptoms of cervical stenosis include neck pain, arm pain, and motor weakness of the upper extremities.

▶ **HINT:** Hand numbness and tingling, especially associated with neck pain, should increase suspicion of cervical stenosis.

## DIAGNOSIS

- *What is the primary diagnostic technique used to determine the presence of TN?*
- Pain history

TN is a primary pain syndrome. There is no diagnostic test that can definitively diagnose it. The diagnosis of TN is made based on pain history. TN can be difficult to diagnose due to the multiple possible causes of facial pain and may be misdiagnosed for years after the pain begins.

▶ **HINT:** One of the difficulties in diagnosing of TN is the pain typically comes and goes (relapses and remissions).

- *How are benign headaches diagnosed?*
- By exclusion

The primary diagnosis of benign headaches is made by exclusion. Diagnostic imaging with CT scans and MRIs is used to identify organic brain disease such as a brain tumor or cerebral hemorrhage. No evidence of organic disease leads to the diagnosis of a benign headache.

▶ **HINT:** A new or different headache, focal neurological signs, or seizures could indicate a pathological cause of the headache.

- *What is the definitive diagnosis of AD?*
- Autopsy

The definitive diagnosis of AD is on biopsy or autopsy only. Histological study of brain tissue will reveal plaque formation and neurofibrillary tangles, which confirm the diagnosis. There are many different causes of dementia, and AD is just one of those causes. A probable diagnosis is made based on history and physical, diagnostic tests, cognitive testing, and mental status evaluation.

# 1. CHRONIC NEUROLOGICAL DISORDERS

▶ **HINT:** Diagnostic tests are used to rule out other causes of dementia and assist diagnosis of AD.

■ *Which diagnostic test can identify amyloid deposits in the brain?*
■ **Pittsburgh compound B (PiB) PET scan**

PiB PET scans use tracers, which bind selectively to A-beta-amyloid deposits. This diagnostic test is 80% accurate in predicting which person with mild cognitive impairment will develop AD within 2 years. This test has a 92% accuracy in ruling out the likelihood to develop AD.

▶ **HINT:** Volumetric MRI can detect changes in volume size in the different regions of the brain. It measures the atrophy in the hippocampal area to determine the progress of AD.

■ *What is the definitive diagnosis of PD?*
■ **Lewy bodies present on autopsy**

The definitive diagnosis of PD is the finding of Lewy bodies in the midbrain on autopsy. PD tends to be a clinical diagnosis based on presentation and symptoms.

▶ **HINT:** PET scans may be used to identify abnormalities of dopamine in the brain and decreased activity in the basal ganglia.

■ *What is the primary diagnostic tool used to diagnose hydrocephalus?*
■ **Brain MRI**

Hydrocephalus can be identified on the brain via CT or MRI. The determination between increased pressure and NPH is based on the presenting symptoms. Cisternography uses a radioactive isotope injected into the subarachnoid space in the lumbar region, which allows for evaluation of absorption rates.

▶ **HINT:** Remember: NPH presents with the symptoms: *wobbly, wet,* and *wacky.*

■ *What is the method used to determine the need for ventriculoperitoneal (VP) shunt placement in patients with NPH?*
■ **Drainage of CSF**

The evaluation process for NPH includes removal of CSF to evaluate for improvement in the patient's gait. This can be accomplished with a lumbar puncture and removal of CSF one time or placement of a lumbar drain. The lumbar drain allows for the drainage of CSF over a 72-hour period.

▶ **HINT:** If the patient's gait improves after the CSF is removed, the patient is a possible candidate for the placement of a VP shunt.

■ *Which diagnostic examination can visualize compression of individual nerve roots?*
■ **Myelogram**

Myelography provides a view of the central canal and the lateral recesses and visualizes compression of individual nerve roots (Box 1.22).

> ▶ **HINT:** Myelogram studies are superior to MRI studies of the spine in identifying spinal nerve compression and identifying patients who may benefit from surgery.

**Box 1.22** Spine Diagnostic Studies

| Plain radiographics | Disc degeneration |
| --- | --- |
| | Facet hypertrophy |
| | Subluxation |
| | Intralaminal narrowing |
| Flexion extension x-rays | Indicates segmental instability and subluxation |
| Myelography | Provides a view of the central canal and the lateral recesses |
| | Visualizes compression of individual nerve root |
| CT scan | Allows visibility of bony structures |
| MRI | Identifies lateral recess stenosis and soft-tissue injury |

## MEDICAL MANAGEMENT

- *What class of medication is considered the first-line treatment of neuropathic pain?*
- **Anticonvulsants**

Anticonvulsants, such as gabapentin (Neurontin), are considered the first drug of choice in managing neuropathy pain (Box 1.23). Opioids are not as effective in managing neuropathic pain.

The overall goal in managing neuropathic pain is to stabilize the CNS, preventing or limiting aberrant remodeling and the potential development of chronic neuropathic pain.

> ▶ **HINT:** The second line of therapy for neuropathic pain is tricyclic antidepressants.

**Box 1.23** Medications Commonly Used in Managing Neuropathic Pain

| Anticonvulsants | Gabapentin (Neurontin) |
| --- | --- |
| | Lyrica (Pregabalin) |
| | Carbamazepine (Carbatol, Tegretol) |
| | Oxcarbazepine (Trileptal) |
| | Clonazepam (Klonopin) |
| Tricyclic antidepressants | Amitriptyline |
| SNRIs | Venlafaxine |
| NSAIDs | Tramadol |
| 5% lidocaine patch | |

NSAID, nonsteroidal anti-inflammatory drug; SNRI, serotonin–norepinephrine reuptake inhibitor.

- *What complementary approach may be used to treat neuropathic pain?*
- **Acupuncture**

Acupuncture is one of many complementary approaches used to manage neuropathic pain. Complementary approaches are often used in addition to traditional pain management techniques (Box 1.24).

> ▶ **HINT:** Typical analgesics and opioids are not usually helpful in treating the sharp, recurring pain caused by neuropathies, including TN.

**Box 1.24** Complementary Techniques Used for Pain Management

| |
|---|
| Acupuncture |
| Biofeedback |
| TENS |
| Nutritional and vitamin supplements |
| Imagery |
| Meditation |

TENS, transcutaneous electrical stimulation.

- **When managing benign headaches, would the use of triptans be considered an abortive or preventive treatment?**
- **Abortive**

Management techniques for benign headaches can be divided into preventive and abortive techniques. Abortive techniques are used to treat a current headache and commonly use the serotonin 5HT-1-B and 1-D receptor agonists, such as the class of drugs known as *triptans*. Most of the abortive drugs are *habituating*, meaning they lead to chronic drug abuse, and are not recommended on a regular basis.

> ▶ **HINT:** Antiemetics may be used to prevent the nausea and vomiting associated with migraines.

- **When administering dihydroergotamine mesylate (DHE) intravenously (IV), what is a common side effect?**
- **Nausea and vomiting**

DHE can be used in intractable migraine pain. It is most commonly administered via IV and can cause nausea and vomiting. An antiemetic is recommended prior to the administration of DHE.

> ▶ **HINT:** DHE should also be used with caution in patients with significant coronary artery disease or peripheral vascular disease due to its potential vasoactive effects.

- **What is a common class of medications used to prevent migraine pain?**
- **Tricyclic antidepressants**

Tricyclic antidepressants, such as amitriptyline, are commonly the first-line drugs used to prevent chronic benign headaches (Box 1.25). Other medications include beta-blockers, calcium channel blockers, and anticonvulsants.

▶ **HINT:** Opioids are not recommended to manage benign headaches.

**Box 1.25** Indications for Preventive Management of Benign Headaches

| |
|---|
| Frequent headaches (three to four headaches per month or more) |
| Headaches of severe intensity |
| Long duration (two severe headaches lasting 4 days or more per month) |
| Extent and tolerability of side effects caused by abortive medications |

■ *What is the most common medication used to treat the vertigo in Ménière's disease?*
■ **Meclizine (Antivert)**

Meclizine (Antivert) is an antihistamine and is the most commonly used medication to treat vertigo. Antihistamines are effective in treating motion sickness and disequilibrium, or vertigo. Other classes of medications used to treat vertigo include anticholinergics and antiemetics.

▶ **HINT:** Medical management treats the symptoms, not the actual disease process.

■ *What is the primary medication classification approved to manage AD?*
■ **Acetylcholinesterase inhibitors**

Four of the five approved drugs for AD include acetylcholinesterase inhibitors. Cholinesterase is an enzyme that breaks down acetylcholine (ACh) after it crosses the neuromuscular synapse. These drugs suppress this enzyme so that acetylcholine will not be broken down as readily, thus increasing the concentration of ACh. In AD, there is a decrease in activity of cholinergic neurons; thus, these medications can increase this activity. The other approved drug is NMDA (N-methyl-D-aspartate), a receptor antagonist.

▶ **HINT:** This may temporarily slow the rate of decline in memory and thinking ability in early stages but does not reverse the process.

■ *Which class of Parkinson's drugs converts to dopamine in the dopaminergic neurons by decarboxylase?*
■ **Dopaminergic agents**

Levodopa, a dopaminergic agent, is converted into dopamine in dopaminergic neurons by the enzyme decarboxylase. This increases dopamine in the CNS and the peripheral nervous system (PNS). Levodopa is frequently combined with carbidopa, which is a peripheral decarboxylase inhibitor.

It prevents metabolism of levodopa in the PNS before it reaches dopaminergic receptors in the CNS.

▶ **HINT:** The addition of carbidopa increases bioavailability and lowers the side effects of levodopa.

■ *What is the severe side effect of levodopa that can limit usage of the medication?*
■ **Dyskinesia**

# 1. CHRONIC NEUROLOGICAL DISORDERS

Dyskinesia can limit the utilization of levodopa in the treatment of PD. The severe complication of dyskinesia may delay the initial use of levodopa in the treatment of Parkinson's symptoms.

> ▶ **HINT:** Sudden withdrawal of levodopa can cause neuroleptic malignant syndrome, also called *parkinsonism–hyperpyrexia syndrome*.

- **Which class of Parkinson's medications acts directly on the postsynaptic dopamine receptors and bypasses the nigral dopaminergic pathways?**
- **Dopamine agents**

Dopamine agents improve the effect of dopamine by acting directly on the postsynaptic dopamine receptors and bypassing the nigral dopaminergic pathways (Box 1.26).

> ▶ **HINT:** Know the different mechanisms of these two major classes of medications in managing the symptoms of Parkinson's disease.

**Box 1.26** Side Effects of Parkinson's Disease Medications

| Dopaminergic Agents | Dopamine Agonists |
| --- | --- |
| Dyskinesia | Orthostatic hypotension |
| Orthostatic hypotension | Confusion |
| Confusion and agitation | Hallucinations |
| Hallucinations and psychosis | Mental clouding |
| Nausea | |

## SURGICAL MANAGEMENT

- **How can opioids and local anesthetics be delivered in the CNS to assist with neuropathic pain management?**
- **Intrathecally or intraventricularly**

Opioids and local anesthetics can be delivered directly to the vicinity of the neural tissue via the epidural, subarachnoid (intrathecal), or intraventricular spaces. This route of drug delivery should be used when severe pain cannot be controlled with systemic drugs because of dose-limiting side effects. Epidural or subarachnoid drug administration may be used with percutaneous catheterization, reservoir, or implantation of a catheter and pump.

> ▶ **HINT:** Intrathecal and intraventricular routes for administering pain medications are called the *neuraxial* route of delivery.

- **What surgical treatment for managing pain involves the nerve root?**
- **Sympathectomy**

Sympathectomy is a type of neuroablation therapy involving the destruction of the nerve root or nerve and can be accomplished with chemical, thermal (heat ablation), cryoanalgesia (cold), or surgical destruction of neural tissue. When systemic therapies have failed, neuroablative techniques should be initiated to provide adequate pain control or when adverse side effects from systemic therapies are unacceptable (Box 1.27).

▶ **HINT:** Neural tissue can regenerate, so the procedure may have to be repeated.

**Box 1.27** Invasive Management of Neuropathic Pain Syndromes

| Class | Technique | Clinical Situation |
|---|---|---|
| Regional anesthesia | Spinal opioids and/or local anesthetics | Preserves sensation, strength, sympathetic function |
| Sympathetic blockade and neurolysis | Celiac plexus block | Refractory malignant pain involving upper abdominal viscera |
| | Lumbar sympathetic blockade | Includes upper retroperitoneum, liver, small bowel, and proximal colon |
| | Stellate ganglion blockade | Sympathetically maintained pain involving legs |
| | | Sympathetically maintained pain involving head, neck, and arms |
| Somatic neurolysis | Chemical rhizotomy | Refractory brachial plexopathy or arm pain, intercostal nerve pain (chest pain), refractory pelvic pain |
| | Trigeminal neurolysis | Refractory unilateral facial pain |
| | Transacral neurolysis | Refractory pain limited to peritoneum |
| | Cordotomy | Refractory unilateral pain in torso or lower extremity |
| High center ablation | Cingulotomy (rare) Pituitary ablation | Refractory multifocal pain |

■ *A stimulator that delivers a continuous low-voltage electrical current can be placed that blocks pain sensation and assists with managing neuropathic pain. Where is this stimulator most commonly placed?*

■ **Spine**

Spinal stimulation is commonly used to manage unresponsive neuropathic pain and may be effective in treating pain from prior back surgeries (failed back syndrome), chronic sciatica, nerve damage, and peripheral vascular disease.

▶ **HINT:** Deep brain stimulation (DBS) is a newer technique and works by delivering a continuous electrical pulse to regions of the brain involved in the processing of pain signals.

■ *What surgical technique is used to remove vascular compression of the trigeminal nerve?*

■ **Microvascular decompression (MVD)**

MVD removes vascular compression from the trigeminal nerve. The surgical access is through the posterior fossa. Radiosurgery may also be used as a minimally invasive technique.

# 1. CHRONIC NEUROLOGICAL DISORDERS  23

▶ **HINT:** Potential complications of posterior fossa access for neurosurgical procedures are CSF leaks and CNS infections.

### What is the microsurgical intervention for Ménière's disease?
### Vestibular nerve section

The acoustic cranial nerve has two components: the vestibular portion (equilibrium) and the cochlear portion (hearing). A surgical technique that can treat the vertigo and attempt to prevent hearing loss is the sectioning of the vestibular portion of the cranial nerve, sparing the cochlear portion. This is a posterior fossa approach.

▶ **HINT:** Postoperatively, the patient may still have disequilibrium but not the severe episodes of vertigo.

### What is the most common surgical management of Parkinson's disease and other motor disorders?
### DBS

DBS is the placement of pacemaker wires into the deep structures of the brain that are connected to a generator box; target areas include the thalamus, globus pallidus, or subthalamic nucleus. DBS is indicated for motor complications refractory to the best medical treatment.

▶ **HINT:** This is often called a *brain pacemaker*.

### What surgical management is recommended for managing hydrocephalus?
### VP shunt

A flexible tube placed into the ventricular system shunts CSF to another area of the body. The most commonly used shunt is a VP shunt, in which the CSF is shunted into the peritoneum. CSF can also be shunted into the right atrium or pleural cavity.

▶ **HINT:** VP shunts can adjust the amount of CSF drained from the ventricles into the peritoneum.

### What type of spine surgery is used most frequently to treat spinal stenosis from degeneration?
### Laminectomy

Central stenosis is commonly treated with laminectomy and medial facetectomy is used to relieve symptoms. Surgical management of lateral recesses includes laminectomy, facetectomy, and foraminotomy.

▶ **HINT:** Most surgical procedures used to open the space in the central canal are unilateral procedures.

## COMPLICATIONS

### What psychological complication accompanies chronic neuropathic pain?
### Depression

Depression and anxiety commonly accompany chronic neuropathic pain. Depression can further result in avoidant behavior patterns that contribute to the feelings of isolation.

> ▶ HINT: It is difficult for the patient and family to understand neuropathic pain because the injury is not visible or has obvious tissue damage.

■ **What is a common complication of postural instability and retropulsion in PD?**
■ **Falls**

Postural instability and retropulsion are common problems with PD and frequently result in falls. Retropulsion occurs when the patient may reach for something (i.e., a door) but continues to fall backward or adjusts by using excessive forward movement. The complications of frequent falls tend to limit the person's mobility and activity level.

> ▶ HINT: Physical therapy (PT) plays an important role in teaching gait safety, fall prevention, and fall recovery.

■ **In PD, patients may develop hypotension. What is the physiologic cause for the hypotension?**
■ **Autonomic dysfunction**

Autonomic dysfunction is a complication of PD (Box 1.28), characterized by orthostatic hypotension and bladder abnormalities such as urinary hesitancy and frequency.

> ▶ HINT: The dopaminergic drugs used to treat PD may contribute to the orthostatic hypotension and bladder abnormalities.

**Box 1.28** Symptoms of Autonomic Dysfunction in Parkinson's Disease

| |
|---|
| Orthostatic hypotension |
| Constipation |
| Difficulty with temperature regulation |
| Drooling |
| Erectile dysfunction |
| Changes in sensation |
| Dysphagia |
| Hypophonia |
| Masked face |
| Swelling |
| Loss of appetite |

■ **What is the most common VP shunt complication found within the first month of placement?**
■ **Infection**

The greatest incidence of shunt infection occurs early, typically within 1 month of shunt placement or revision (Box 1.29). The infection is commonly caused by skin pathogens such as Gram-positive bacteria. Signs of fever, swelling, or redness along the shunt site may indicate an infection. Management includes antibiotics and possibly temporary externalization of the shunt or shunt removal.

▶ **HINT:** To culture the CSF, obtain the CSF sample directly from the shunt (if possible).

**Box 1.29** Complications of VP Shunts

| |
|---|
| Shunt obstruction |
| Shunt infection |
| Shunt malfunction |
| Overdrainage of CSF |
| Intraventricular hemorrhage |
| Bowel perforation |
| Peritonitis |

CSF, cerebrospinal fluid; VP, ventriculoperitoneal.

# Sample Exam Questions

1. Your patient was diagnosed with Parkinson's disease 2 years prior and is developing subcortical dementia. He would most commonly present with worsening of which of the following?
   A. Significant short-term memory losses
   B. Tasks take longer and have errors in routine tasks
   C. Expressive aphasia and word finding
   D. Alteration in personality

2. Which of the following best describes normal-pressure hydrocephalus (NPH)?
   A. NPH is a noncommunicating hydrocephalus with relative normal opening pressures
   B. Obstruction of the aqueduct resulting in enlarged lateral ventricles
   C. Congenital hydrocephalus
   D. NPH is a communicating hydrocephalus caused by decreased reabsorption of cerebrospinal fluid

3. Which of the following neurological disease processes has been found to be most amendable to deep brain stimulation?
   A. Parkinson's disease
   B. Normal-pressure hydrocephalus
   C. Migraine headaches
   D. Myasthenia gravis

4. Where is the most common placement of the terminal wire of a deep brain stimulator for treatment of Parkinson's disease?
   A. Subthalamic nucleus
   B. Pituitary area
   C. Substantia nigra
   D. Midbrain

5. Late-stage deterioration in patients with Parkinson's disease is most commonly caused by which of the following?
   A. Development of Alzheimer's disease
   B. Flaccidity of muscles
   C. Levodopa-induced dyskinesia
   D. Complication of an ischemic stroke

## BIBLIOGRAPHY

Cristal, A., Chen, K., Hernandez, N., Litvak, P., Clark, L., Ottman, R., & Louis, E. (2018). Knowledge about essential tremor: A study of essential tremor families. *Frontiers in Neurology, 9*, 27. doi:10.3389/fneur.2018.00027

Epstein, N., & Hollingsworth, R. (2017). Nursing review section of Surgical Neurology International: Part 1 lumbar disc disease. *Surgical Neurology International, 8*(35), 301. doi:10.4103/sni.sni_151_17

Ferguson, B., & Parsh, B. (2017). Understanding Tourette syndrome. *Nursing2019, 47*(5), 67.

Freidman, B. W. (2017). Managing migraine. *Annals of Emergency Medicine, 69*(2), 202–207. doi:10.1016/j.annemergmed.2016.06.023

Freidman, B. W., & Grosberg, B. M. (2009).Diagnosis and management of the primary headache disorders in the emergency department setting. *Emergency Medicine Clinics of North America, 27*(1), 71–87. doi:10.1016/j.emc.2008.09.005

Galluzzi, K. (2005). Management of neuropathic pain. *Journal of the Osteopathic Association, 105,* S12–S19.

Gay, P. C. (2008). Complex sleep apnea: It really is a disease. *Journal of Clinical Sleep Medicine, 4,* 403–405.

Jinnah, H. (2015). Diagnosis and treatment of dystonia. *Neurologic Clinics, 33*(1), 77–100. doi:10.1016/j.ncl.2014.09.002

Lindauer, A., Sexson, K., & Harvath, T. A. (2017). Medication management for people with dementia. *American Journal of Nursing, 117*(5, Suppl. 1), S17–S21. doi:10.1097/01.NAJ.0000516389.35634.84

Long, B. J., & Koyfman, A. (2018). Benign headache management in the emergency department. *Journal of Emergency Medicine, 54*(4), 58–468. doi:10.1016/j.jemermed.2017.12.023

Marmarou, A., Bergsneider, M., Relkin, N., Klinge, P., & Black, P. M. (2005). Development of guidelines for idiopathic normal-pressure hydrocephalus: Introduction. *Neurosurgery, 57*(Suppl. 3), S1–S3. doi:10.1227/01.neu.0000168188.25559.0e

Metzgar, R. L. (2016). Evidence-based practice guidelines for the diagnosis and treatment of lumbar spinal conditions. *Nurse Practitioner, 41*(12), 30–37. doi:10.1097/01.NPR.0000508169.67852.bb

Pfeifer, G. (2017). Can dementia be prevented? *American Journal of Nursing, 117*(11), 15. doi:10.1097/01.NAJ.0000526734.90904.0d

Poetzsch, B., & Smith, J. (2012). Ménière disease. *Journal of the American Academy of Physician Assistants, 25*(1), 62.

Pullen, R. L. Jr. (2017). Navigating the challenges of Ménière disease. *Nursing, 47*(7), 38–45. doi:10.1097/01.NURSE.0000520504.06428.ce

Rizzoli, P., & Mullally, W. J. (2018). Headache. *American Journal of Medicine, 131*(1), 17–24. doi:10.1016/j.amjmed.2017.09.005

Shin, J. Y., & Habermann, B. (2016). Initiation of medications for Parkinson's disease: A qualitative description. *Journal of Clinical Nursing, 25*(1), 127–133. doi:10.1111/jocn.13009

Shin J. Y., & Hendrix, C. C. (2013). Management of Parkinson's disease. *Nurse Practitioner, 38*(10), 34–45. doi:10.1097/01.NPR.0000434090.96229.5c

Skirton, H. (2005). Huntington's disease: Nursing perspective. *Medsurg Nursing, 14*(3), 167–172.

Taverner, T. (2014). Neuropathic pain: An overview. *British Journal of Neuroscience Nursing, 10*(3), 116–123. doi:10.12968/bjnn.2014.10.3.116

Thompson, S. (2017). An introduction to hydrocephalus: Types, treatments, and management. *British Journal of Neuroscience Nursing, 13*(1), 36–40. doi:10.12968/bjnn.2017.13.1.36

Volland, J., & Fisher, A. (2014). Best practices or engaging patients with dementia. *Nursing, 44*(11), 44–50. doi:10.1097/01.NURSE.0000454951.95772.8d

Williams, M. A., & Relkin, N. R. (2013). Diagnosis and management of idiopathic normal-pressure hydrocephalus. *Neurology Clinical Practice, 3*(5), 375–385. doi:10.1212/CPJ.0b013e3182a78f6b

Wolkove, N., Elkholy, O., Baltzan, M., & Palayew, M. (2007). Sleep and aging: 1. Sleep disorders commonly found in older people. *Canadian Medical Association Journal, 176,* 1299–1304. doi:10.1503/cmaj.060792

# 2

# Cerebrovascular Disorders

## INTRODUCTION

- **What are brief episodes of neurological dysfunction resulting from focal cerebral ischemia called?**
- **Transient ischemic attacks (TIAs)**

A stroke occurs following the loss of cerebral blood flow to the brain, resulting in ischemic injuries and permanent cerebral infarction. TIAs are brief episodes of neurological dysfunction resulting from focal cerebral ischemia not associated with permanent cerebral infarction.

> ▶ **HINT:** Neurological symptoms do not have to persist greater than 24 hours to be called a stroke. The symptoms need to be persistent.

- **What are the two major classifications of stroke?**
- **Ischemic and hemorrhagic**

Ischemic strokes are attributed to vascular occlusion, resulting in a lack of distal blood flow. The lack of perfusion causes an ischemic stroke. Hemorrhagic strokes are caused by a ruptured blood vessel, resulting in intracerebral blood.

> ▶ **HINT:** Types of strokes
>
> | Ischemic | Hemorrhagic |
> |---|---|
> | Thrombotic | Intracerebral |
> | Embolic | Subarachnoid |

- **Plaque formation in the cerebral arteries can result in which type of stroke?**
- **Thrombotic stroke**

Thrombotic strokes are due to plaque formation. Atherosclerosis narrows the lumen size and unstable plaque ruptures, allowing a clot to form, obstructing blood flow. TIA frequently precedes thrombotic strokes.

> ▶ **HINT:** Neurological deficits commonly increase in severity over time.

■ *What type of stroke commonly results from atrial fibrillation?*
■ **Cardioembolic stroke**

A cardioembolic stroke occurs when a clot is dislodged from the left atrium and travels to the anterior cerebral circulation (Box 2.1). Atrial fibrillation is the most common cause of cardioembolic strokes and is the most preventable class of stroke. Other causes of embolic strokes include patent foramen ovale (PFO) and endocarditis.

> ▶ **HINT:** Left atrial appendage is the origination of the clot in cardioembolic strokes in atrial fibrillation patients.

**Box 2.1** Comparison of Thrombotic and Embolic Strokes

|  | Thrombotic | Embolic |
| --- | --- | --- |
| Cause | Atherosclerotic plaque narrows lumen of the cerebral vessel; plaque ruptures and causes thrombus to form, obstructing blood flow distally. | The clot typically originates in the heart and is thrown to the cerebral circulation; the clot obstructs smaller vessels, resulting in loss of blood flow distally; the most common location is MCA. |
| Presentation | Tends to have a progressive worsening of symptoms. | Typically has abrupt onset without the progression of symptoms. |
| Timing | May occur at rest or upon awakening. | May occur following activity or exercise. |

MCA, middle cerebral artery.

■ *What is the most reversible risk factor for both ischemic and hemorrhagic strokes?*
■ **Hypertension**

Hypertension is a known risk factor for both ischemic and hemorrhagic strokes (Box 2.2). It is considered one of the most reversible risk factors with blood pressure (BP) management. Recommended BP in nondiabetic patient is less than 140 mmHg systolic and 90 mmHg diastolic. A diabetic should have stricter BP parameters. They are recommended to be under 130/85 mmHg.

> ▶ **HINT:** Lowering BP with lifestyle changes and/or BP medications has been found to decrease the risk of stroke.

**Box 2.2** Risk Factors of Stroke

| |
| --- |
| Smoking |
| Hypertension |
| Hyperlipidemia |
| Atrial fibrillation |
| Age above 65 years |
| Diabetes mellitus |
| Sedentary lifestyle |

■ *When would secondary stroke prevention strategies be utilized?*
■ **After the initial stroke**

Primary stroke prevention means one attempts to prevent a first stroke from occurring. Secondary stroke prevention attempts to prevent a stroke patient from having a reoccurring stroke.

▶ **HINT:** Recommendations for stroke prevention may be different for primary versus secondary stroke prevention.

■ *What medications are recommended in primary prevention of thrombotic strokes?*
■ **An aspirin (81–100 mg) a day and an HMG-CoA (β-Hydroxy β-methylglutaryl-CoA) reductase inhibitor (statin) medication**

The recommendation is an aspirin (81–100 mg) a day for high-risk patients. Aspirin is not recommended for low-risk patients. An HMG-CoA reductase inhibitor (statin) medication is also recommended in patients with heart disease or other certain high-risk people (i.e., diabetics).

▶ **HINT:** Prevention of thrombotic strokes involves antiplatelet medications.

■ *What class of medication is most commonly recommended in secondary thrombotic stroke prevention?*
■ **Antiplatelet medications**

Antiplatelet drugs are preferred to oral anticoagulation therapy. The recommendation for antiplatelet therapy includes aspirin monotherapy, combination aspirin/dipyridamole (Aggrenox) therapy, or clopidogrel (Plavix) monotherapy. Statin therapy is also recommended.

▶ **HINT:** Antihypertensive medications are recommended in hypertensive patients.

■ *What class of medication is most commonly recommended in secondary prevention of cardioembolic strokes in patients with atrial fibrillation?*
■ **Antithrombotic agents**

Antithrombotic agents are recommended over antiplatelet therapy in preventing secondary strokes due to nonvalvular atrial fibrillation. Warfarin (Coumadin), a vitamin K antagonist, is the most commonly used antithrombotic agent. Direct thrombin inhibitors (i.e., dabigatran [Pradaxa]) and factor Xa inhibitors may also be used to prevent cardioembolic stroke.

▶ **HINT:** Questions on the exam may include how to monitor the anticoagulation effect of these medications and recognize side effects of hemorrhagic stroke (intracerebral hemorrhage).

■ *When cerebral aneurysm ruptures, what is the most common finding on a noncontrast CT scan?*
■ **Subarachnoid hemorrhage (SAH)**

SAH is commonly caused by an aneurysm or arteriovenous malformation. Hemorrhagic strokes are classified as intracerebral hemorrhage or SAH (Box 2.3). This is initially differentiated by the location of the blood on a noncontrast CT scan.

▶ **HINT:** Trauma can also result in an SAH.

**Box 2.3** Quick Comparison: Intracerebral and Subarachnoid Hemorrhage

|  | **Intracerebral** | **Subarachnoid** |
| --- | --- | --- |
| Cause | Hypertension | Oral anticoagulation therapy |
| Most common causes | Coagulopathies | Rupture of aneurysm or AVM |
| Location of bleed | Primarily goes into brain tissue (parenchyma) and ventricles (called *extension*) | Primarily goes into subarachnoid space and intraventricularly |
| Presentation | Headache, vomiting, hypertension, decreased level of consciousness, seizures | "Worst headache of one's life," vomiting, focal neurological deficits, decreased level of consciousness |

AVM, arteriovenous malformation.

- **What is the most common area of the brain to experience an intracerebral hemorrhage (ICH)?**
- **Basal ganglia**

The subcortical region of the basal ganglia is the most common site for an ICH (Box 2.4). ICH is commonly a result of chronic hypertension, which causes damage to the smaller, perforating vessels.

> ▶ **HINT:** The vessels involved are the same ones that cause lacunar ischemic stroke.

**Box 2.4** Common Sites of Intracerebral Hemorrhage

| |
| --- |
| Basal ganglia (putamen area) |
| Thalamus |
| Lobar |
| Pons |
| Cerebellum |

- **What is the most common risk factor for hemorrhagic stroke?**
- **Hypertension**

Hypertension, both chronic and acute, is the most common cause for hemorrhagic stroke (Box 2.5). Chronic hypertension causes damage to the lacunar vessels (small vessels) and commonly results in basal ganglia hemorrhage. Acute hypertensive bleeds can occur anywhere within the brain but commonly occur as a lobar hemorrhage.

> ▶ **HINT:** Anticoagulation therapy is another significant cause of intracerebral hemorrhage.

**Box 2.5** Causes of Intracerebral Hemorrhage

| |
| --- |
| Hypertension |
| Anticoagulation therapy |
| Coagulopathy |

*(continued)*

**Box 2.5** Causes of Intracerebral Hemorrhage *(continued)*

| |
|---|
| Vasculitis |
| Cerebral venous thrombosis |
| Sympathomimetic drugs |
| Trauma |
| Brain tumors |

- **What is the most common type of intracerebral aneurysm?**
- **Saccular aneurysm**

Saccular or "berry" aneurysms have a neck or stem. They frequently occur at bifurcations. Their size can range from 1 mm to 5 cm or greater. Fusiform aneurysms are an outputting of the vascular wall and do not have a "neck" like saccular aneurysms.

> ▶ **HINT:** Giant intracerebral aneurysms measure 2.5 cm or greater and can present as a space-occupying lesion.

- **What is the type of intracranial aneurysm caused by septic emboli commonly associated with bacterial endocarditis?**
- **Mycotic aneurysm**

Mycotic aneurysm is caused by septic emboli, which separate the endothelial lining (septic degeneration), forming an aneurysm. It is typically associated with bacterial endocarditis.

> ▶ **HINT:** Traumatic injury can also cause a shearing of the endothelial lining, resulting in formation of an aneurysm.

- **A system of dilated vessels that shunt arterial blood directly into the venous system without the capillary network is called what?**
- **Arteriovenous malformation (AVM)**

AVM is a high-pressure system (arteries) that feeds directly into a low-pressure system (venous) without capillaries in between. AVMs are composed of a nidus, which is a fairly well-circumscribed center, as well as the feeding arteries and draining veins.

> ▶ **HINT:** Rupture of the AVM results in bleeding primarily into the subarachnoid space but it can also bleed into subdural or intracerebral tissue. Presentation is similar to an aneurysm rupture.

## PATHOPHYSIOLOGY

- **What is the term used in strokes to indicate the ischemic or reversible injury zone?**
- **Penumbra**

*Penumbra* refers to the reversible injury (ischemic zone) in an ischemic stroke (Box 2.6). The core is the irreversible area of infarction. Therapy is aimed at reperfusing the penumbra, reversing the injury, and limiting the infarction size.

> ▶ **HINT:** The primary goal for treatment in ischemic strokes is to reverse the penumbra, or reperfuse the ischemic zone.

**Box 2.6** Zones of Injury in Ischemic Stroke

| |
|---|
| Core (irreversible injury) |
| Penumbra (reversible injury) |
| Hyperperfusion (localized edema) |

■ *What is hemorrhagic transformation in ischemic stroke?*
■ **Bleeding into the ischemic core**

Hemorrhagic transformation is considered a natural evolution of an ischemic stroke and is usually asymptomatic. CT scans obtained following an acute ischemic stroke and potentially after reperfusion may demonstrate hemorrhage in the infarcted area of the brain. This is called *transformation*.

> ▶ **HINT:** Hemorrhagic transformation frequently occurs within the infarcted zone, which is the irreversible injury area and is usually asymptomatic.

■ *Which cerebral artery is most commonly involved in embolic strokes?*
■ **Middle cerebral artery (MCA)**

The MCA is predominantly affected in embolic strokes. The carotid artery feeds directly into the MCA, and the MCA is the largest vessel in the circle of Willis. A clot flows more readily into the MCA.

> ▶ **HINT:** An embolic stroke presents with an abrupt onset of symptoms and is not usually preceded by TIAs.

■ *Which hemisphere is considered to be the dominant hemisphere in the majority of the people?*
■ **Left hemisphere**

The dominant hemisphere is the hemisphere that contains the language centers (Broca's and Wernicke's). The dominant hemisphere is predominantly the left hemisphere in the majority of people.

> ▶ **HINT:** Left hemispheric strokes are typically considered "devastating" due to the loss of language (expressive and/or receptive).

■ *Following an intracerebral hemorrhage from acute hypertension, does the clot remain the same size or expand?*
■ **Expand**

Rupture of cerebral artery leads to accumulation of blood in the parenchyma of the brain with substantial increases in hematoma size up to 12 hours post initial bleed. This increase in clot volume has been shown to be associated with clinical neurological deterioration.

> ▶ **HINT:** It is common for neurological status to deteriorate rapidly in the first few hours after the bleed, which is associated with a decrease in the Glasgow Coma Scale (GCS) score.

## 2. CEREBROVASCULAR DISORDERS

■ *What is the primary physiologic cause of brain tissue damage in ICH?*
■ **Space-occupying lesion**

The ICH clot damages the brain tissue, displaces the structure of the brain, and dissects the tissue (Box 2.7). After hours to days, extracellular (vasogenic) edema develops in the periphery of the hematoma. Shifts and herniation syndrome can occur.

▶ **HINT:** ICH is considered a space-occupying lesion. The larger clot causes a greater amount of damage and herniation.

**Box 2.7** Intracerebral Hemorrhage Physiology

| Cerebral edema |
| --- |
| Disruption of brain tissue |
| Compression of adjacent tissue |
| Intracranial pressure elevation |
| Herniation syndromes |

■ *What is an aneurysm rupture frequently associated with?*
■ **Increase in BP**

A sudden increase in BP is often associated with the rupture of an aneurysm. The activities that increase BP may vary but are commonly seen with exercise or physical activity, stress, sexual activity, or use of sympathomimetic drugs and alcohol.

▶ **HINT:** The most common presentation is the sudden onset of headache associated with these activities.

■ *What portion of the cerebral circulation experiences the most intracerebral aneurysms?*
■ **Circle of Willis**

The most common location is the anterior circulation with 85% to 90% of the aneurysms found in the Circle of Willis. Intracerebral aneurysms are found in the branches or bifurcations of the cerebral circulation (Box 2.8). The Circle of Willis contains multiple bifurcations.

▶ **HINT:** The Circle of Willis sits adjacent to the third ventricle. It is common for the rupture of an aneurysm to cause IVH as well as SAH.

**Box 2.8** Common Locations of Cerebral Aneurysms

| Intracranial internal carotid artery |
| --- |
| Posterior communicating artery |
| Anterior communicating artery |
| Middle cerebral artery |
| Anterior cerebral artery |
| Basilar tip |
| Posterior inferior cerebellar artery |

■ **What scale is used to grade the severity of the SAH?**
■ **Hunt and Hess**

The SAH is graded based on the presenting signs and symptoms, which determine the severity and outcomes of the SAH. Grade I is the least severe and grade V represents the worst clinical presentation and predicted outcome (Box 2.9).

▶ **HINT:** Grade 0 is an unruptured aneurysm found incidentally.

**Box 2.9** Hunt and Hess Grading System for Subarachnoid Hemorrhage Severity

| Grade I | Asymptomatic, mild headache, slight nuchal rigidity |
|---|---|
| Grade II | Moderate to severe headache, nuchal rigidity, no neurologic deficit other than cranial nerve palsy |
| Grade III | Drowsiness/confusion, mild focal neurologic deficit |
| Grade IV | Stupor, moderate to severe hemiparesis |
| Grade V | Coma, decerebrate posturing |

## SYMPTOMS/ASSESSMENT

■ **Which population is more likely to present with nontraditional symptoms?**
■ **Women**

Women are 60% more likely than men to present with one of the nontraditional symptoms. These include sudden face, arm, or leg pain, mental status changes, generalized neurological symptoms (hiccupping, nausea and vomiting), sudden chest pain or palpitations, sudden tiredness, or shortness of breath.

▶ **HINT:** Mental status changes are most often associated with stroke in women.

■ **A patient presents with facial droop and upper extremity weakness. Which vessel is most likely involved?**
■ **MCA**

The MCA perfuses the portion of the motor strip responsible for movement of the upper extremities and face. Common presentation of MCA occlusion is unilateral upper extremity weakness/paralysis and facial droop (Box 2.10).

▶ **HINT:** Remember, motor symptoms are contralateral to the site of the injury/infarction in the cerebral cortex.

**Box 2.10** Stroke Syndromes of Anterior Circulation

| Anterior Cerebral Artery | Middle Cerebral Artery | Internal Carotid Artery |
|---|---|---|
| Impaired gait | Hemiplegia contralateral to upper extremity | Hemiplegia contralateral to upper and lower extremity |
| Paresis/paralysis contralateral lower extremity | Sensory impairment contralateral upper to extremity | Sensory impairment contralateral to upper and lower extremity |

*(continued)*

**Box 2.10** Stroke Syndromes of Anterior Circulation *(continued)*

| Anterior Cerebral Artery | Middle Cerebral Artery | Internal Carotid Artery |
|---|---|---|
| Flat affect | Aphasia (dominant hemisphere) | Homonymous hemianopsia |
| Impaired mentation | Hemineglect (nondominant hemisphere) | Aphasia (dominant hemisphere) |
| Gaze deviation toward affective side | Gaze deviation toward affective side | Agnosia |
| Aphasia (dominant hemisphere) | Dysarthria | Hemineglect |
| Urinary incontinence | | Amaurosis fugax |

- *Occlusion of which of the cerebral vessels can cause locked-in syndrome?*
- Basilar artery

The basilar artery supplies blood to the ventral portion of the pons. This is the location of the motor pathway. An occlusion of the basilar artery can result in the complete loss of motor control called *locked-in syndrome* (Box 2.11).

▶ **HINT:** The basilar artery is a component of the posterior circulation.

**Box 2.11** Stroke Syndromes of Posterior Circulation

| Posterior Cerebral Artery | Vertebral Basilar Arteries | Cerebellar Arteries | Basilar Artery |
|---|---|---|---|
| Contralateral homonymous hemianopsia | Impaired mentation/ loss of consciousness | Nausea and vomiting | Quadraplegia |
| Visual deficits | Cranial nerve deficits | Vertigo | Locked-in syndrome |
| Memory deficits | Dysarthria | Nystagmus | Weakness of face, tongue, and pharyngeal muscles |
| Receptive aphasia | Dysphagia | Ataxia | |
| | Ipsilateral Horner's syndrome | Dysphagia | |
| | Nystagmus | Dysarthria | |
| | Dizziness/vertigo | Contralateral loss of pain and temperature | |
| | Nausea and vomiting | Ipsilateral Horner's syndrome | |
| | Ataxia | | |
| | Contralateral paresis or paralysis extremities | | |
| | Ipsilateral face sensory abnormalities | | |

■ *What symptom is considered a red flag for a patient experiencing an ICH?*
■ **Sudden-onset headache associated with nausea and vomiting**

The classic clinical presentation of ICH includes the onset of a sudden focal neurological deficit, commonly a headache or altered level of consciousness, which progresses over minutes to hours. Other symptoms include nausea and vomiting, seizures, and focal neurological deficits. Onset usually occurs with activity and rarely occurs at night.

> ▶ **HINT:** Vomiting is more common with ICH than with either ischemic stroke or SAH.

■ *What is the most common presentation of patients with SAH from an aneurysm rupture?*
■ **Worst headache of one's life**

One of the most common presentations of an SAH is the "worst headache of my life" (Box 2.12). Sudden-onset headache is often associated with activities that can increase blood pressure.

> ▶ **HINT:** Headache in combination with vomiting is a strong indicator for potential SAH.

**Box 2.12** Symptoms of Subarachnoid Hemorrhage

| |
|---|
| Headache |
| Vomiting |
| Nuchal rigidity |
| Focal neurological deficits |
| LOC |
| CN deficits (especially CN III) |
| Pupillary changes |
| Visual disturbances |
| Low-grade fever |

CN, cranial nerve; LOC, loss of consciousness.

## DIAGNOSIS

■ *Which radiographic study is considered the gold standard for initial diagnostic study of ischemic stroke?*
■ **Noncontrast CT scan**

Even though the actual infarct may not be recognized on CT scan until 12 to 24 hours after the infarct, the scan is used to rule out hemorrhagic strokes and other causes of neurological deterioration that can mimic a stroke (Box 2.13).

> ▶ **HINT:** Newer multimodal CT and MRI scans are available in some centers that will identify ischemic strokes earlier and have the ability to differentiate between reversible and irreversible injury.

**Box 2.13** Stroke Mimics

| |
|---|
| Postictal state |
| CNS infections |
| Intracerebral tumors |
| Toxic–metabolic encephalopathy |
| Hypoglycemia or hyperglycemia |
| Subdural hematoma |
| Migraines |

CNS, central nervous system.

- **When obtaining a recent history of symptoms, what is the single most important historical information to obtain?**
- **Time of onset of symptoms**

The most important assessment is last known normal (LKN) to determine indications of thrombolytic therapy. The clock starts for determining indications for intravenous thrombolytic therapy and intervention when the patient was at his or her previous baseline or symptom free; this is termed *last known normal*.

> ▶ **HINT:** If a patient wakes up with symptoms of a stroke, the LKN is the time he or she went to sleep in a normal neurological state.

- **A patient awakens with facial drop and slurred speech. Is this patient a candidate for intravenous thrombolytic therapy?**
- **No**

Symptoms of a stroke found upon awakening are called a *wake-up stroke* and are not considered appropriate for intravenous thrombolytics because of the time window. The actual time of onset (or LKN) is not known.

> ▶ **HINT:** If the patient has a wake-up stroke but presents with a large-vessel obstruction, he or she may be a candidate for intraarterial thrombolysis or thrombectomy.

- **A patient presents with symptoms of a stroke, which have resolved completely in the ED. About 1 hour later, the patient's symptoms reoccur. Is this a potential case for intravenous (IV) thrombolytic therapy?**
- **Yes**

If a patient's symptoms completely resolve and return at a later time, he or she is a potential candidate for IV thrombolytics. The time window for therapy is reset if the patient returns to normal again.

> ▶ **HINT:** The time is not reset if the symptoms are "resolving" but patient is not completely back to normal.

- **What is the most commonly used stroke assessment tool to determine the severity of the stroke?**

## The National Institutes of Health Stroke Scale (NIHSS)

The NIHSS is the most commonly utilized stroke assessment tool. It is used to determine the severity of the stroke and can be used for ischemic and hemorrhagic strokes.

> ▶ **HINT:** The NIHSS is not as effective in identifying posterior strokes as anterior.

## What is the most important laboratory result to have before administering alteplase?
## Glucose level

A glucose test is recommended on every patient prior to the administration of alteplase. Hypoglycemia is a stroke mimic. If the patient is hypoglycemic, administer glucose and continue to assess the patient's neurological status. If symptoms do not resolve and the patient is normoglycemic, it still may be a stroke.

> ▶ **HINT:** An international normalized ratio (INR) is important and required prior to alteplase administration in patients on a vitamin K antagonist (VKA).

## What associated finding on the CT scan would indicate a poor prognosis in patients with ICH?
## Intraventricular extension

Intraventricular extension occurs when the artery ruptures near the ventricles and the tissue loss occurs through the wall of the ventricular system. Bleeding then occurs into the ventricular system, resulting in damage to the ventricles and the development of hydrocephalus.

> ▶ **HINT:** The combination of ICH and IVH offers a poor prognosis.

## When an SAH is identified on a plain CT, what further diagnostic study is recommended?
## Cerebral angiogram

A cerebral angiogram is recommended to identify the presence of an aneurysm or arteriovenous malformation, location, and size. The angiogram can be performed initially with CT angiogram (CTA) or MR angiogram as a screening tool. The most definitive diagnostic tool is an invasive digital subtraction arteriogram (DSA).

> ▶ **HINT:** A DSA can identify an aneurysm smaller than 4 mm, which the CTA may not be able to identify.

# MEDICAL MANAGEMENT

## What systolic pressure needs to be treated if an ischemic stroke patient is NOT a candidate for thrombolytic therapy?
## Pressure greater than 220 mmHg

If the patient is not a candidate for thrombolytic therapy and has ruled out a hemorrhagic stroke, then the recommendation is to not treat the BP unless the systolic reading is greater than 220 mmHg or the diastolic is greater than 120 mmHg.

> ▶ **HINT:** If the patient is a candidate for thrombolytic therapy, then systolic BP is kept below 180 mmHg.

## 2. CEREBROVASCULAR DISORDERS

■ *Within how many hours from onset of symptoms, is it recommended to administer an IV thrombolytic in an ischemic stroke patient?*

■ **3 hours**

Based upon the American Heart Association (AHA)/American Stroke Association (ASA) recommendations, the time can be expanded to 4.5 hours in some patients, but the goal is still within 3 hours of onset. The earlier the blood clot is dissolved and reperfusion is established, the better the neurological outcomes.

▶ **HINT:** Administration beyond the 4.5 hours from LKN can increase the risk of bleeding.

■ *When administering IV alteplase for an ischemic stroke, the BP should be less than?*

■ **185/110 mmHg**

The recommendation of administering IV alteplase only when the BP is less than 185/110 mmHg is to lower the risk of the bleeding complications of alteplase. This BP management can be done with any antihypertensive if needed, but being able to titrate to prevent hypotension is suggested. Hypotension can worsen neurological outcomes.

▶ **HINT:** Once the alteplase is administered, it is recommended the BP remains less than 180/105 mmHg.

■ *What is considered the most definitive contraindication for administering alteplase to a patient with stroke symptoms?*

■ **Hemorrhagic stroke**

Any signs of blood on plain CT scan on patients with stroke-like symptoms are an absolute contraindication to administering a thrombolytic. Other contraindications include, but are not limited to novel anticoagulant administration within 48 hours, INR >1.7, platelet count <100,000 mcL and recent history of significant high-risk surgery for bleeding, gastrointestinal bleeding, traumatic brain injury, and spinal surgeries.

▶ **HINT:** Age and a low NIHSS score are no longer contraindications for thrombolytics.

■ *When caring for a patient with an ischemic stroke in the ICU, the following vital signs were obtained: BP is 172/82 mmHg, heart rate (HR) is 85 beats/minute, respiratory rate (RR) of 18 breaths/minute, $SaO_2$ of 99%, and temperature of 38.2°C. Which of these vital signs would be a concern to the ICU nurse?*

■ **Temperature**

Fever following a stroke can increase the risk for a poor neurological outcome. Following a stroke, patients should be monitored closely for fever, and the temperature should be managed immediately. The goal is to maintain a stroke patient within the normal body temperature range.

▶ **HINT:** Currently, there is insufficient evidence to recommend hypothermia for treatment of patients with acute stroke.

■ **Which electrolyte abnormality can worsen neurological outcomes and should be corrected?**

■ **Hyperglycemia**

Hyperglycemia causes worsening neurological outcomes. Stroke patient's glucose level should be monitored frequently, and hyperglycemia should be treated. The mechanism of the worsening of the neurological outcomes may include alteration in anaerobic metabolism and damage to the blood–brain barrier, contributing to cerebral edema. Hyperglycemia may be associated with risk of hemorrhagic transformation of the infarction and increased bleed risk following administration of thrombolytics.

> ▶ **HINT:** Hyperglycemia is not an absolute contraindication to administration of alteplase, but it should be corrected appropriately.

■ **What medication is recommended initially in ischemic stroke patients with contraindications for thrombolytics?**

■ **Aspirin**

An aspirin is recommended initially in patients who are not candidates for thrombolytics. If a patient receives a thrombolytic, aspirin should not be administered until 24 hours after the thrombolytic.

> ▶ **HINT:** Aspirin is recommended as secondary prevention for an ischemic stroke patient.

■ **What should be performed prior to administration of oral intake, including oral medications?**

■ **Bedside swallow screen**

Prior to administering oral intake, including oral medications, a bedside swallow screen should always be performed on stroke patients or patients with stroke-like symptoms

> ▶ **HINT:** Aspirin can be administered rectally if an ischemic stroke patient is unable to pass the bedside swallow test.

■ **A patient with an ischemic stroke has a low-density lipoprotein (LDL) level of 110. What class of medication is recommended?**

■ **Statin**

High LDL is a risk factor for stroke, and a statin is recommended. An LDL level should be obtained on stroke patients and managed according to current guidelines for use of statins.

> ▶ **HINT:** Patients diagnosed with an ischemic stroke who are already on a statin, may require a high-intensity statin.

■ **What is the priority of care in patients with ICH?**

■ **Airway and breathing**

ICH commonly presents with a loss of consciousness (LOC). An LOC results frequently in loss of airway and ineffective breathing. Airway and breathing are always the priorities of care in stroke patients.

> ▶ **HINT:** Airway is more important than noncontrast CT scans and stroke treatments, especially if the patient has an LOC.

## 2. CEREBROVASCULAR DISORDERS

■ *Following an intracerebral hemorrhage, what is the goal for BP management?*
■ **Systolic BP less than 160 mmHg**

The level of BP control has not been established, but a decrease in systolic BP to less than 160 mmHg is reasonable. The systolic BP may be frequently maintained in the range of 130 to 150 mmHg. This range may decrease risk of hypertensive extension of the bleed and allows for adequate cerebral perfusion.

> ▶ **HINT:** BP is frequently controlled with a titratable agent to balance the risk of hypertension-related rebleeding and maintenance of cerebral perfusion (Box 2.14).

**Box 2.14** Intravenous Medications for Management of an Intracerebral Hemorrhage

| Drug | Bolus | Continuous Infusion |
| --- | --- | --- |
| Labetalol | 5–20 mg every 15 min | 2 mg/min (maximum 300 mg/d) |
| Nicardipine | NA | 5–15 mg/h |
| Esmolol | 250 mcg/kg IVP loading dose | 25–300 mcg/kg/min |
| Enalapril | 1.25–5 mg IVP every 6 h | NA |
| Hydralazine | 5–20 mg IVP every 30 min | 1–5 mg/hr |
| Nipride | NA | 0.1–10 mcg/kg/min |
| Nitroglycerin | NA | 0–400 mcg/min |

IVP, intravenous push; NA, not applicable.

■ *It has been determined that the cause of the acute ICH was anticoagulation therapy with warfarin and an elevated INR greater than 4. What would you expect the patient to receive?*
■ **Prothrombin complex concentrate (PCC)**

PCC reverses the INR more rapidly than vitamin K and fresh frozen plasma (FFP). Patients with ICH will have rapid extension of the bleed if allowed to remain anticoagulated. Administering PCC will correct the INR and decrease the hematoma expansion.

> ▶ **HINT:** Vitamin K is still administered with the PCC due to the shorter half-life of the PCC.

## SURGICAL MANAGEMENT

■ *Obstruction of which cerebral vessels is considered a large vessel obstruction (LVO)?*
■ **MCA**

Obstruction of the MCA is considered an LVO and is recommended to be treated with endovascular thrombectomy and/or an intra-arterial thrombolytic. If there are no contraindications to an IV thrombolytic, it is recommended it be administered before an intervention.

> ▶ **HINT:** Small vessel obstructions are treated with IV thrombolytics if within the time window and no contraindications exist.

- **If a patient with an LVO is on a novel anticoagulant, is he or she a candidate for interventional thrombectomy?**
- **Yes**

Patients with LVO are candidates for interventional thrombectomy even though they may be on an anticoagulant or have an elevated INR. They would NOT be candidates for an IV thrombolytic prior to the procedure.

▶ **HINT:** Potentially, LVO patients may be candidates for interventional procedures even up to 24 hours from LKN.

- **What is the recommended thrombectomy device to be used as the first deployment device in interventional treatment?**
- **Stent retriever**

Stent retrievers are the recommended thrombectomy devices to be deployed initially during interventional thrombectomy. Other devices may be used during the clot retrieval.

▶ **HINT:** Intraarterial thrombolysis can be used in combination with clot retrieval devices.

- **When considering surgical evacuation of an intracerebral hemorrhage, which location of the clot is recommended for surgery?**
- **Cerebellum**

The current recommendation is to perform clot evacuation in symptomatic cerebellar hemorrhage within 24 to 48 hours. Surgery is not recommended to evacuate deep or large clots in the supratentorial area.

▶ **HINT:** CT-guided aspiration or minimally invasive endoscopic surgery for clots close to the surface is being performed to evacuate hematomas.

## COMPLICATIONS

- **What is a potentially life-threatening complication of alteplase, besides bleeding?**
- **Angioedema**

Bleeding is a potential complication of alteplase, but another potential complication is angioedema. Angioedema is potentially life-threatening due to airway swelling. It is typically managed with antihistamines and steroids.

▶ **HINT:** The examination is more likely to ask about angioedema as a complication of alteplase.

- **What is the most life-threatening complication of an SAH that occurs within the first 24 hours following an aneurysm rupture?**
- **Rebleed**

Rebleed following the initial aneurysm rupture has the highest mortality rate. The peak incidence of a rebleed is within the first 24 to 48 hours. Prior to securing the aneurysm, the patient's blood pressure needs to be lowered and interventions implemented to lower the risk of a rebleed. These interventions are called *subarachnoid precautions* (Box 2.15).

▶ **HINT:** The best method to use to lower the risk of a rebleed is to secure the aneurysm with either surgical clips or endovascular coiling.

**Box 2.15** Subarachnoid Precautions: Interventions to Lower the Risk of Rebleeds in Patients With Subarachnoid Hemorrhage

| |
|---|
| Lower blood pressure (<120–140 mmHg). |
| Avoid straining or Valsalva maneuvers. |
| Maintain dark, quiet room. |
| Maintain bed rest. |
| Decrease physical stimulation. |
| Manage pain. |
| Manage anxiety. |

■ *Your patient is 7 days post SAH. During the day, the patient has a sudden decrease in LOC. Which complication is the most likely cause of the LOC?*

■ **Vasospasm (VS)**

VS is defined as the focal narrowing of the cerebral arteries. It most commonly occurs within 7 to 10 days following the SAH. Symptoms of VS can be ANY neurological deficit. Diagnosis is screened using transcranial Doppler (TCD) and confirmed with angiography.

▶ **HINT:** The examination question frequently uses the number of days after an SAH to determine the cause of a neurological change.

■ *What primary treatment is used to improve perfusion during VS?*

■ **Hypertension**

Hypertension and optimization of hemodynamics are used in an attempt to open the vessel in VS and perfuse the brain distally. Hypertension is the mainstay of treatment of VS. Blood pressure is usually driven above 160 mmHg.

▶ **HINT:** "Triple H" therapy used to be initiated (hypertension, hypervolemia, hemodilution) to treat VS but is no longer recommended due to complications of volume overload.

■ *What is the primary function of the calcium channel blocker nimodipine (Nimotop), administered from the time of admission until 14 to 21 days after admission?*

■ **It is a neuroprotectant.**

Nimodipine has been found to improve neurological outcomes through neuroprotection. It has been shown to improve collateral circulation and protect the brain tissue during ischemia. It has been found to improve neurologic outcomes.

▶ **HINT:** Interventions may involve angioplasty and intraarterial antihypertensives to open the vessels in vasospasm and reperfuse the brain.

■ *What is the most common electrolyte abnormality in patients with SAH?*

■ **Hyponatremia**

Sodium abnormalities are common following any neurological insult. SAH patients frequently experience hyponatremia. This can be attributed to syndrome of inappropriate antidiuretic hormone (SIADH) and cerebral salt wasting syndrome (CSWS).

> ▶ **HINT:** Other complications of SAH include hydrocephalus, cerebral edema, and increased intracranial pressure (ICP).

# Sample Exam Questions

1. A patient is brought into the emergency room with right-sided weakness and facial droop. A noncontrast brain CT scan is obtained. The brain CT results are negative. Which of the following is the most accurate statement regarding this patient?

    A. This patient should be diagnosed as having a transient ischemic attack.
    B. A negative CT brain scan indicates the stroke age is undetermined.
    C. The brain CT scan ruled out hemorrhagic stroke only.
    D. The patient did not have an ischemic stroke.

2. Which of the following is a potential complication of intravenous alteplase?

    A. Angioedema
    B. Thrombocytopenia
    C. Leukocytosis
    D. Hypotension

3. How long should nimodipine be administered in aneurysm-ruptured subarachnoid hemorrhage?

    A. 48 hours
    B. 1 year
    C. 21 days
    D. 3 months

4. Which of the following diagnostic studies is frequently used to screen for the occurrence of vasospasm following a subarachnoid hemorrhage?

    A. PET scan
    B. Noncontrast CT scan
    C. Cerebral angiograms
    D. Transcranial Doppler

5. If the right side (nondominant hemisphere) is affected by the stroke, the patient will most likely demonstrate which of the following?

    A. Neglect of unaffected side
    B. Neglect of affected side
    C. Aphasia
    D. Ipsilateral hemiplegia

6. Which of the following vessels involved in an ischemic stroke is most likely to result in incontinence of the patient?

    A. Anterior cerebral artery
    B. Middle cerebral artery
    C. Posterior cerebral artery
    D. Vertebral artery

## BIBLIOGRAPHY

Albers, G. W., Thijs, V. N., Wechsler, L., Kemp, S., Schlaug, G., Skalabrin, E., ... DEFUSE Investigators. (2006). Magnetic resonance imaging profiles predict clinical response to early reperfusion: The diffusion and perfusion imaging evaluation for understanding stroke evolution (DEFUSE) study. *Annals of Neurology, 60*(5), 508–517. doi:10.1002/ana.20976

Bader, M. K., & Palmer, S. (2006). What's the "hyper" in hyperacute stroke? Strategies to improve outcomes in ischemic stroke patients presenting within 6 hours. *AACN Advanced Critical Care, 17*(2), 194–214.

Furie, K. L., Kasner, S. E., Adams, R. J., Albers, G. W., Bush, R. L., Fagan, S. C., ... American Heart Association Stroke Council, Council on Cardiovascular Nursing, Council on Clinical Cardiology, and Interdisciplinary Council on Quality of Care and Outcomes Research. (2011). Guidelines for the prevention of stroke in patients with stroke or transient ischemic attack: A guideline for healthcare professionals from the American Heart Association/American Stroke Association. *Stroke, 42*(1), 227–276. doi:10.1161/STR.0b013e3181f7d043

Hacke, W., Kaste, M., Bluhmki, E., Brozman, M., Dávalos, A., Guidetti, D., ... ECASS Investigators. (2008). Thrombolysis with alteplase 3 to 4.5 hours after acute ischemic stroke. *New England Journal of Medicine, 359*(13), 1317–1329. doi:10.1056/NEJMoa0804656

January, C. T., Wann, L. S., Alpert, J. S., Calkins, H., Cigarroa, J. E., Cleveland, J. C., ... ACC/AHA Task Force Members. (2014). 2014 AHA/ACC/HRS guideline for the management of patients with atrial fibrillation: Executive summary: A report of the American College of Cardiology/American Heart Association Task Force on practice guidelines and the Heart Rhythm Society [published correction appears in *Circulation,* 2014; 130: e270–271]. *Circulation, 130,* 2071–2104. doi:10.1161/CIR.0000000000000040

Middleton, S., Grimley, R., & Alexandrov, A. W. (2015). Triage, treatment, and transfer: Evidence-based clinical practice recommendations and models of nursing care for the first 72 hours of admission to hospital for acute stroke. *Stroke, 46*(2), e18–e25. doi:10.1161/STROKEAHA.114.006139

Powers, W., Rabenstein, T., Adeoye, O., Bambakidis, K., Becker, K., Biller, J., ... American Heart Association Stroke Council. (2018). 2018 Guidelines for the early management of patients with acute ischemic stroke: A guideline for healthcare professionals from the American Heart Association/American Stroke Association. *Stroke, 49*(3), e46–e99. doi:10.1161/STR.0000000000000158

Smith, E. E., Kent, D. M., Bulsara, K. R., Leung, L. Y., Lichtman, J. H., Reeves, M. J., ... American Heart Association Stroke Council. (2018). Accuracy of prediction instruments for diagnosing large vessel occlusion in individuals with suspected stroke: A systematic review for the 2018 guidelines for the early management of patients with acute ischemic stroke: A guideline for healthcare professionals from the American Heart Association/American Stroke Association. *Stroke, 49*(3), e111–e122. doi:10.1161/STR.0000000000000160

Sturgeon, J. D., Folsom, A. R., Longstreth, W. T., Jr., Shahar, E., Rosamond, W. D., & Cushman, M. (2007). Risk factors for intracerebral hemorrhage in a pooled prospective study. *Stroke, 38,* 2718–2725. doi:10.1161/STROKEAHA.107.487090

Towfighi, A., Ovbiagele, B., El Husseini, N., Hackett, M., Jorge, R., Kissela, B., ... Council on Quality of Care and Outcomes Research. (2017). Poststroke depression: A scientific statement for healthcare professionals from the American Heart Association/American Stroke Association. *Stroke, 48*(2), e30–e43. doi:10.1161/STR.0000000000000113

Yaghi, S., Willey, J. Z., Cucchiara, B., Goldstein, J. N., Gonzales, N. R., Khatri, P., ... Council on Quality of Care and Outcomes Research. (2017). Treatment and outcome of hemorrhagic transformation after intravenous alteplase in acute ischemic stroke: A scientific statement for healthcare professionals from the American Heart Association/American Stroke Association. *Stroke, 48*(12), e343–e361. doi:10.1161/STR.0000000000000152

# 3

# Tumors of the Brain and Spinal Cord

## INTRODUCTION

- *A brain tumor that originates in the central nervous system (CNS) and consists of CNS cells is called?*
- **Primary brain tumor**

A primary brain tumor originates in the CNS and is composed of CNS cells. A secondary brain tumor is a metastatic tumor. Metastatic brain tumors originate outside of the CNS and spread to the CNS (Box 3.1).

> ▶ **HINT:** Lung cancer (especially non-small cell) frequently spreads to the brain and is one of the most common causes of secondary brain tumors.

**Box 3.1** Common Locations of Metastasis

| Lung (non-small cell) |
|---|
| Skin (melanoma) |
| Breast |
| Renal |
| Colon |

- *What is the most recognized environmental exposure known to cause primary brain tumors?*
- **Ionizing radiation**

Many studies have been done on potential environmental exposures for risk factors that cause primary brain tumors. Of all of these environmental potential risk factors, exposure to ionizing radiation has been recognized to increase the risk of developing a primary brain tumor. Other potential exposures may include cigarette smoking, residential power-line exposure, and consumption of nitrites in food.

> ▶ **HINT:** Genetic predisposition is another known risk factor for the development of brain tumors.

■ *What is the autosomal-dominant disorder that is characterized by the development of tumors along the nerve sheath?*
■ **Neurofibromatosis type I**

Neurofibromatosis type I is a genetic disorder that affects *NF1* gene, which is responsible for the production of a protein that suppresses tumor cells along nerves (Box 3.2). Diagnosis of this genetic abnormality usually occurs in the pediatric population. Neurofibromas develop along peripheral and CNS nerves, with the most common CNS tumor being optic pilocytic astrocytoma.

> ▶ **HINT:** Neurofibromatosis type II frequently presents with bilateral vestibular schwannomas.

**Box 3.2** Genetic Syndromes That Increase Risk of Brain Tumors

| |
|---|
| Cowden syndrome |
| Gorlin syndrome |
| Li-Fraumeni syndrome |
| Neurofibromatosis type I |
| Tuberous sclerosis |
| Turcot syndrome |
| Von Hippel–Lindau disease |

■ *Which of the glial cells line the ventricles in the brain?*
■ **Ependymal cells**

Ependymal cells line the ventricles and the central canal of the spinal cord. Tumors arising from the ependymal cells are called *ependymomas*.

> ▶ **HINT:** An ependymoma commonly presents with obstructive (noncommunicating) hydrocephalus.

■ *Which of the glial cells form the blood–brain barrier (BBB)?*
■ **Astrocyte cells**

Astrocyte cells are small glial cell bodies that extend into the piaglial membrane next to the subarachnoid space. They form the BBB. The astrocytes also proliferate to fill the spaces left by the death of neurons in the scarring process.

> ▶ **HINT:** An astrocytoma is a type of glioma.

■ *Which of the glial cells are responsible for the formation and repair of the myelin sheaths that surround the neurons?*
■ **Oligodendrocytes**

Oligodendrocytes are smaller than astrocyte cells and are found in rows along the nerve fibers. They are responsible for myelin formation and maintenance.

> ▶ **HINT:** Pure oligodendrioglioma is not common. Typically the tumor contains astrocyte cells.

### 3. TUMORS OF THE BRAIN AND SPINAL CORD

■ *Which of the glial cells do not multiply to form a tumor?*
■ **Microglial cells**

Microglial cells are the smallest of the brain cells. They are macrophages in the brain that migrate to the sites of inflammation, degeneration, and injured brain cells.

▶ **HINT:** This is the only glial cell that is not at risk of becoming a tumor.

■ *Which is the most common location for a CNS tumor to be found?*
■ **Meninges**

Of the CNS tumors, brain tumors account for about 80%, whereas 20% of these tumors are located in the spine (Box 3.3). The most common location for a CNS tumor is in the meninges, and this tumor is called a *meningioma*. These are typically nonmalignant and classified as extra-axial tumors (intracranial tumors not located in brain tissue).

▶ **HINT:** The most common malignant CNS tumor is a glioma.

**Box 3.3** Locations of Central Nervous System Tumors

| |
|---|
| Meninges |
| Pituitary |
| Pineal |
| Lobes of brain (frontal, parietal, occipital, temporal) |
| Cerebrum (including subcortical areas) |
| Cerebellum |
| Ventricles |
| Brainstem |
| Cranial nerves |
| Spinal cord and cauda equina |

■ *When a tumor is termed* extra-axial, *where is it located?*
■ **Outside of brain tissue**

Extra-axial tumors originate outside of the actual brain tissue (glial cells). These tumors originate in the meninges, cranial nerves, and pituitary gland, whereas intra-axial tumors originate from the glial cells and are more destructive and invasive.

▶ **HINT:** Extra-axial tumors are more amendable to surgical excision than are intra-axial tumors.

■ *Is a grade I–II tumor benign or malignant?*
■ **Benign**

The grading of tumors is determined by the microscopic evaluation of the cells. Grades I and II are the least abnormal under the microscope and are considered benign based on cellular appearance and growth. Grades III and IV are abnormal cells that experience rapid growth and cell division. These are considered to be malignant.

- **If a spinal tumor is described as intramedullary, where would the tumor be located?**
- **Within the spinal cord**

Intramedullary tumors are located within the spinal cord and are commonly found in the cervical region. The tumors are derived from the glial cells, most often astrocytes or ependymal cells. Extradural tumors (located outside the spinal cord) are usually the result of metastatic disease.

▶ **HINT:** The most common site of metastatic spine tumor origination is bone.

## PATHOPHYSIOLOGY

- **Primary brain tumors are classified based on the type of cell from which they originate. A glial cell can develop into which type of primary brain tumor?**
- **Glioma**

Glial cells are the support cells of the brain. They are like the "glue" of the brain tissue. Glial cells include astrocytes, oligodendrocytes, microglial cells, and ependymal cells (Box 3.4).

▶ **HINT:** The only glial cell that does not develop into a tumor is the microglial cell.

**Box 3.4** Primary Gliomas

| Brain Cells | Tumor | Function |
| --- | --- | --- |
| Astrocyte cell | Astrocytoma | Form the BBB and primary brain tissue |
| Oligodendrocyte | Oligodendroglioma | Form and maintain the myelin sheath |
| Ependymal | Ependymoma | Line the ventricles and facilitate movement of CSF |
| Microglial | None | Migrate to the site of inflammation, degeneration, and injury and clean up the site |

BBB, blood–brain barrier; CSF, cerebrospinal fluid.

- **Where is the most common location in the brain for a glioma to develop?**
- **Frontal lobe**

The majority of primary, intra-axial brain tumors develop in the four lobes of the brain. The most common lobe for a glioma is the frontal lobe, and the least common is the occipital lobe.

▶ **HINT:** Nursing assessment is directed by the location of the tumor.

- **As indicated previously, brain tumors are classified based on the type of brain cell from which they arise. What is a tumor originating from neurons commonly called?**
- **Neuroma**

Neurons are the brain cells responsible for the impulses in the brain. If a tumor arises from the neuron cells, the tumor is generally classified as a neuroma.

> ▶ **HINT:** If the tumor is invading the peripheral nerve sheath, it is called a schwannoma.

- *What grade of glioma tumor is called an anaplastic tumor?*
- Grade III

Grade I and II gliomas are considered to be benign tumors. An anaplastic tumor is a grade III glioma (Box 3.5). And a grade IV glioma is called a glioblastoma multiform (GBM) tumor. Grades III and IV are considered malignant tumors.

> ▶ **HINT:** The terms *malignant* and *nonmalignant* are not as meaningful when discussing brain tumors.

**Box 3.5** Terminology Grade of Gliomas

| Grade of the Astrocytoma | Name of Astrocytoma |
|---|---|
| Grade I | Pilocytic astrocytoma |
| Grade II | Diffuse astrocytoma |
| Grade III | Anaplastic astrocytoma |
| Grade IV | Gliobastoma |

- *Brain tumors cause injury and symptoms through several mechanisms. What is the primary mechanism for the complication of hydrocephalus with brain tumors?*
- Obstruction of cerebropinal fluid (CSF) flow

A brain tumor can invade the ventricles or compress the ventricular system, resulting in hydrocephalus (Box 3.6). Obstruction of CSF flow results in the hydrocephalus being classified as noncommunicating.

> ▶ **HINT:** A common CNS tumor that produces hydrocephalus is an ependymoma.

**Box 3.6** Mechanisms of Brain Injury With Tumors

| |
|---|
| Infiltration of brain tissue |
| Compression of adjacent tissue |
| Producing cerebral edema |
| Obstructing flow of CSF |
| Creating vessels that hemorrhage (vascular tumor) |
| Shifting and herniating brain tissue |

CSF, cerebrospinal fluid.

■ **What is the most common location of a tumor that results in seeding of the tumor cells throughout the CNS?**

■ **Leptomeninges**

Tumors located in the leptomeningeal area and subarachnoid space are most likely to spread throughout the CNS. The spread occurs in the CSF with colonizing of tumor cells in the regions of slow-moving CSF. Invasion of the leptomeninges can occur through arterial venous dissemination or lymphatic spread.

▶ HINT: Leptomeningeal tumors are often metastasized from breast, lung, or melanoma.

■ **What is the most common CNS neuroma?**

■ **Acoustic neuroma**

Acoustic neuromas are benign tumors that invade the myelin sheath of the acoustic nerve (cranial nerve [CN] VIII). It may also involve CN V and VII due to the close proximity of the nerves. Tumor growth may also compress the fourth ventricle, resulting in hydrocephalus.

▶ HINT: A tumor involving a nerve sheath is called a *neuroma*.

■ **Which area of the brain does a craniopharyngioma commonly affect?**

■ **Hypothalamus**

A craniopharyngioma is commonly located in the intrasellar region and involves the hypothalamus. It is typically a benign tumor found in the pediatric population. Symptoms include headache, visual impairment, decreased growth, polyuria, and polydipsia.

▶ HINT: Symptoms are caused by the compression of the tumor on the optic chiasm and pituitary gland.

## SYMPTOMS/ASSESSMENT

■ **Symptoms of brain tumors can be generalized or localized. Would a patient presenting with hemiparesis be considered to have generalized or localized symptoms?**

■ **Localized**

Generalized symptoms of brain tumors include seizures, altered level of consciousness (LOC), and cognitive or behavioral changes (Box 3.7). Symptoms of an increased intracranial pressure include headache, altered LOC, vomiting, and papilledema.

▶ HINT: The triad of headache, vomiting, and focal deficits, frequently leads to the diagnosis of a brain tumor.

**Box 3.7** Localized Symptoms of Brain Tumors

| Tumor Location | Associated Symptoms |
|---|---|
| Frontal lobe | Altered mental status<br>Inappropriate behavior<br>Emotional lability<br>Apathy/depression<br>Inability to concentrate<br>Altered speech<br>Motor dysfunction<br>Hemiparesis/hemiparalysis<br>Bowel and bladder dysfunction<br>Conjugate eye deviation<br>Impairment of recent memory |
| Parietal lobe | Sensory deficits<br>Agnosia<br>Paresthesia<br>Tactile inattention<br>Apraxia<br>Hyperesthesia<br>Motor dysfunction<br>Psychomotor seizures<br>Loss of right/left discrimination<br>Agraphia (inability to write)<br>Visual field deficits |
| Temporal lobe | Visual field deficits<br>Memory losses<br>Speech and language deficits (especially Wernicke's aphasia)<br>Psychomotor seizures<br>Personality changes<br>Ataxia<br>Conjugated eye deviation |
| Occipital lobe | Visual field deficits<br>Headache<br>Visual agnosia<br>Cortical blindness<br>Visual hallucinations<br>Seizures (focal or generalized) |

■ *Symptoms of brainstem lesions commonly involve which set of CNS nerves?*
■ **CNs**

The majority of the CNs originate in the brainstem (10 of the 12 CNs). Brainstem tumors commonly present with symptoms of CN involvement (Box 3.8).

▶ **HINT:** CN III and IV originate in the midbrain. CN V, VI, VII, and VIII originate in the pons, and CN IX, X, XI, and XII originate in the medulla.

**Box 3.8** Symptoms of Brainstem Tumors

| |
|---|
| Cranial nerve palsies |
| Dizziness/vertigo |
| Vomiting |
| Nystagmus |
| Gait disturbances |
| Motor and sensory deficits |
| Headache |

- *A patient presents in the emergency department with the appearance of being "drunk" and has been diagnosed with a brain tumor. Which is the most likely location of the tumor?*
- **Cerebellum**

The cerebellum is responsible for coordination of movement, fine motor control, and gait. Tumors located in the cerebellum cause symptoms of unsteady gait, ataxia, falling, incoordination, and slurred speech.

> ▶ **HINT:** Motor abnormalities and tremors occur ipsilateral to the tumor site in the cerebellum. It is ipsilateral because the cerebellum affects motor impulses after they cross the brainstem.

- *A pituitary tumor often presents with visual deficits. Is the medial or lateral vision most likely affected in both eyes?*
- **Lateral vision**

The pituitary gland lies in close proximity to the optic chiasm. Visual fields are divided between medial (middle of the eyes to the nose) and lateral (middle of the eyes outward) vision. Lateral vision in both eyes cross to the opposite side to travel to the occipital lobe. Compression or injury of the optic chiasm causes a loss of lateral vision bilaterally (Box 3.9).

> ▶ **HINT:** Medial vision remains on the same side (ipsilateral), and lateral vision crosses to the opposite side (contralateral).

**Box 3.9** Signs of Pituitary Adenomas

| |
|---|
| Loss of lateral vision bilaterally |
| Hormonal dysfunction |
| Headache |
| Water imbalances (DI/SIADH) |
| Sleep pattern disruption |

DI, diabetes insipidus; SIADH, syndrome of inappropriate antidiuretic hormone.

- *Which hormone produced by the pituitary gland can result in acromegaly in a pituitary adenoma?*
- **Growth hormone**

## 3. TUMORS OF THE BRAIN AND SPINAL CORD 57

Pituitary adenoma can be a secreting or nonsecreting tumor. A pituitary tumor that secretes growth hormone can cause gigantism (before adolescence) or acromegaly (after adolescence; Box 3.10). Craniopharyngiomas are benign tumors found near the pituitary gland that present with visual changes and slow growth.

▶ **HINT:** Multidisciplinary involvement with a pituitary adenoma includes a neurosurgeon, endocrinologist, and neuroophthalmologist.

**Box 3.10** Secreting Pituitary Adenomas

| Growth hormone | Gigantism (if present before puberty) or acromegaly (if present after puberty) |
|---|---|
| Prolactin | Lack of menstruation in women, gynecomastosis, inappropriate breast milk production |
| ACTH | Cushing's disease (elevated cortisol levels) |

ACTH, adrenocorticotropic hormone.

- **What is commonly the first presentation of an acoustic neuroma?**
- **Dizziness/vertigo**

An acoustic neuroma involves the myelin sheath of CN VIII, which has both a vestibular and cochlear component. The vestibular component involves balance, whereas the cochlear component involves hearing (Box 3.11). Vestibular involvement is typically the initial presentation with signs of dizziness, imbalance, and vertigo.

▶ **HINT:** May also involve CN V (trigeminal nerve) and VII (facial nerve) so symptoms depend on the size of the tumor.

**Box 3.11** Signs and Symptoms of Acoustic Neuroma

| |
|---|
| Tinnitus |
| Dizziness |
| Vertigo |
| Loss of balance |
| Loss of facial sensation |
| Unilateral hearing loss |
| Nystagmus |
| Loss of corneal reflex |
| Facial weakness |
| Unsteadiness of gait |
| Visual deficits (diplopia) |
| Dysphagia |
| Dysarthria |
| Seizures |

■ **A patient presents with symptoms of nausea/vomiting, headache, and mental status changes. The CT scan found a leptomeningeal tumor. What is the most likely cause of the patient's symptoms?**
■ **Hydrocephalus**

Leptomeningeal tumor is present within the meninges and subarachnoid space. The tumor can affect the flow of the cerebrospinal fluid, resulting in hydrocephalus. The symptoms include headache, nausea/vomiting, gait disturbances, altered mental status, and diplopia.

▶ **HINT:** The patient's presentation (headache, nausea/vomiting, altered mentation) includes the common triad of symptoms for hydrocephalus of any cause.

■ **An 8-year-old child presents with nausea and vomiting, listlessness, morning headaches, and ataxia. What is the most likely location and type of tumor?**
■ **Posterior fossa; medulloblastoma**

Posterior fossa tumors typically present with symptoms of hydrocephalus (nausea and vomiting and headaches). Medulloblastoma is a tumor located between the brainstem and the cerebellum (present in the posterior fossa), which has an incidence of about 20% in young children (Box 3.12).

▶ **HINT:** Brainstem tumors frequently result in hydrocephalus and present with typical signs of hydrocephalus.

**Box 3.12** Symptoms of Medulloblastoma

| |
|---|
| Lethargic; listless |
| Nausea and vomiting |
| Morning headaches |
| Stumbling gait |
| Limb ataxia |
| Dizziness |
| Nystagmus |
| Visual alterations (not as common) |

■ **What is a unique symptom of a brain tumor in an infant who still has open cranial fontanels?**
■ **Tense and bulging anterior fontanel**

Symptoms of increased intracranial pressure (ICP) and tumor growth depend on the age of the child and whether the cranial fontanels have closed (Box 3.13). If the infant still has open fontanels, the presentation of a tense or bulging anterior fontanel would be a sign of increased ICP.

▶ **HINT:** Persistent lethargy, especially without fever, in an infant should be considered a neurological sign.

**Box 3.13** Signs of Increased Intracranial Pressure in Infants

| |
|---|
| Lethargy |
| High-pitched cries |
| Irritability |
| Anorexia |
| Failure to thrive |
| Developmental delays or regressions |
| Tense and bulging anterior fontanel (only in infants with open fontanels) |

■ *What is the most common symptom of a patient with a spinal tumor?*
■ Pain

Pain is the most common presentation of spinal tumors and is usually present months before signs of neurological involvement (Box 3.14). Causes of pain include spinal cord compression, vertebral body instability, vertebral bone destruction, and spinal nerve injury.

> ▶ **HINT:** Treatment of the tumor (surgery, radiation, or chemotherapy) may worsen the pain due to the development of neuropathic pain syndrome.

**Box 3.14** Signs of Spinal Tumors

| |
|---|
| Neck or back pain |
| Radiculopathy |
| Motor weakness or paralysis |
| Bowel or bladder dysfunction |
| Altered sensation or loss of sensation |

## DIAGNOSIS

■ *Which radiographic diagnostic examination is commonly ordered initially in an acute setting?*
■ CT

An initial brain CT scan without contrast may be ordered in an acute setting to rule out hemorrhage. If a mass lesion is identified, a contrast CT scan is typically obtained. MRI is recommended following the CT if an abnormality is recognized and there are no contraindications.

> ▶ **HINT:** Ferrous-containing implants are contraindications for MRI and may include pacemakers and automatic implantable cardioverters/defibrillators.

■ *What is the "gold standard" radiographic study used to identify the tumor location, characteristics, and mass effect?*
■ MRI

The gold standard for CNS tumor identification, localization, and determining characteristics is an MRI. MRI is also primarily used to follow up with the tumor's response to surgical resection or treatment. A CT may be used if an MRI is contraindicated.

▶ HINT: Both T1- and T2-weighted sequences are recommended.

■ **Which advanced MRI imaging can be used to map eloquent areas of the brain prior to brain tumor surgical resection?**
■ **Functional magnetic resonance imaging (fMRI)**

An fMRI may be used preoperatively to identify eloquent areas of the brain specific to functions such as speech, language, and motor. This can assist the surgeon in resecting the tumor with minimal damage to the eloquent areas of the brain.

▶ HINT: Intraoperative MRI can be used to permit real-time imaging to improve the tumor resection and minimize damage to eloquent areas of the brain.

■ **What is a potential complication of the use of gadolinium contrast in the MRI imaging?**
■ **Acute kidney injury (AKI)**

Gadolinium, used in MRI with contrast, can cause nephrogenic fibrosis and AKI. The half-life in patients with normal renal function is about 2 hours, but in patients with renal dysfunction, the half-life may be as long as 120 hours.

▶ HINT: Monitoring serum creatinine and blood urea nitrogen (BUN) levels is recommended in patients receiving contrast for CT or MRI scans.

■ **Which diagnostic study measures glucose uptake of the brain tissues?**
■ **PET**

PET scans use radiolabel tracers to provide information on the uptake of glucose, differentiating normal brain tissue from brain tumors. Increased glucose uptake indicates higher malignancy.

▶ HINT: PET scan is used more to identify recurrence or residual tumor more than diagnosis.

■ **Tumors located in the sellar region require which diagnostic test to evaluate the hypothalamic–pituitary axis?**
■ **Laboratory results**

Endocrine laboratory tests are obtained when patients are found to have a tumor in the sellar region of the brain, commonly a pituitary tumor (Box 3.15). These endocrine labs are used to evaluate the hypothalamic–pituitary axis.

▶ HINT: The sellar area of the brain is where the pituitary gland is located.

**Box 3.15** Laboratory Tests for Pituitary Tumors

| |
|---|
| ACTH |
| Cortisol |
| Prolactin |
| Growth hormone |
| Growth factor |
| Thyroid studies (T3, T4, TSH) |
| Testosterone |
| Follicular stimulating hormone |
| Luteinizing hormone |

ACTH, adrenocorticotropic hormone; TSH, thyroid-stimulating hormone.

- *Which is the most diagnostic for determining the brain tumor type and classification?*
- **Brain biopsy**

Radiographic studies, such as CT and MRI, are highly sensitive in recognizing a mass or tumor but are not specific in identifying the type or origin of the tumor. Brain biopsy is the "gold standard" for the diagnosis and determination of the type of brain tumor.

> ▶ **HINT:** Gross total resection, if feasible, is the best method used to obtain a biopsy of the tumor. Stereotactic biopsy requires an adequate amount of tumor tissue for pathology identification.

- *What is the CSF result that would be considered the gold standard for establishing the presence of leptomeningeal tumor?*
- **Presence of malignant cells in CSF**

The presence of malignant tumor cells in the CSF is considered a positive diagnosis for leptomeningeal tumor. Other CSF results are nonspecific such as leukocytosis, elevated opening pressures, elevated proteins, and decrease in glucose.

> ▶ **HINT:** Larger CSF samples (>10 mL) and processing within 30 minutes of obtaining the sample will improve sensitivity of the CSF analysis.

## MEDICAL MANAGEMENT

- *What lab value should be monitored closely when a patient is on a steroid?*
- **Serum glucose levels**

Steroids are commonly used to manage cerebral edema in patients with brain tumors. Steroids have multiple side effects, which should be monitored and managed (Box 3.16). Hyperglycemia and steroid-induced diabetes are common side effects that are monitored with frequent blood glucose checks.

> ▶ **HINT:** Gastrointestinal (GI) prophylaxis is recommended in patients on steroids to prevent GI distress.

**Box 3.16** Complications of Steroids

| |
|---|
| Hyperglycemia/steroid-induced diabetes |
| GI distress/gastric ulceration |
| Immunosuppression |
| Fluid retention |
| Weight gain |
| Proximal myopathy |
| Insomnia |
| Behavioral changes |

GI, gastrointestinal.

■ *In high-grade gliomas, radiation therapy is commonly used in conjunction with which modality of medical management?*

■ **Chemotherapy**

Radiation therapy may be used only in the management of brain tumors or in conjunction with chemotherapy as medical management. High-grade gliomas may require radiation with chemotherapy.

▶ HINT: Focused stereotactic radiosurgical techniques, including proton beams and the Gamma Knife, can be used on some tumors.

■ *What chemotherapy delivery system is used to deliver the chemotherapy drug carmustine directly to the tumor bed?*

■ **Wafers**

Wafers can be surgically placed after the complete resection of the glioblastoma. These wafers release the chemotherapy drug carmustine. The wafer then dissolves over time. This may extend the life expectancy in high-grade gliomas.

▶ HINT: Oral chemotherapy in addition to use of the wafers may be recommended. Side effects may increase with the combination therapy.

■ *A leptomeningeal tumor may be treated with IV chemotherapy drugs used to treat the original tumor cell type. What is different in these tumors regarding the ability to use a larger variety of systemically administered chemotherapy drugs than when treating a glioma?*

■ **Disruption of the BBB**

Leptomeningeal tumors are typically enhanced by contrast and receive blood flow indicating a disruption of the BBB. This allows for a greater chance of systemic distribution to reach the tumor bed. If the BBB is intact, the drug must be able to cross the BBB if administered systemically.

▶ HINT: The presence of elevated protein in the CSF of patients with leptomeningeal tumor is another indication of the disruption of the BBB.

### What medical management is used to treat a prolactinoma?
### Dopamine agonist therapy

A prolactinoma is a pituitary tumor that secretes prolactin, which accounts for a large percentage of the pituitary tumors. Medical management is recommended to "shrink" the size of the tumor. Dopamine is the primary inhibitor of prolactin secretion, so dopamine agonist therapy has been found to effectively decrease the size of the prolactinoma.

> ▶ HINT: Pituitary tumor is also called pituitary adenoma.

## SURGICAL MANAGEMENT

### What preoperative intervention may be used in highly vascular tumors to lower the risk of hemorrhage during surgical resection of the tumor?
### Embolization

Embolization involves using agents that clot or obstruct blood flow through selective arteries supplying blood to the highly vascular tumor. This decreases blood supply to the tumor with the goal of decreasing intraoperative blood loss during the surgical resection. Embolization is performed by interventional radiologists or neurologists and guided by cerebral angiography.

> ▶ HINT: Postprocedural frequent neurological assessments and groin/pulse checks are recommended to identify complications.

### What is the purpose of performing an awake craniotomy and cortical brain mapping?
### To identify eloquent areas of brain

The use of an fMRI or awake craniotomy is to map the brain for eloquent areas and avoidance of those areas during brain tumor surgical resection (Box 3.17).

> ▶ HINT: Awake craniotomies and fMRI are used to map the brain of eloquent areas in attempt to avoid injury to those areas during the resection of the tumor.

**Box 3.17** Examples of Eloquent Areas of the Brain

| |
|---|
| Motor cortex |
| Sensory cortex |
| Basal ganglia |
| Language cortex |
| Internal capsule |

### What surgical approach is used to remove a pituitary tumor?
### Transphenoidal surgery

The surgical management of a pituitary tumor is resection or removal of the tumor through the transphenoidal approach. The potential complications include CSF leak and CNS infection.

> ▶ **HINT:** Postoperative nursing care includes assessing for CSF leak, avoiding packing of the nasal passages, and instructing patients not to blow their nose.

- **What is a potential reason for an incomplete surgical excision of a tumor?**
- **Invasion into an eloquent area of brain**

The eloquent area of the brain is an area with a specific function, such as language. The outcome of surgically excising the eloquent area is compared with the outcome for an incomplete resection, determining risk versus benefit. Other reasons for incomplete resections include if the tumor is located in the brainstem and invasion into the base of the skull.

> ▶ **HINT:** Recognition and mapping of the eloquent areas of the brain is assisted by fMRI.

- **What is the primary recommendation for a patient presenting with an acute loss of motor function due to a spinal tumor?**
- **Surgical resection of the tumor**

The best prognosis for being able to ambulate following acute cord compression is surgical resection or decompression of the spinal cord. Spinal compression and spine instability are indications for immediate surgical intervention in patients with acute presentation of motor loss.

> ▶ **HINT:** The goal of surgical management is to preserve neurological function and reduce pain.

## COMPLICATIONS

- **What is a common complication of a posterior fossa surgery for tumor resection?**
- **CSF leak**

Surgical procedures involving the posterior fossa or transphenoidal approach have the postoperative risk of CSF leak. It is more difficult to obtain a watertight dural seal in the area of the posterior fossa. The longer the duration of the CSF leak, the greater the risk of CNS infection.

> ▶ **HINT:** Assessment for a CSF leak includes "watery" drainage from the nose (rhinorrhea) or from the ears (otorrhea).

- **Surgical resection of a tumor adjacent to Broca's area can result in which deficit?**
- **Expressive aphasia**

Broca's area in the dominant frontal lobe controls one's ability to speak. Resection near the Broca can result in expressive aphasia (Box 3.18).

> ▶ **HINT:** Neurological deficits following surgical resection depend on the location of the brain tumor.

**Box 3.18** Complications of Surgical Resections

| | |
|---|---|
| Frontal lobe: Motor strip | Motor weakness/paralysis |
| Frontal lobe: Broca's area | Expressive aphasia |
| Frontal lobe | Memory and personality changes |
| Temporal lobe: Wernicke's area | Receptive aphasia |
| Parietal lobe | Sensation and position abnormalities |
| Cerebellum | Balance issues |

▪ *Which of the following tumor locations is more likely to present with seizures: cortical gray matter or deep white matter?*

▪ **Cortical gray matter**

Tumors located in the cortical gray matter (cerebral lobes) are more likely to develop seizures than those in the deeper white matter structures (i.e., thalamus, basal ganglia). A temporal lobe tumor is a common site for seizure complications.

▶ **HINT:** Seizures may be caused by progression of the brain tumor, cerebral edema, or hemorrhage.

▪ *Which type of glial tumor is most likely to develop the complication of hydrocephalus?*

▪ **Ependymoma**

Ependymal cells (which are a type of glial cell) line the ventricles. Tumors, arising from ependymal cells, develop within the ventricular system and are likely to obstruct CSF flow, resulting in hydrocephalus (Box 3.19).

▶ **HINT:** This is called *obstructive* or *noncommunicating hydrocephalus.*

**Box 3.19** Physiology of Hydrocephalus With Brain Tumors

| |
|---|
| Obstruction of the ventricular system |
|    Tumor within the ventricular system |
|    Tumor causing a shift |
|    Tumor in posterior fossa obstructing CSF flow |
| Blood present in the CSF (i.e., postsurgically) |
| Tumor infiltrated in meninges preventing reabsorption of CSF |
| Cerebral edema |

CSF, cerebrospinal fluid.

▪ *A meningioma is most commonly a grade I (benign) tumor. What is the complication of an atypical (grade II) or anaplastic (grade III) meningioma?*

▪ **Brain tissue invasion**

Higher grade meningiomas can erode through bone and invade brain tissue with cerebral edema. If there is invasion in the brain tissue, the tumor is at least a grade II.

▶ **HINT:** Tumor invasion into brain tissue may be difficult to recognize with MRI. Cerebral edema may be present from compression without tissue invasion.

■ *A patient is on the unit following a pituitary adenoma removal using the transphenoidal approach. He develops a sudden increase in urine output. What is the most likely complication experienced by this patient?*

■ **Diabetes insipidus (DI)**

DI is a potential complication of a pituitary tumor resection by the transphenoidal route. Postoperative management includes strict intake and output to recognize the onset of DI and rapid management of the complication.

▶ **HINT:** The symptoms of DI include increased urine output, hypernatremia, serum hyperosmolality, and decrease in urine specific gravity.

■ *What complication can occur with a tumor causing spinal nerve root compression?*

■ **Bladder dysfunction**

Bladder dysfunction is a potential complication of spinal tumors and compression of either the upper motor or lower motor neurons (Box 3.20). Bladder incontinence or retention can occur depending on the location of the compression.

▶ **HINT:** Commonly, cauda equina injuries produce bladder and bowel incontinence.

**Box 3.20** Complications of Spinal Compression

| |
|---|
| Bowel dysfunction (ileus, bowel obstruction) |
| Bladder dysfunction (urinary incontinence or retention) |
| Sensory alteration (skin breakdown/pressure sores) |
| Paresis or paralysis |
| Sexual dysfunction |

# Sample Exam Questions

1. A patient presents with vertigo, hearing loss, and new-onset visual changes. The patient is diagnosed with neurofibromatosis type II. Which of the following best describes this type of tumor?

   A. Neuroendocrine tumor
   B. Primary central nervous system lymphoma
   C. Bilateral acoustic neuroma
   D. Embryonal tumor

2. A patient who presents with a recent history of behavior and mood changes, short-term memory deficits, and gait abnormality is diagnosed with a brain tumor. Which of the following is the most likely site of the tumor?

   A. Hypothalamus
   B. Occipital lobe
   C. Pons
   D. Frontal lobe

3. A tumor in the right cerebellar lobe will present with which of the following symptoms?

   A. Cranial nerve deficits
   B. Contralateral sensory deficit
   C. Ipsilateral ataxia
   D. Contralateral motor weakness

4. Which of the following statements is <u>incorrect</u> regarding the diagnostic workup for a brain tumor?

   A. PET may be used to differentiate tumor versus radiation necrosis.
   B. A functional MRI can be used to map the eloquent areas of the brain.
   C. An MRI is the diagnostic test of choice for identifying brain masses.
   D. A serum marker is available to assist with the diagnosis of a primary brain tumor.

5. Which of the following is the gold standard for diagnosing a spinal tumor?

   A. Spine x-rays
   B. Myelogram
   C. MRI
   D. CT scan

6. Which of the following is the best diagnostic tool to use to recognize and diagnose primary central nervous system lymphoma?

   A. Steroid trial with glucocorticoids
   B. Brain biopsy
   C. CT scan
   D. Cerebrospinal fluid analysis

## BIBLIOGRAPHY

Amid, A., Keene, D. L., & Johnston, D. L. (2015). Presentation of central nervous system tumors. In K. Scheinemann & E. Bouffet (Eds.), *Pediatric neuro-oncology*. New York, NY: Springer Publishing Company.

Armstrong, T., Vera-Bolanos, E., Beleke, N., Aldape, K., & Gilbert, M. (2010). Adult ependymal tumors: Prognosis and the M. D. Anderson Cancer Center experience. *Neuro-Oncology, 12*(8), 862–870. doi:10.1093/neuonc/noq009

Blissitt, P. (Ed.). (2014). *Care of the pediatric patient with a brain tumor: AANN Clinical Practice Guideline Series*. Chicago, IL: American Association of Neuroscience Nurses.

Cahill, J., & Armstrong, T. (2011). Caring for an adult with a malignant primary brain tumor. *Nursing, 41*(6), 28–33. doi:10.1097/01.NURSE.0000397930.50420.c6

Crawford, J. (2013). Childhood brain tumours. *Pediatrics in Review, 34*, 63–78. doi:10.1542/pir.34-2-63

Davis, M. (2016). Gliobastoma: Overview of diseases and treatments. *Clinical Journal of Oncology Nursing, 20*(5), S2–S8. doi:10.1188/16.CJON.S1.2-8

Ginsberg, D. (2013). The epidemiology and pathophysiology of neurogenic bladder. *American Journal of Managed Care, 19*(10), 191–196.

Guerrero, D. (2003). Caring for patients with central nervous system metastases. *Nursing Times, 99*(8), 30–32.

Kaplow, R., & Iyere, K. (2016). Understanding spinal cord compression. *Nursing, 46*(9), 44–51. doi:10.1097/01.NURSE.0000490208.81425.19

Kreiner, D. S., Shaffer, W. O., Baisden, J. L., Gilbert, T. J., Summers, J. T., Toton, J. F., ... North American Spine Society. (2013). An evidence-based clinical guideline for the diagnosis and treatment of degenerative lumbar spinal stenosis (update). *Spine Journal, 13*(7), 734–743. doi:10.1016/j.spinee.2012.11.059

Louis, D., Perry, P., Reifenberger, G., von Deimling, A., Figarella-Branger, D., Cavenee, W., ... Ellison, D. (2016). The 2016 World Health Organization classification of tumors of the central nervous system: A summary. *Acta Neuropathologica, 131*(6), 803–820. doi:10.1007/s00401-016-1545-1

Lovely, P., Stewart-Amidei, C., Arzbaecher, J., Bell, S., Maher, M. E., Maida, M., ... Nicolaseau, G. (2014). Care of the adult patient with a brain tumor. *Journal of Neuroscience Nursing, 46*(6), 367–368.

Raj, V., & Edeker, J. (2013). Neoplasm of the spinal cord: Implications for clinical care to improve symptom management and functionality. *Clinical Nursing Studies, 1*(2), 1–26. doi:10.5430/cns.v1n2p14

Riblet, N., Schlosser, E., Snide, J., Ronan, L., Thorley, K., Davis, M., ... Fadul, C. E. (2016). A clinical pathway to improve the acute care of patients with glioma. *Neuro-Oncology Practice, 3*(3), 45–153. doi:10.1093/nop/npv050

Roberts, T. T., Leonard, G. R., & Cepela, D. J. (2017). Classifications in brief: American Spinal Injury Association (ASIA) impairment scale. *Clinical Orthopaedics and Related Research, 475*(5), 1499–1504. doi:10.1007/s11999-016-5133-4

# 4

# Immune Infections, Part 1

## INTRODUCTION

- *What is a central nervous system (CNS) infection called that is located within the meninges?*
- **Meningitis**

Meningitis is an infection within the meninges, or the protective covering of the brain. Any microorganism can cause meningitis, but the most common cause is bacterial. Encephalitis, on the other hand, is an infection within the brain tissue itself and is typically caused by a viral infection.

> ▶ **HINT:** Viral meningitis is more self-limiting and less severe than bacterial meningitis.

- *Which neurological infection is caused by the larval stage of pig tapeworm?*
- **Neurocysticercosis**

Neurocysticercosis is the most common parasitic infection of the CNS worldwide. The infection is caused by the larval stage of the pig tapeworm (*Taenia solium*).

> ▶ **HINT:** Neurocysticercosis is most commonly found in Mexico and developing countries. Cases in the United States are typically caused by immigration of carriers and the people they infect.

- *What is it called when the inflammation or infection is present throughout the brain tissue (not just localized in the meninges)?*
- **Encephalitis**

Encephalitis is the inflammation or infection of parenchymal tissue. It is commonly caused by viral infections or is an extension of the bacterial meningitis (Box 4.1). Identification of its potential etiology includes obtaining history of recent infection, travel, occupational or recreational exposure, vaccination status, or animal contact.

> ▶ **HINT:** Encephalitis can be a result of bacterial, viral, or fungal causes; protozoa; or prions.

**Box 4.1** Common Etiologies of Viral Encephalitis

| |
|---|
| Herpes simplex |
| West Nile virus |
| Enterovirus |
| Polio |
| St. Louis encephalitis |
| Cytomegalovirus |
| Rabies |

■ *Which etiology of viral encephalitis is the most common cause of sporadic, fatal encephalitis?*
■ **Herpes simplex encephalitis (HSE)**

Herpes simplex is common worldwide. About 70% to 95% of humans are seropositive for herpes simplex virus by adulthood, and humans are its only reservoir. The virus lies dormant in neurons and ganglia until triggered. It is the most common cause of sporadic fatal encephalitis.

▶ **HINT:** HSE most commonly affects the temporal lobe.

■ *How is the West Nile virus (WNV) transmitted to humans?*
■ **By mosquito**

The transmission of WNV is by mosquito, with birds as amplifying host. There is not a human vaccination to prevent WNV, so prevention is to avoid mosquito-infested areas and wear protection.

▶ **HINT:** Motor neuron damage is seen with WNV encephalitis and can present with new-onset movement disorders due to the involvement of basal ganglia.

■ *What is the cause of transmissible spongiform encephalopathy (TSE)?*
■ **Prions**
■ **TSEs are known as** *prion diseases.*

They are rare degenerative brain disorders characterized by tiny holes that give the brain a "spongy" appearance. Prion diseases are invariably fatal brain disorders.

▶ **HINT:** "Mad cow" disease (bovine spongiform encephalopathy [BSE]) is a type of prion disease.

■ *What is the most common human form of the prion diseases?*
■ **Creutzfeldt–Jakob disease (CJD)**

CJD is a prion disease that can affect humans. It is rare, only affecting around one person per million per year, which accounts for about 400 people in the United States annually.

▶ **HINT:** Another type of CJD is called *variant CJD (vCJD)* and is a result of consumption of beef from cattle infected with bovine spongiform encephalopathy or "mad cow disease."

# PATHOPHYSIOLOGY

▪ *A patient with a recent episode of sinusitis begins to complain of headache, fever, and nuchal rigidity. What is the most likely cause?*
▪ Meningitis

Sinusitis is a source of bacterial entry into the meninges, resulting in CNS infection. There are multiple sources and routes of entry for bacterial meningitis (Box 4.2).

> ▶ **HINT:** The triad of symptoms (headache, fever, and nuchal rigidity) is a commonly used clue for the answer of meningitis.

**Box 4.2** Routes of Entry for Bacterial Meningitis

| |
|---|
| Bloodstream |
| Sinuses |
| Middle ear |
| Direct entry (via facial or cranial fracture, penetrating injury, post craniotomy, ventriculostomy) |
| CSF (CSF leak, basal skull fracture) |
| Extension (microorganisms follow along peripheral, cranial, or spinal nerves such as rabies) |
| Mouth/nose droplets |

CSF, cerebrospinal fluid.

▪ *Which of the bacterial agents causes meningococcal meningitis?*
▪ *Neisseria meningitidis*

*Neisseria meningitidis* is the causative agent for meningococcal meningitis and is a Gram-negative diplococcus. It is one of the causes of bacterial meningitis that can be spread by airborne droplet and close contact (Box 4.3). It can cause epidemics if spread through close living quarters. It is spread through carriers that colonize in the nasopharynx.

> ▶ **HINT:** A meningococcal meningitis vaccination is available against certain strains of the disease and is recommended if people live in close quarters (e.g., dorms, military barracks).

**Box 4.3** Examples of Causative Bacteria of Meningitis

| |
|---|
| *Haemophilus influenzae* |
| *Neisseria meningitidis* |
| *Streptococcus pneumoniae* |
| *Listeria* |
| Pneumococcus (most common in adults) |
| Group B Streptococcus (more common neonates) |

▪ *In meningitis, what layers of the meninges are involved with the infection?*
▪ Pia and arachnoid layer

The two meningeal layers involved in the infection of meningitis are the pia and arachnoid layers. This involves the subarachnoid space. The purulent drainage spreads rapidly through the cerebrospinal fluid (CSF) pathway. The exudate can extend along cranial nerves, entering perivascular space and causing encephalitis.

> ▶ HINT: The ventricles accumulate the exudate causing hydrocephalus.

■ **Which of the white blood cells (WBCs) will elevate in viral meningitis?**
■ **Lymphocytes**

During viral infections, including viral meningitis, lymphocytes are the primary WBCs to increase and can be found elevated on the differential. Viral meningitis has been called *benign lymphocytic meningitis*. Bacterial infections will elevate neutrophils.

> ▶ HINT: The type of elevated WBC can assist with the differential diagnosis between bacterial and viral meningitis.

■ **What is the primary cause of the cerebral edema that accompanies bacterial meningitis?**
■ **Release of inflammatory cytokines**

The elevated neutrophils in bacterial meningitis release proinflammatory cytokines and cellular toxins. This results in a combination of cytotoxic and vasogenic cerebral edema.

> ▶ HINT: Increased intracranial pressure can complicate meningitis due to the cerebral edema.

■ **What is an encapsulated mass of infection in brain tissue called?**
■ **Abscess**

Brain abscess is an encapsulated mass of infection with varying degrees, or stages, of infection (Box 4.4). Initially, brain tissue softens, and WBCs infiltrate. Over time, brain tissue separates into layers, creating a well-defined abscess. A wall of fibroblasts seal off the infection.

> ▶ HINT: Varying degrees of wall thickness can occur with an abscess. Thin walls can rupture, spreading infection throughout the cranial nerve, leading to encephalitis.

**Box 4.4** Locations of Brain Abscesses

| |
|---|
| Intraparenchymal space |
| Subdural space |
| Epidural space |

■ **What is the "carrier" of the CNS infection called neurocysticercosis?**
■ **Humans**

Humans eating undercooked pork carrying the tapeworm (*Taenia solium*) can acquire the tapeworm larvae and become a carrier. The larvae attach to the intestinal wall and grow into tapeworms that lay eggs in the human carrier's intestines. The eggs are expelled in the feces, and improper handwashing can pass the eggs to another human. The eggs can penetrate the intestinal mucosa, entering lymphatics and mesenteric vasculature, and eventually enter muscle, tissue, spinal cord, eyes, and brain tissue. Once inside the brain, they can can remain as live, active larvae or walled off cystic larvae (called *cysticerci*).

▶ **HINT:** Proper handwashing could eradicate the CNS infection of neurocysticercosis.

### The classification of CJD is a prion disorder. What is a prion?
### Abnormal protein

Prion diseases are caused by an abnormal version of a protein called a *prion*. Prion is an abbreviation of *proteinaceous infectious particle*. Prion proteins occur in both a normal form (harmless protein) found in the body's cells, and an infectious form that is disease causing. Once the protein becomes "abnormal," it creates a cascade effect, converting normal proteins to prions.

▶ **HINT:** Prions are not microorganisms, such as bacteria or viruses, but are the body's own proteins.

### What is the most prominent change that occurs in the brain with CJD?
### Neuronal tissue loss

There are significant neuronal changes that occur in the brain with prion diseases. The most prominent change is the loss of neuronal tissue (brain mass). There are a triad of histological changes that occur, including spongiform vacuolation, neuronal loss, and astroglial proliferation with and without amyloid plaque.

▶ **HINT:** On autopsy, the appearance of a brain with prion disease is of a sponge with holes (vacuoles) throughout.

### How is CJD transmitted from one person to another?
### Exposure to infected tissue or fluid

There are three ways a person can develop CJD: sporadic, inherited, and transmitted from infected individuals. Transmission is through exposure to tissue, fluid, and medical equipment infected with the prion (Box 4.5). CJD cannot be transmitted through air or most forms of casual contact. Variant CJD is transmitted through consumption of beef containing an abnormal prion.

▶ **HINT:** Contaminated medical equipment should be destroyed. Normal sterilization procedures, such as boiling or irradiating materials, do not prevent transmission of prions.

**Box 4.5** Known Routes of Creutzfeldt–Jakob Disease Transmission

| |
|---|
| Contaminated medical equipment |
| Corneal transplants |
| Dural grafts |
| Growth hormones prepared from pooled cadaver pituitary glands |
| Pituitary hormones |
| Blood transfusion (vCJD) |

vCJD, variant Creutzfeldt–Jakob disease.

## SYMPTOMS/ASSESSMENT

- **What symptoms comprise the triad of symptoms of bacterial meningitis?**
- **Headache, fever, and nuchal rigidity**

Headache is typically the initial sign of meningitis and is described as severe. This is caused by irritation of the pain-sensitive dura and vascular pressure. The fever is usually high, greater than 38°C. Nuchal rigidity is present in both passive and active flexion.

> ▶ HINT: Fever tends to be higher in bacterial meningitis than in viral meningitis.

- **What is the "sign" when the hips or knees flex automatically in response to passive flexion of the neck?**
- **Brudzinski's sign**

Brudzinski's sign is positive when hips or knees flex in response to passive flexion neck. This is due to inflammation in the meninges and spinal nerve roots. The other sign of meningeal irritation is Kernig's sign. This is tested by flexing the leg at the hip to a 90° angle and then extending the knee. Positive Kernig's sign is pain and/or spasm of the hamstring.

> ▶ HINT: Brudzinki's and Kernig's signs are not always present with meningitis, but are assessed to assist with the diagnosis (Box 4.6).

**Box 4.6** Signs of Meningitis

| |
|---|
| Headache |
| Fever |
| Nuchal rigidity |
| Positive Brudzinski's sign |
| Positive Kernig's sign |
| Photophobia |
| Altered mentation |
| Cranial nerve dysfunction |

- **Which of the cranial nerves (CNs) is most commonly affected in children with bacterial meningitis?**
- **CN VIII (acoustic)**

CN VIII (acoustic) is commonly involved with children and some adults with bacterial meningitis. This produces hearing losses that can become permanent after the resolution of the meningitis (Box 4.7).

> ▶ HINT: Steroids are commonly used to prevent hearing loss in children with bacterial meningitis.

**Box 4.7** Commonly Affected Cranial Nerves in Meningitis

| | |
|---|---|
| CN VIII (acoustic) | Hearing loss |
| CN II (optic) | Visual acuity changes |
| CN III (oculomotor), IV, and VI | Dysconjugate gaze |

CN, cranial nerve.

### 4. IMMUNE INFECTIONS, PART 1    75

■ *What is the most common type of meningitis that presents with petechiae and cutaneous hemorrhage?*
■ **Meningococcal meningitis**

Meningococcal meningitis presents with the triad of symptoms, but the symptoms are often accompanied by petechiae and cutaneous hemorrhage (Box 4.8). Meningococcal meningitis can result in thrombophlebitis and tissue necrosis.

> ▶ **HINT:** A complication of meningococcal meningitis is amputation resulting from thrombophlebitis and tissue necrosis.

**Box 4.8** Symptoms Specific to Meningitis Types

| | |
|---|---|
| *Haemophilus influenzae* meningitis | Acute mania |
| | Prodrome fever |
| | Otitis media |
| | Pharyngitis |
| | Rash (sometimes) |
| | May be associated with subdural effusions |
| *Listeria monocytogenes* | Diffuse encephalitis |
| | Localized brain abscesses in either hemisphere, thalamus, and brainstem |
| | Cerebritis with focal neurological deficits |
| Tuberculosis meningitis | Multiple CN dysfunctions |
| | May have tuberculomas of brain and spinal cord |

CN, cranial nerve.

■ *What is a common sign of meningitis in an infant?*
■ **Lethargy**

Infants are not able to communicate complaints of the headache commonly found with meningitis. They frequently present with lethargy or irritability (Box 4.9).

> ▶ **HINT:** Infants who present with fever, lethargy, and high-pitched cries should be suspected to have a CNS infection.

**Box 4.9** Common Symptoms of Meningitis in Pediatric Patients

| |
|---|
| Lethargy |
| Irritability |
| Unable to be consoled |
| Vomiting |
| Fever |
| Poor feeding |
| Nuchal rigidity |
| Bulging fontanels |
| Dysconjugate gaze |

■ *What is the most common presentation of a patient infected with neurocysticercosis?*
■ **Seizure**

Seizure is the most common presentation of patients infected with neurocysticercosis making it one of the most common causes of epilepsy in developing countries (Box 4.10). Cysts may be asymptomatic and found incidentally.

> ▶ **HINT:** Cysts present within the ventricular system can result in the patient presenting with symptoms of hydrocephalus.

**Box 4.10** Symptoms of Neurocysticercosis

| |
|---|
| Seizures |
| Mass effect of cysts |
| Inflammation |
| Hydrocephalus |
| Stroke |
| Headache |
| Encephalopathy |
| Back pain and radiculopathy |
| Presence of nodule in subcutaneous tissue |
| Myositis with fever |

■ **What is the most common presentation of viral encephalitis?**
■ **Altered mental status (AMS)**

Altered mentation is the most common presentation of patients with viral encephalitis. The nonspecific symptoms of viral encephalitis, commonly delay the diagnosis (Box 4.11).

> ▶ **HINT:** Recent history indicating potential exposure to viral infections known to cause encephalitis is important in increasing suspicion of encephalitis.

**Box 4.11** Symptoms of Viral Encephalitis

| |
|---|
| Altered mental status |
| Change in personality |
| Decreased level of consciousness |
| Fever |
| Headache |
| Papilledema |
| Nausea and vomiting |
| Focal neurological findings |
| Seizures |

■ **What is the most common initial presentation of a patient with CJD?**
■ **Abnormal movement**

Lack of coordination and/or an unsteady gait (cerebral ataxia) is commonly the initial presentation of CJD (Box 4.12). Personality changes and psychiatric problems often accompany the neurological changes. Symptoms progress rapidly to a state of akinetic mutism (severe mental impairment and loss of ability to move or speak) and death.

▶ **HINT:** Variant CJD presents with the psychological changes first, followed by the neurological changes of abnormal movement.

**Box 4.12** Symptoms of Creutzfeldt–Jakob Disease

| Neurological Symptoms | Psychiatric Symptoms |
| --- | --- |
| Lack of coordination | Personality changes |
| Unsteady gait | Depression |
| Myoclonus movement | Memory lapses |
| Rigidity in limbs | Mood swings |
| Incontinence | Psychosis |
| Abnormal sensations in face and limbs | Insomnia |
| Dysphagia | Confusion |
| Mutism | Hallucinations |
|  | Progressive dementia |
|  | Severe mental impairment |

## DIAGNOSTICS

■ *While obtaining the history of a patient presenting with fever, headache, and nuchal rigidity, the nurse discovers the patient has recently had sinusitis. What is important about the discovered current history?*

■ **Potential source of meningitis**

Obtaining recent histories from patients suspected of having meningitis is important to assist with identifying the potential source of the meningitis. Recent histories of sinus, ear, and upper respiratory infection are potential sources for seeding of bacteria or exposure to a viral source of the meningitis.

▶ **HINT:** Blood cultures; nose and throat cultures; and skull, chest, and sinuses radiographs are frequently obtained in patients with meningitis to identify the source of the infection.

■ *What is the difference in the CSF glucose level between bacterial and viral meningitis?*

■ **It is decreased in bacterial meningitis.**

The CSF glucose levels are decreased in bacterial meningitis and tend to remain normal in viral meningitis (Box 4.13). A normal CSF glucose level is two-thirds that of the patient's serum glucose level. False results of CSF glucose may be due to administration of D50 resulting in a rapid increase of blood glucose levels with a delay in CSF glucose response.

▶ **HINT:** A "traumatic tap" can result in WBCs being introduced into the CSF, resulting in a falsely elevated WBC count.

**Box 4.13** Comparison of CSF Findings in Bacterial and Viral Meningitis

| Bacterial Meningitis | Viral Meningitis |
| --- | --- |
| Turbid, cloudy | Cloudy |
| WBC >12,000 | WBC >12,000 |
| Increase in PMN and neutrophils | Increase in lymphocytes |
| Increased protein (>150 mg/dL) | Increased protein (<150 mg/dL) |
| Decreased glucose (<40 mg/dL)—ratio of CSF to glucose <0.3–0.4 | Normal glucose |
| Increased lumbar pressures (>180 mmH$_2$O) | Normal to slightly elevated lumbar pressures |
| Positive Gram stain and culture | Negative Gram stain and culture |
| Increased lactate levels (>4 mmol/L) | Normal lactate levels |

CSF, cerebrospinal fluid; PMN, polymorphonuclear leukocyte; WBC, white blood cell.

- **What is a contraindication to performing a diagnostic lumbar puncture (LP)?**
- **Increased intracranial pressure (ICP)**

Performing an LP on a patient with an elevated ICP can result in herniation syndromes (Box 4.14). The negative pressure created by the LP with the elevated ICP can herniate brain tissue.

> ▶ **HINT:** Frequently, a CT scan is performed before an LP to identify mass lesions or cerebral edema.

**Box 4.14** Contraindications and Relative Contraindications to Lumbar Puncture

| |
| --- |
| Elevated ICP |
| Infection at the site of the needle puncture |
| Anticoagulation therapy |
| Antiplatelet therapy |
| Intracranial mass lesion |
| Cardiovascular compromise in a neonate |

ICP, intracranial pressure.

- **What is the cardinal sign of an abscess on contrast CT or MRI?**
- **Hyperdense ring**

A hyperdense ring surrounds the brain abscess on contrast CT or MRI scans. It is a capsular ring of 1 to 3 mm in diameter and is considered the cardinal sign of an abscess.

> ▶ **HINT:** The fiberblasts that form the wall of the abscess are hyperdense to brain tissue and appear white.

- **What is the most common diagnostic radiograph used to identify neurocysticercosis cystic lesions?**
- **MRI**

Contrast CT scans can identify cystic lesions, but MRI has an increased sensitivity and accuracy, especially with intraventricular cystic lesions. Multiple lesions at different stages, active larvae, and walled-off cysts are commonly identified on MRI.

> ▶ HINT: The use of contrast with CT and MRI may result in ring enhancement similar to that in brain abscesses.

### Which WBCs are commonly found in the CSF of patients infected with neurocysticercosis?
### Eosinophils

CSF of patients infected with neurocysticercosis presents with pleocytes and elevated eosinophils (Box 4.15).

> ▶ HINT: WBC differential is commonly used to differentiate among bacterial, viral, and parasitic infections.

**Box 4.15** Cerebrospinal Fluid Analysis of Neurocysticercosis

| |
|---|
| Elevated eosinophils |
| Presence of pleocytes |
| Elevated protein |
| Increased IgG levels |
| Low glucose |
| Increased lumbar pressures |

IgG, immunoglobulin G.

### What is the primary diagnostic procedure used to diagnose encephalitis?
### MRI of the brain

An MRI of the brain is primarily used to recognize changes that indicate the presence of encephalitis. The T2-weighted brain MRI will show hyperintensities and enhancements in more than 90% of patients. It is uncommon to find signs of encephalitis on CT scan. An EEG will show nonspecific findings with spikes and slow activity. CSF has limited diagnostic capabilities with encephalitis but may identify bacterial or fungal infections (Box 4.16). The "gold standard" is brain biopsy for a definitive diagnosis, but it is not recommended and is infrequently performed.

> ▶ HINT: Positive blood cultures may indicate systemic infection caused the encephalitis, not a virus.

**Box 4.16** CSF Analysis of Encephalitis

| |
|---|
| Opening pressures normal |
| RBC normal to elevated |
| Elevated protein (about 50% of the time) |
| Elevated WBC<br>  Predominantly lymphocyte elevation<br>  Mild mononuclear pleocytosis |
| Glucose normal |

CSF, cerebrospinal fluid; RBC, red blood cell; WBC, white blood cell.

■ *What diagnostic procedure is most definitive in diagnosing CJD?*
■ **Brain biopsy**

A brain biopsy is considered the most definitive test for CJD, but it is not typically recommended. An MRI demonstrating an increased signal in the basal ganglia may be useful, along with the history and patient presentation. Serum lab work, EEG, and CSF analysis are also used in the diagnosis of CJD.

> ▶ HINT: Brain biopsy of suspected CJD requires strict adherence to protocols to prevent transmission of CJD to healthcare providers and other patients through contaminated instruments.

## MEDICAL MANAGEMENT

■ *What is the primary treatment of bacterial meningitis?*
■ **Antibiotic therapy**

Antibiotic therapy is an important component in treating bacterial meningitis. Survival and morbidity are affected by length of time until administration of the first dose of antibiotics after the onset of signs of meningitis. Initially, broad-spectrum antibiotics are recommended until culture results with sensitivities are available.

> ▶ HINT: Supportive therapy (i.e., antipyretics, analgesics, hydration) is recommended for viral meningitis.

■ *What pharmacological management is used to prevent hearing loss in pediatric patients with bacterial meningitis?*
■ **Steroids**

Acoustic nerve injury can occur with bacterial meningitis, resulting in long-term hearing loss. Steroids have been used to limit hearing loss, particularly in the pediatric population. It is recommended that the steroid be administered before or with an antimicrobial in the pediatric population. Steroids are most effective as an antiinflammatory in adults with pneumococcal meningitis.

> ▶ HINT: Reduction of fever in the pediatric population has been found with steroid therapy as well.

■ *What is the treatment for pig tapeworm larvae found in the CNS that present with symptoms?*
■ **Cysticidal medications**

Cysticidal medications damage the parasite and release antigens, triggering an inflammatory reaction. There may be a period of decompensation following the initial dose. Examples of the cysticidal medications include albendazole and praziquantel.

> ▶ HINT: Steroids are used to decrease the inflammation and limit side effects of the cysticidal medications.

■ *What is the medical management of HSE?*
■ **Acyclovir**

Acyclovir is the antiviral medication used to treat herpes simplex virus. It may be administered in higher doses and for a longer duration to prevent relapses of HSE.

Acyclovir can be started empirically during suspected encephalitis until specific results are obtained.

> **HINT:** Most viral infections involve supportive therapy only.

## SURGICAL MANAGEMENT

- *What is the recommended treatment of an empyema, or brain abscess?*
- **Surgical drainage**

Brain abscesses are encapsulated infectious lesions requiring surgical drainage. Antibiotic therapy is included but has limited efficacy as a sole treatment. Surgical drainage can be through burr holes, craniotomy, or CT-guided aspiration.

> **HINT:** Brain abscess can be a complication of bacterial meningitis.

## COMPLICATIONS

- *What potential complication of the ventricles can occur with bacterial meningitis?*
- **Hydrocephalus**

Bacterial meningitis causes purulent drainage in the subarachnoid space. The drainage is thicker than CSF and causes the arachnoid villi to obstruct. This blocks the reabsorption of CSF and results in hydrocephalus (Box 4.17).

> **HINT:** Another potential complication involving the ventricles is ventriculitis, or infection in the ventricles.

**Box 4.17** Complications of Meningitis

| |
|---|
| Ventriculitis |
| Hydrocephalus |
| Encephalitis |
| Brain abscess |
| Sepsis |
| Cerebral edema |
| Increased intracranial pressure |
| Hearing loss |
| Multisystem organ failure |

- *What is the complication of cysticercosis (multiple cysts) with diffuse inflammation in patients with neurocysticercosis?*
- **Cysticercosis encephalopathy**

Cysticercosis encephalopathy is associated with the CNS infection neurocysticercosis (Box 4.18). The encephalopathy is caused by the presence of multiple cysts, resulting in severe, diffuse inflammation.

▶ **HINT:** Frequently diagnosed with CT to identify the cysts.

**Box 4.18** Complications of Neurocysticercosis

| |
|---|
| Seizure |
| Ischemic stroke |
| Headache |
| Hydrocephalus |
| Encephalopathy |
| Radiculopathy (spinal cysts) |
| Myositis |
| Ophthalmic cysticercosis |

## BIBLIOGRAPHY

Angulo, M., & Babcock, E. (2015). Bell palsy. *Journal of the American Academy of Physician Assistants, 28*(10), 1. doi:10.1097/01.JAA.0000470511.20862.36

Burnet, S., Huntley, A., & Kemp, K. (2007). Meningitis: inflamed brain. *Nursing Critical Care, 2*(4), 36–47.

Linder, T. E., Abdelkafy, W., & Cavero-Vanek, S. (2010). The management of peripheral facial nerve palsy: "Paresis" versus "paralysis" and sources of ambiguity in study designs. *Otology & Neurotology, 31*(2), 319–327. doi:10.1097/MAO.0b013e3181cabd90

Roman, C., & Manning, K. (2017). Treatment and disease management of multiple sclerosis patients: A review for nurse practitioners. *Journal of the American Association of Nurse Practitioners, 29*(10), 629–638. doi:10.1002/2327-6924.12514

Strunk, J., & Rocchiccioli, J. (2010). Meningococcal meningitis: An emerging infectious disease. *Journal of Community Health Nursing, 27*(1), 51–58. doi:10.1080/07370010903466197

Torpy, J. M., Lynm, C., & Glass, R. M. (2007). JAMA patient page. Meningitis. *Journal of the American Medical Association, 297*(1), 122. doi:10.1001/jama.297.1.122

VanDemark, M. (2013). Acute bacterial meningitis. *Critical Care Nursing Clinics of North America, 25*, 351–361. doi:10.1016/j.ccell.2013.04.004

# 5

# Immune Infections, Part 2

## INTRODUCTION

- **What is the neurological disorder that is an immune-mediated, chronic, demyelinating disease of the central nervous system (CNS)?**
- **Multiple sclerosis (MS)**

MS is a progressive demyelinating disease that is an immune-mediated disorder.

Demyelination of nerve fibers is the primary injury and can result in partial or total loss of the myelin sheath. From the damage to the nerve fibers, speed of conduction along nerve fibers is impaired.

▶ HINT: MS affects the upper motor neurons (UMNs) (Box 5.1).

**Box 5.1** Comparison of Upper and Lower Motor Neurons

| Upper Motor Neurons | Lower Motor Neurons |
| --- | --- |
| Begin in the motor cortex of the brain, travel through to the spinal cord, and terminate at the lower motor neuron | Begin in anterior nerve roots or the cranial nerve nuclei of the brainstem and travel through the peripheral nerve to muscle |
| Motor spasticity | Flaccid paralysis |
| Hyperreflexia | Hyporeflexia |
| Minimal muscle atrophy | Muscle atrophy |

- **What is the primary characteristic of the clinical presentation of MS?**
- **Remission and relapse**

There are several presentation types of MS, but the most common is remission and relapse (Box 5.2). This presentation involves the symptoms of MS. During remissions, the symptoms may disappear or remain consistent without worsening. Relapses occur when symptoms worsen or progress.

▶ HINT: The remission-and-relapse presentation is considered the most characteristic presentation of MS.

**Box 5.2** Types of Multiple Sclerosis

| |
|---|
| Relapsing and remitting |
| Primary progressive |
| Secondary progressive |
| Progressive relapsing |

■ *What exposure is most likely a trigger of MS?*
■ **Viral infections**

Viral infections are believed to be a trigger for development of MS. Different viruses are considered possible risks, including Epstein–Barr and human herpes virus. Allergies, living with dogs or small animals, and experiencing physical trauma have been dispelled as possible causes of MS.

▶ **HINT:** There is increasing evidence that reduced exposure to sunshine and vitamin D is linked to MS.

■ *What neurological disease is a chronic autoimmune disorder affecting the neuromuscular junction causing fatigable muscle weakness?*
■ **Myasthenia gravis (MG)**

MG is an autoimmune disorder that is characterized by a worsening of motor fatigability during exercise with improvement at rest. In this neuromuscular disorder, the immune system attacks the acetylcholine receptors. The actual trigger for the development of MG is relatively unknown.

▶ **HINT:** MG is commonly associated with other autoimmune disorders (Box 5.3).

**Box 5.3** Associated Autoimmune Disorders With Myasthenia Gravis

| |
|---|
| Thyroid abnormality |
| Systemic lupus erythematosus |
| Rheumatoid arthritis |
| Vitamin B12 deficiency |

■ *How is the neurological disorder of amyotrophic lateral sclerosis (ALS) classified?*
■ **Motor neuron disease**

ALS is classified as a motor neuron disease affecting both upper and lower motor neurons. It is a progressive, chronic, degenerative paralyzing disease. The word *amyotrophic* refers to muscle atrophy, and *lateral sclerosis* is the scarring of the lateral aspect of the spinal cord (corticospinal tract).

▶ **HINT:** ALS is also called *Lou Gehrig's disease*.

■ *What is best described as a generalized cortical dysfunction?*
■ **Encephalopathy**

*Encephalopathy* is defined as generalized cortical dysfunction. Additional descriptions of encephalopathy include cognitive changes that cannot be fully explained by preexisting or evolving dementia.

▶ **HINT:** Encephalopathy is not a disease or a disorder, but rather a syndrome of symptoms.

■ *A patient presents with altered mental status (AMS) and visual changes. He or she has a history of uncontrolled hypertension. What is the most probable type of encephalopathy?*

■ **Posterior reversible encephalopathy syndrome (PRES)**

PRES is the syndrome caused by hypertension (Box 5.4). Malignant hypertension causes transient neurological symptoms in a hypertensive crisis. Acute hypertension increases cerebral perfusion causing a loss of integrity in the blood–brain barrier with cerebral edema as a complication.

▶ **HINT:** Hypertensive encephalopathy is now called *PRES* because it is usually reversible if the blood pressure is normalized and it most commonly affects the occipital lobes.

**Box 5.4** Causes of Encephalopathy

| |
|---|
| Alcohol-induced encephalopathy |
| Hypertensive encephalopathy |
| Anoxic/hypoxic encephalopathy |
| Wernicke's encephalopathy |
| Hepatic encephalopathy |
| AIDS encephalopathy |
| Toxic/metabolic encephalopathy |
| Hashimoto's encephalopathy |
| Infectious encephalopathy |
| Chronic traumatic encephalopathy |
| Drug-induced encephalopathy |
| Uremic encephalopathy |

■ *Which encephalopathy is caused by thiamine (vitamin B1) deficiency?*

■ **Wernicke's encephalopathy**

Wernicke's encephalopathy is a disorder caused by thiamine (vitamin B1) deficiency (Box 5.5). It is more often seen in alcoholics, as alcohol affects thiamine uptake and utilization. It may be associated with acute alcohol withdrawal, Wernicke–Korsakoff's syndrome, and congestive heart failure (CHF).

▶ **HINT:** Many factors will interact to reduce the supply of thiamine; thiamine deficiency can result in brain damage.

**Box 5.5** Causes of Wernicke's Encephalopathy

| |
|---|
| Malnutrition or prolonged starvation (reduced thiamine absorption) |
| Alcoholism |
| Bariatric surgery (malabsorption of thiamine) |
| HIV/AIDS patients |
| Dialysis patients in ESRD (dialysis water-soluble thiamine) |

ESRD, end-stage renal stage.

## PATHOPHYSIOLOGY

▪ *What does the immune system destroy in patients with MS?*
▪ **Myelin**

Myelin covers the nerve fibers, allowing nerve impulses to travel at faster speeds. In MS, the immune system (macrophages) destroys the myelin, oligodendrocytes, and nerve fibers (Box 5.6). T cells become sensitized to the proteins in the central nervous system (CNS) causing inflammation. Damage to the nerve fibers causes plaque to form and can be identified on MRI. Remyelination can occur but will be incomplete with chronic injury.

> ▶ HINT: Oligodendrocytes are the glial cells that produce myelin. Chronic lesions become hyperplasic and decrease the number of oligodendrocytes.

**Box 5.6** High-Risk Nerves at Risk for Demyelinating in Multiple Sclerosis

| |
|---|
| Optic nerve |
| Optic chiasm |
| Periventricular regions |
|   Brainstem |
|   Cerebellum |
|   Cerebrum |

▪ *What do the antibodies attack in the chronic, autoimmune disorder myasthenia gravis?*
▪ **Acetylcholine receptors on postsynaptic muscle**

Antibodies destroy the acetylcholine receptors at the postsynaptic muscle membrane, which decreases the effect of acetylcholine (Ach). Ach is released normally, but the effect on the end-plate receptors is diminished. Affected junctions will have 70% to 80% fewer receptors on the muscle side (Box 5.7).

> ▶ HINT: During repetitive firing of the muscle, the muscle gets weaker each time until it is unable to contract.

**Box 5.7** Examples of Repetitive Muscle Contractions Affected in Myasthenia Gravis

| |
|---|
| Eyelid opening |
| Blinking |
| Chewing |
| Swallowing |
| Speaking |
| Smiling |
| Movement of limbs |
| Maintaining neck upright |

■ **What type of daily pattern does a patient with MG experience in regard to strength?**
■ **Diurnal pattern**

Patients with MG experience a diurnal pattern of return of strength during the day, with the morning being the strongest. By evening, patients are weaker and can experience a greater incidence of MG crisis.

> ▶ **HINT:** There are many situations and factors that can influence the strength of patients with MG (Box 5.8).

**Box 5.8** Factors That Can Worsen Myasthenia Gravis

| |
|---|
| Emotional upset |
| Systemic illness |
| Hypothyroidism or hyperthyroidism |
| Pregnancy |
| Menstrual cycle |
| Certain medications |

■ **What neurological disease process is an acute inflammatory demyelinating polyneuropathy (AIDP)?**
■ **Guillain–Barré (GB)**

GB is an acute immune-mediated process that is characterized by demyelination of the cranial and spinal nerves. It is classified as a polyneuropathy and involves the lower motor neurons (LMNs).

> ▶ **HINT:** MS and GB both demyelinate nerves, but MS affects the upper motor neuron (UMN) and GB affects the LMN (Box 5.9).

**Box 5.9** Comparison of Multiple Sclerosis and Guillain–Barré

| Multiple Sclerosis | Guillain–Barré |
|---|---|
| Chronic | Acute |
| Immune mediated | Immune mediated |
| Trigger: Viral | Trigger: Viral or immunizations |
| Affects UMN (cerebral motor tracts to the spinal cord) | Affects LMN (spinal nerve to peripheral nerves) |

LMN, lower motor neuron; UMN, upper motor neuron.

■ **GB is most commonly an acute process that resolves over time. What is the difference between the inflammatory demyelination resulting in an acute versus chronic progressive process of MS?**
■ **Peripheral nerves are involved**

GB affects the peripheral nerves or LMNs. Peripheral nerves are more likely to remyelinate and recover normal to near normal conduction of impulses (Box 5.10). MS affects the CNS or UMNs and have less regeneration capability. The complete process of regeneration and recovery of GB may take up to 6 months to 2 years.

> ▶ HINT: Some patients with GB do develop a chronic form of GB called *chronic inflammatory demyelinating polyneuropathy (CIDP)* syndrome.

**Box 5.10** Peripheral Nerves Involved in Guillain–Barré

| |
|---|
| Cranial nerves |
| Ventral and dorsal nerve roots |
| Dorsal root ganglia |
| Entire length of the peripheral nerves |
| Autonomic nervous system |

■ *What is the most common "trigger" for the onset of GB?*
■ **Viral infection**

A large percentage of the cases of GB report a history of respiratory or gastrointestinal infection 1 to 3 weeks before the onset of the symptoms.

> ▶ HINT: Obtaining the recent history (e.g., viral infection or vaccination) is important in determining the diagnosis of GB (Box 5.11).

**Box 5.11** Triggers for Guillain–Barré

| |
|---|
| Viral infection |
|    *Campylobacter jejuni* |
|    Zika virus |
|    Cytomegalovirus |
|    Epstein–Barr virus |
|    Influenza A virus |
| Immunizations |
|    Flu vaccination |
|    Rabies vaccination |
|    Pneumococcal vaccination |
| Surgical procedures |
| Malignant disease |

■ *ALS is a motor neuron disease that affects which of the following: CNS, peripheral nervous system (PNS), or both?*
■ **Both CNS and PNS**

Motor neuron diseases affect the motor neurons of the CNS and the PNS. Lower extremity symptoms are most common in patients, followed by UMN symptoms

> ▶ HINT: ALS is the degeneration that results from the loss of both UMNs (which is considered the CNS) and LMNs (considered the PNS).

▪ *What portion of the spinal cord is involved in ALS?*
▪ **Corticospinal tract**

The spinal cord shows evidence of anterior horn cells and corticospinal tract degeneration. When the spinal cord is involved, it is considered to be an upper motor neuron (UMN) injury. The myelin sheath begins to deteriorate in ALS, leaving sclerotic scar tissue and resulting in significant muscle atrophy.

> ▶ **HINT:** An easy way to determine where the spinal tract begins and ends is to look at the name. The first part of the word is where the tract originates, the second part is where it terminates. For example, corticospinal tract begins in the cortical region and ends in the spinal cord. This is a descending tract.

▪ *What is the most identifiable risk for the development of ALS?*
▪ **Laborers engaged in agricultural work**

There are no definitively known causes of ALS at this time. There are a couple of established known risks, including history as a laborer engaged in agricultural work (Box 5.12).

> ▶ **HINT:** Neurotoxin exposure (i.e., lead, mercury) has been highly suspected but is not a known risk.

**Box 5.12** Known Risks for Amyotrophic Lateral Sclerosis

| |
|---|
| Laborers engaged in the following: |
|    Agricultural work |
|    Factory work |
|    Heavy manual labor |
|    Welding |
| Repetitive muscle use |
| Athleticism |
| Trauma |
| Electrical shock |

▪ *A patient recovers from a near-drowning but has significant altered mentation afterward. What type of encephalopathy is this patient experiencing?*
▪ **Ischemic–hypoxic encephalopathy**

Hypoxic–ischemic encephalopathy is a syndrome of acute global brain injury resulting from a critical loss of blood supply to the brain (Box 5.13). Following a near-drowning, the brain can sustain a significant lack of blood flow, resulting in severe hypoxia to the brain.

> ▶ **HINT:** The triad of symptoms involved with ischemic–hypoxic encephalopathy includes unresponsiveness (vegetative state), myoclonus activity, and seizures.

**Box 5.13** Etiology of Encephalopathies

| | |
|---|---|
| Hypertensive encephalopathy | History of hypertension<br>Current hypertensive crisis<br>Chronic renal disease<br>Acute glomerulonephritis<br>Pheochromocytoma<br>Sympathomimetic agents<br>Eclampsia and preeclampsia<br>Encephalitis and meningitis |
| Wernicke's encephalopathy | Alcoholism<br>Malnutrition or prolonged starvation<br>Bariatric<br>HIV/AIDS patients<br>Hemodialysis patients in ESRD |
| Hypoxic–ischemic encephalopathy | Cardiopulmonary arrest<br>Near-drowning<br>Asphyxia<br>Carbon monoxide poisoning<br>Profound anemia<br>Severe hypotension or hypovolemic shock |
| Hepatic encephalopathy | Hepatic dysfunction or failure |

ESRD, end-stage renal disease.

## SIGNS AND SYMPTOMS

▪ *Which cranial nerve (CN) is initially involved in MS?*
▪ **CN II (optic nerve)**

CN II is commonly involved in MS patients, and frequently, blurred vision is the first presentation of MS. Other symptoms of cranial nerve involvement include diplopia, facial weakness, and dysphagia.

▸ **HINT:** The upper motor portion of the cranial nerves are affected in MS.

▪ *MS patients can experience pain sensations and Lhermitte's sign. What is Lhermitte's sign?*
▪ **Electric shock-like sensations**

MS affects motor neurons and has a sensory component (Box 5.14). The pain is neuropathic pain, and patients commonly experience Lhermitte's sign. These electric shock-like sensations can radiate down the spine and extremities.

▸ **HINT:** Neuropathic pain is managed differently than other types of pain.

**Box 5.14** Symptoms of Multiple Sclerosis

| | |
|---|---|
| Motor symptoms | Weakness<br>Spasticity<br>Paralysis |

*(continued)*

**Box 5.14** Symptoms of Multiple Sclerosis *(continued)*

| Cranial nerve symptoms | Blurred visions<br>Diplopia<br>Facial weakness<br>Dysphagia |
|---|---|
| Cerebellar symptoms | Dysarthria<br>Tremors<br>Incoordination<br>Ataxia<br>Vertigo |
| Brainstem | Nystagmus<br>Dysarthria |
| Bowel and bladder | Incontinence<br>Retention |
| Cognitive dysfunction | Short-term memory deficits<br>Word-finding abnormalities<br>Short attention span<br>Mood alteration |

▪ *Which signs are most commonly the first reported symptoms of MG?*
▪ **Ocular signs**

Ocular signs are typically the first reported symptoms of MG (Box 5.15). Ptosis and diplopia are the hallmark signs of MG. These signs are due to ptosis caused by the fatigable eyelid muscle and diplopia caused by extraocular muscles.

▶ **HINT:** Patients with MG report diurnal fluctuations in strength, with normal strength in the morning and severe weakness in the evening.

**Box 5.15** Signs of Myasthenia Gravis

| Ocular signs | Ptosis<br>Diplopia<br>Unable to completely close eyelids<br>Blurred vision |
|---|---|
| Bulbar (brainstem) signs | Dysarthria<br>Dysphagia<br>Dysphonia |
| Trunk signs | Weak neck flexor muscles |
| Facial signs | Unable to maintain a smile ("myasthenia snarl")<br>Nasal, weak speech<br>Difficulty chewing |
| Limb strength | Difficulty holding hands over head, performing repetitive deep-knee bends, and stair climbing |

▪ *What is the hallmark sign of GB?*
▪ **Ascending bilateral paralysis**

The hallmark presentation of a patient with GB is bilateral ascending paralysis (Box 5.16). It has an abrupt onset and is progressive. The severity depends on the type of GB. It can ascend to affect respiratory muscles and the diaphragm, requiring intubation and ventilation.

> ▶ HINT: The resolution of the paralysis occurs in a descending fashion, opposite of its onset.

**Box 5.16** Cardinal Symptoms of Guillain–Barré

| |
|---|
| Abrupt and progressive onset |
| Bilateral, symmetrical symptoms |
| Descending return of function |
| No atrophy |
| Associated with pain |

- **A patient with GB presents with postural hypotension and tachycardia. What is the physiological cause for these symptoms in GB?**
- **Autonomic involvement**

Autonomic nervous system (ANS) involvement with GB patients can result in hypotension and tachycardia. The ANS contains some of the peripheral nerves involved in demyelination, so GB can present with ANS symptoms.

> ▶ HINT: GB typically presents with lower extremity weakness and gait abnormalities, which progress to upper trunk and neck weakness (Box 5.17).

**Box 5.17** Other Symptoms of Guillain–Barré

| | |
|---|---|
| Motor symptoms | Bilateral ascending paralysis<br>No atrophy<br>Hypotonia<br>Loss of superficial and deep tendon reflexes |
| Pain symptoms | Discomfort<br>Increased sensitivity<br>Increased tenderness<br>"Crawling sensations" |
| Bulbar (brainstem) symptoms | Bilateral facial weakness<br>Loss of neck flexor muscles<br>Eye movement weaknesses<br>Dyspnea<br>Dysphagia<br>Dysarthria |
| Autonomic manifestations | Postural hypotension<br>Heart block or bradycardia<br>Tachycardia<br>Inverted T waves<br>Bladder atony<br>Life-threatening arrhythmias<br>Facial flushing<br>Anhydrosis<br>GI dysmotility |

GI, gastrointestinal.

■ *CNs III, IV, and VI can be involved in GB. How would the patient present if these CNs are involved?*
■ **With diplopia and abnormal gaze**

CNs III, IV, and VI are commonly involved in GB. These CNs innervate the ocular muscles and are responsible for extraocular eye movement (EOM). Symptoms include dysconjugate gaze and diplopia.

> ▶ **HINT:** CNs responsible for swallow and gag reflex (CN IX, X, XII) are also commonly affected in GB patients.

■ *What is the hallmark sign of the motor dysfunction in ALS?*
■ **Asymmetry**

In ALS, there is asymmetrical motor dysfunction in which distal weakness is greater than proximal weakness. It is a progressive, degenerative neurological disorder characterized by muscle atrophy of the hands, forearms, and legs. ALS is a terminal disease that is eventually fatal.

> ▶ **HINT:** There are no known causes, no specific treatments, no patterns of progression, and no method of prevention for ALS.

■ *Which CNs are spared in ALS?*
■ **CNs III, IV, and VI**

ALS affects motor CNs except CNs III, IV, and VI. These are spared in patients with ALS. These cranial nerves affect EOM. Eye movement is the primary movement preserved in patients with ALS.

> ▶ **HINT:** Motor CNs commonly affected by ALS include CNs V, VII, IX, X, and XII.

■ *What is one of the initial presenting signs of ALS?*
■ **Clumsy hands and gait**

Typical initial complaints of patients developing ALS include clumsy and weak hands, shoulders, and upper arms with a tendency to drop things (Box 5.18). They also report a heavy feeling in the legs, which causes stumbling and a clumsy gait. Cramping can also be a first sign of ALS.

> ▶ **HINT:** In ALS patients, mental capacity is intact until death in most patients.

**Box 5.18** Symptoms of Amyotrophic Lateral Sclerosis

| Upper motor neuron symptoms | Muscle weakness<br>Decreased strength<br>Spasticity<br>Loss of voluntary movement<br>Hyperreflexia |
|---|---|

*(continued)*

**Box 5.18** Symptoms of Amyotrophic Lateral Sclerosis *(continued)*

| Lower motor neuron symptoms | Muscle weakness<br>Paralysis<br>Muscle atrophy of arms and legs<br>Flaccidity<br>Areflexia |
|---|---|
| Cranial nerve involvement | Difficulty with swallow<br>Dysphagia<br>Aspiration risks |
| Bulbar symptoms | Altered speech (nasal monotone)<br>Inability to elevate palate, chew, suck, swallow, or cough<br>Loss of salivary control |
| Generalized symptoms | Fatigue<br>Inappropriate weeping and laughing<br>Behavioral improvement |

- **What is the most common characteristic of encephalopathy?**
- **AMS**

Encephalopathy is characterized by fluctuations in level of consciousness, poor attention span (inattentive), frequent hallucinations and delusions, and changes in psychomotor activity (hyper- or hypoactivity).

> ▶ **HINT:** There are multiple different causes of encephalopathy that can present with symptoms similar to AMS.

- **What is the characteristic symptom of encephalopathy?**
- **Altered level of consciousness (LOC)**

The onset of encephalopathy is acute to subacute (hours to days). Encephalopathy is characterized by fluctuations or alterations in LOC, poor attention span (inattentive), frequent hallucinations and delusions, and changes in psychomotor activity.

> ▶ **HINT:** The definition of *encephalopathy* is similar to that of *dementia*, but in encephalopathy cognitive changes cannot be fully explained by preexisting or evolving dementia in acute situations.

- **What is the triad of symptoms in Wernicke's encephalopathy?**
- **Confusion, ataxia, and ophthalmoplegia**

A triad of symptoms, including confusion, ataxia, and ophthalmoplegia, characterizes Wernicke's encephalopathy (Box 5.19). The confusion involves disinterest, inattention, and agitation. Ophthalmoplegia includes nystagmus, bilateral lateral rectus palsies, and conjugate gaze palsies.

> ▶ **HINT:** Peripheral neuropathies are commonly associated with Wernicke's encephalopathy.

**Box 5.19** Symptoms of Common Encephalopathies

| Types of Encephalopathy | Common Symptoms |
|---|---|
| Hypertensive encephalopathy | Progressive headache<br>Nausea<br>Confusion<br>Visual disturbances<br>Papilledema |
| Wernicke's encephalopathy | Confusion<br>Ataxia<br>Ophthalmoplegia<br>Hypotension<br>Hypothermia<br>Lactic acidosis<br>Peripheral neuropathy |
| Hypoxic–ischemic encephalopathy | Coma or vegetative state<br>Myoclonus activity<br>Seizures |
| Hepatic encephalopathy | Personality changes<br>Apathy<br>Irritability<br>Disinhibition<br>Alterations in consciousness<br>Alterations in motor function<br>Disturbances of sleep–wake cycles (excessive daytime sleeping)<br>Hallucinations<br>Coma |

■ *A patient presents with inappropriate behavior and asterixis. At what grade of hepatic encephalopathy (HE) would this patient most likely be classified in?*
■ **Grade II**

Overt HE is seen when the patient develops onset of disorientation, inappropriate behavior, or asterixis ("liver flap"). These symptoms indicate that the patient is classified as a grade II HE (Box 5.20).

▶ **HINT:** Poor handwriting is another common sign of HE.

**Box 5.20** Grading of HE

| HE Grading | |
|---|---|
| Minimal | Psychometric or neuropsychological alterations seen in tests exploring psychomotor speed/executive functions or neurophysiological alterations without clinical evidence of mental change |
| Grade I | Trivial lack of awareness<br>Euphoria or anxiety<br>Short attention span<br>Impairment of addition/subtraction ability<br>Altered sleep patterns |

*(continued)*

**Box 5.20** Grading of Hepatic Encephalopathy *(continued)*

| Grade II | Lethargy or apathy |
| --- | --- |
| | Disorientation of time |
| | Obvious personality change |
| | Inappropriate behavior |
| | Asterixis |
| Grade III | Somnolence or near stupor |
| | Responsive to stimuli |
| | Confused |
| | Gross disorientation |
| | Bizarre behavior |
| Grade IV | Coma |

HE, hepatic encephalopathy.

# DIAGNOSIS

■ *Which diagnostic examination is considered to be the best in diagnosing MS?*

■ **T2-weighted MRI**

The T2-weighted MRI is used to assist with the diagnosis of MS. T1-weighted images are less sensitive for detecting lesions and those that appear are hypointensities or "black holes." Multiple focal periventricular areas of increased signal with irregular-shaped lesions are indicative of MS. The diagnosis of MS is based on lesions disseminating over time and involving multiple, discrete anatomic areas within the white matter of the CNS. The patient can be diagnosed with one attack if diagnostic criteria are met. MS is a disease of exclusion.

▶ **HINT:** CSF analysis and visual evoked potentials are used to support a diagnosis of MS (Box 5.21).

**Box 5.21** Characteristics of CSF in MS

| Elevated IgG levels |
| --- |
| Positive for oligoclonal bands |
| Normal opening pressures |
| Mildly elevated WBCs |
| Mild elevation proteins |
| Increase MBP |

CSF, cerebrospinal fluid; IgG, immunoglobulin G; MBP, myelin basic protein; MS, multiple sclerosis; WBCs, white blood cells.

■ *What diagnostic test is used to assist with the diagnosis of MG in patients presenting with progressive muscle weakness and fatigue?*

■ **Electromyography (EMG)**

Progressive muscle weakness and fatigue are the cardinal presentations of MG. EMG testing in patients with MG demonstrates a rapid reduction of amplitude, or delay or failure of transmission in pairs of muscle fibers.

▶ **HINT:** Lab work is also utilized in the diagnosis of MG with elevated levels of serum acetylcholine receptor (AchR) antibodies found in the majority of cases.

- **What pharmacological test can be utilized to assist with the diagnosis of MG?**
- **Cholinergic drug test**

Cholinergic drug testing can be performed to assist with the diagnosis, including tensilon (Reversol), neostigmine (Prostigmin), or edrophonium tests. These are short-acting anticholinesterase drugs that will increase the neurotransmission. MG patients will exhibit an abrupt improvement of their muscular weakness within 5 to 10 minutes of administration of the tensilon.

▶ **HINT:** Tensilon is most effective on ocular and cranial nerve weakness, and neostigmine is primarily effective with limbs and respiratory muscles.

- **What is the most prominent finding used to diagnose GB?**
- **Symptoms and history**

GB is commonly diagnosed with presentation of common symptoms such as ascending paralysis and history of recent viral infection or immunizations. Diagnostic tests frequently used to assist with the diagnosis of GB include lumbar puncture with CSF analysis and EMG or nerve conduction velocity (NCV) studies (Box 5.22).

▶ **HINT:** Sensory symptoms of numbness and tingling of the fingers and feet or pain in an ascending pattern may accompany the motor involvement.

**Box 5.22** CSF Analysis of Guillain–Barré

| |
|---|
| Increased protein |
| Normal mononuclear cell count |
| Pleocytosis |
| Albuminocytologic dissociation |

CSF, cerebrospinal fluid.

- **In patients with ALS undergoing neurological testing, does the EMG testing demonstrate muscle or nerve dysfunction?**
- **Muscle dysfunction**

The EMG exam demonstrates denervation of muscles. Other neuromuscular disorders affect nerve innervation. There are no laboratory studies used in the diagnosis of ALS. The diagnosis is made by the characteristics of the disease.

▶ **HINT:** Muscle biopsy is more definitive than EMG.

- **Which cerebral lobe is most commonly affected in HE?**
- **Occipital lobe**

Hypertensive encephalopathy (also called *posterior reversible encephalopathy syndrome*) most commonly affects the occipital lobe. MRI demonstrates bilateral occipital involvement.

▶ **HINT:** Blood pressure management can reverse the process, and that is why it is called *reversible encephalopathy*.

■ **What laboratory test is most commonly ordered in suspected HE?**
■ **Ammonia level**

The diagnosis of HE is made with the exclusions of other causes of AMS and the history of acute liver failure (ALF) or chronic liver disease (CLD). High ammonia levels alone do not add to the diagnosis of HE, the grading of its severity, or its prognosis. But repeated values may be helpful in determining the effectiveness of ammonia-lowering drugs.

▶ **HINT:** The grading of the severity of HE is dependent on the neurological changes that have occurred.

## MEDICAL MANAGEMENT

■ **What is the class of medications recommended to treat neuropathy pain in MS patients?**
■ **Anticonvulsants**

Neuropathy pain is managed differently than other types of pain. Opioids are not as effective in treating neuropathies. The recommended class of medications for neuropathy pain is anticonvulsants.

▶ **HINT:** Other medications used to manage neuropathy pain include nonsteroid anti-inflammatory drugs (NSAIDs) and tricyclic antidepressants.

■ **What is the primary pharmacological treatment for managing the symptoms in patients with MG?**
■ **Anticholinesterase medications**

The primary medications used to manage the symptoms of MG are anticholinesterase medications (Box 5.23). Corticosteroids and immunosuppressants may also be used to manage the disease process due to the autoimmune etiology.

▶ **HINT:** The anticholinesterase may be taken on an as-needed basis (prior to exercise or meals). In acute situations, if taken too late, the patient may not even be able to swallow the medication.

**Box 5.23** Side Effects of Anticholinesterase Medications

| |
|---|
| Diarrhea |
| Heartburn/belching |
| Nausea/vomiting |
| Abdominal cramping |
| Increased micturition |
| Uterine cramping |
| Increased salivation |

*(continued)*

**Box 5.23** Side Effects of Anticholinesterase Medications *(continued)*

| |
|---|
| Increased bronchial secretions |
| Bradycardia |
| Blurred vision |
| Wheezing |
| Muscle cramping |
| Muscle fasciculations |

■ **What are two common nonpharmacological interventions that can be utilized in acute situations of exacerbation of MG?**
■ **Intravenous immunoglobulin (IVIG) and plasmapheresis**

IVIG is typically administered over 4 to 5 days following acute exacerbation of MG with severe weakness. IVIG is typically the initial treatment in these cases followed by plasmapheresis if improvement is not seen (Box 5.24). Plasmapheresis is the exchange of plasma to remove the inflammatory markers and antibodies.

▶ **HINT:** Respiratory effort is monitored closely during the acute exacerbation of MG throughout the treatments.

**Box 5.24** Complications of IVIG and Plasmapheresis

| IVIG Complications | Plasmapheresis Complications |
|---|---|
| Headache | Cardiac arrhythmias |
| Chills | Nausea |
| Fever | Light-headedness |
| | Chills |
| | Edema |

IVIG, intravenous immunoglobulin.

■ **Which of the following is NOT recommended in the care of GB: steroids, IVIG immunotherapy, or plasmapheresis?**
■ **Steroids**

There is no cure for GB, but IVIG immunotherapy and plasmapheresis have been found to lessen the severity and accelerate recovery. Steroids have not been found beneficial in managing GB and may even have a deleterious effect in GB.

▶ **HINT:** IVIG is frequently the initial treatment of GB because it is less invasive and easier to initiate than plasmapheresis, but both are similar in effectiveness.

■ **What is the currently approved medication for ALS?**
■ **Riluzole (Rilutek)**

Riluzole (Rilutek) is approved by the Food and Drug Administration (FDA) for slowing the ALS disease process and improving survival ranges from several weeks to several years (Box 5.25). The indications include a disease process of less than 5 years' duration, forced vital capacity (FVC) <60%, and no tracheostomy in the patient.

▶ **HINT:** Riluzole (Rilutek) is most effective if started within 5 years of onset of ALS.

**Box 5.25** Management of ALS Symptoms

| | |
|---|---|
| Sialorrhea (drooling) | Anticholinergic agents |
| | Amitriptyline |
| | BOTOX injections into the parotid gland |
| | Low-dose radiation |
| Pseudobulbar symptoms | Mixed-dose combination of DM/quinidine/antidepressants |
| Spasticity | Antispasmodics |
| Weight loss | Enteral nutrition |
| Pulmonary complications | Bronchodilator therapy |
| | Mucomyst |

ALS, amyotrophic lateral sclerosis; DM, dextromethorphan.

■ *Which of the encephalopathies is managed by the administration of thiamine?*
■ **Wernicke's encephalopathy**

Parenteral replacement of thiamine is used in patients with Wernicke's encephalopathy. Rapid resolution of symptoms occurs with thiamine except for impairment of memory and learning.

▶ **HINT:** It is not recommended to administer dextrose in thiamine-deficient patients. The glucose oxidation involves thiamine and can drive thiamine intracellularly, resulting in an acute decrease in thiamine levels, which precipitates neurological injury.

■ *What is the primary pharmacological treatment for HE?*
■ **Lactulose**

Lactulose is the initial treatment for overt HE. It is a nonabsorable disaccharide that binds ammonium and clears it through the gastrointestinal tract.

▶ **HINT:** Side effects of lactulose include dehydration and hypernatremia.

## SURGICAL MANAGEMENT

■ *What surgical procedure has been used to treat MG?*
■ **Thymectomy**

An abnormal thymus is present in most of the acquired MG patients. The relationship is unclear, but the thymus is the central organ for immunological self-tolerance. The abnormality of the thymus can range from a thymic tumor to microscopic changes of hyperplasia.

▶ **HINT:** Thymectomy is controversial, but in some situations it has been found to attain medication-free remission.

# COMPLICATIONS

- **What is the most life-threatening complication of MG?**
- **Ventilatory insufficiency**

Respiratory muscles, including the diaphragm, may be affected in patients with MG, resulting in an inability to ventilate. During an exacerbation of MG, the patient's vital capacity (VC) is monitored closely. A decrease in VC indicates fatigued respiratory muscles and respiratory insufficiency.

> ▶ **HINT:** In severe cases of MG, patients may require intubation to maintain ventilation.

- **What is the complication of severe weakness and bulbar symptoms in MG patients called?**
- **Myasthenia crisis**

Myasthenia crisis is an acute exacerbation of MG. Patients present with severe weakness, severe bulbar symptoms (dysphagia, dysarthria, dystonia), and respiratory failure. These patients may require intubation and ventilation for a short period of time.

> ▶ **HINT:** This crisis is a problem that can occur due to either undermedication or no response to cholinergic treatment at the neuromuscular junction (Box 5.26).

**Box 5.26** Precipitating Factors for Myasthenia Crisis

| |
|---|
| Undermedicated |
| Infection |
| Aspiration |
| Surgery |
| Drug interactions |

- **What is it called when an MG patient presents with symptoms of overmedication with anticholinesterase medications?**
- **Cholinergic crisis**

Cholinergic crisis is a result of overmedication with anticholinesterase medications. Medical interventions to manage the crisis include withholding the anticholinesterase medications and restarting the medications at a lower dose once the symptoms improve.

> ▶ **HINT:** Symptoms of a cholinergic crisis are "wet" symptoms. Use the acronym "SLUD" to remember the primary symptoms (Box 5.27).

**Box 5.27** "SLUD" Acronym for Signs of Cholinergic Crisis

| | |
|---|---|
| S | Salivation, excessive |
| L | Lacrimation |
| U | Urination |
| D | Defecation (diarrhea) |

■ *What is the chronic form of GB called?*
■ **CIPD**

CIPD is considered the chronic form of GB. It is classified as either a chronic progressing or relapsing symmetrical sensorimotor disorder.

> ▶ HINT: CIPD is not always preceded by an infection but involves sensory and motor components similar to the acute process of GB.

■ *What is the complication of Wernicke's encephalopathy?*
■ **Korsakoff's syndrome**

Without treatment, Wernicke's encephalopathy progresses to an irreversible cognitive state, including severe antegrade (inability to assimilate new information) and retrograde amnesia (inability to recall information) memory loss.

> ▶ HINT: Korsakoff's amnestic syndrome is frequently called *Wernicke–Korsakoff syndrome* or *psychosis with confabulation*.

# Sample Exam Questions

1. A patient with history of myasthenia gravis (MG) presents to the ED with ventilatory failure requiring intubation and mechanical ventilation. Which of the following is the reason for the ventilatory failure?

   A. Serotonin syndrome
   B. Refractory MG
   C. Myasthenia crisis
   D. Cholinergic crisis

2. Which of the following surgical procedures is potentially an option in patients with myasthenia gravis who are not improving with medical management?

   A. Thyroidectomy
   B. Adrenalectomy
   C. Thymectomy
   D. Pituitary tumor resection

3. A patient develops bulbar symptoms with the onset of amyotrophic lateral sclerosis. Which of the following are more likely to be the signs the patient presented with?

   A. Tachycardia and miosis
   B. Dysphagia and dysarthria
   C. Anhydrosis and mydriasis
   D. Memory loss and cognitive slowing

4. A patient presents with visual field losses and headache. The MRI shows bilateral occipital involvement, and the patient is diagnosed with posterior reversible encephalopathy syndrome (PRES). What is the underlying etiology for PRES?

   A. Alcohol intoxication
   B. Hypertension
   C. Hepatic failure
   D. Ischemic stroke

5. Which of the following is NOT a component of the triad of symptoms in Wernicke's encephalopathy?

   A. Confusion
   B. Ataxia
   C. Dysphagia
   D. Ophthalmoplegia

6. A patient with chronic hepatic failure and hypertension presents with confusion, asterixis, and abnormal handwriting. Which of the following is the most likely cause of the patient's presentation?

   A. Encephalitis
   B. Uremic encephalopathy
   C. Posterior reversible encephalopathy
   D. Hepatic encephalopathy

## BIBLIOGRAPHY

Abbott, S. A. (2010). Diagnostic challenge: Myasthenia gravis in the emergency department. *Journal of the American Academy of Nurse Practitioners, 22*, 468–473. doi:10.1111/j.1745-7599.2010.00541.x

American Association for the Study of Liver Diseases and European Association for the Study of the Liver. (2014). Clinical guidelines: Hepatic encephalopathy in chronic liver disease: 2014 practice guidelines for European Association for the Study of the Liver and the American Association for the Study of Liver Diseases. *Journal of Hepatology, 61*(3), 642–659. doi:10.1016/j.jhep.2014.05.042

Bellmo, T., & Cichminski, L. (2015). Amyotrophic lateral sclerosis: What nurses need to know. *Nursing, 45*(10), 46–51. doi:10.1097/01.NURSE.0000471410.04013.6d

Benatar, M. (2010). Pearls: Myasthenia. *Seminars in Neurology, 30*(1), 35–37. doi:10.1055/s-0029-1244999

Blisset, P., & Fowler, S. (2013). Care of the patient with myasthenia gravis. *Journal of Neuroscience Nursing, 45*(5), 317.

Boentert, M., Brenscheidt, I., Glatz, C., & Young, P. (2015). Effects of non-invasive ventilation on objective sleep and nocturnal respiration in patients with amyotrophic lateral sclerosis. *Journal of Neurology, 262*(9), 2073–2082. doi:10.1007/s00415-015-7822-4

Bradshaw, M., & Venkatesan, S. (2016). Herpes simplex virus-1 encephalitis in adults: Pathophysiology, diagnosis and management. *Neurotheraputics, 13*(3), 493–508. doi:10.1007/s13311-016-0433-7

Castro, M. (2010). Unraveling Guillain-Barre syndrome. *Nursing Management, 44*(8), 36–39.

Dalakas, M. (2011). Advances in the diagnosis, pathogenesis, and treatment of CIDP. *Nature Reviews Neurology, 7*, 507–517. doi:10.1038/nrneurol.2011.121

Halper, J., & Harris, C. (2016). *Nursing practice in multiple sclerosis, 4th edition: A core curriculum.* New York, NY: Springer Publishing Company.

Harmes, M. (2011). Inpatient management of Guillain-Barré syndrome. *Neurohospitalist, 1*(2), 78–84. doi:10.1177/1941875210396379

Hu, B., Zhou, Y., Lu, X., Xiong, Q., Liu, Q., Qi, X., & Ding, W. (2018). Chronic inflammatory demyelinating polyradiculoneuropathy: A case report. *Medicine (Baltimore), 97*(41), e12469. doi:10.1097/MD.0000000000012469

McNair, N. (2013). Treatment of Guillain-Barré syndrome. *Journal of Infusion Nursing, 36*(6), 397–400. doi:10.1097/NAN.0000000000000011

Miller, R. G., Mitchell, J. D., & Moore, D. H. (2012). Riluzole for amyotrophic lateral sclerosis (ALS)/motor neuron disease (MND). *Cochrane Database of Systematic Reviews, 2012*(3), CD001447. doi:10.1002/14651858.CD001447.pub3

Polman, C. H., Reingold, S. C., Edan, G., Filippi, M., Hartung, H. P., Kappos, L., ... Wolinsky, J. S. (2005). Diagnostic criteria for multiple sclerosis: 2005 revisions to the "McDonald Criteria." *Annals of Neurology, 58*(6), 840–846. doi:10.1002/ana.20703

Vacca, V. M., Jr. (2016). CJD: Understanding Creuzfeldt-Jacob's disease. *Nursing, 46*(3), 36–42. doi:10.1097/01.NURSE.0000480598.84274.0f

Venkatesan, A., & Romergko, G. (2014). Diagnosis and management of acute encephalitis: A practical approach. *Neurology Clinical Practice, 4*(3), 206–215. doi:10.1212/CPJ.0000000000000036

# 6
# Seizures

## INTRODUCTION

- **What is a paroxysmal, uncontrolled, brief event due to abnormal excessive neuronal discharge called?**
- **Epileptic seizure**

An epileptic seizure is a paroxysmal, uncontrolled, brief event due to abnormal excessive neuronal discharge associated with sensory, motor, and/or behavioral changes.

> ▶ **HINT:** Epilepsy involves recurrent epileptic seizure unprovoked by any immediately identifiable cause such as hyponatremia.

- **What is a seizure called when it lasts for longer than 5 minutes?**
- **Status epilepticus (SE)**

SE is a condition of recurrent seizures or continuous seizure activity without the return to normal function. This epileptic activity persists for greater than 5 minutes or occurs repetitively without a complete return to normal function.

> ▶ **HINT:** Refractory SE is an epileptic seizure that persists for greater than 90 minutes even after administration of anticonvulsant medications.

- **When does brain injury begin to occur with epileptic seizure activity?**
- **Within 30 minutes**

Brain damage can result from the excessive electrical activity or from the hypoxemia, metabolic acidosis, and hyperglycemia that occurs. This may start to happen within 30 minutes of the epileptic seizure activity.

> ▶ **HINT:** Rhabdomyolysis can occur with persistent motor seizure activity, leading to acute kidney injury.

## PATHOPHYSIOLOGY

■ *Which of the neurons is most responsive to action potentials and can conduct the impulse rapidly?*
■ **All neurons**

All neurons have the capability of rapid repetitive firing with recurrent membrane depolarization and action potentials. Seizures are a result of abnormally persistent, excessive excitation, or ineffective recruitment of inhibition.

> ▶ **HINT:** Seizures can occur within a focal area of the brain or be widespread throughout the neuronal tissue.

■ *Which excitatory neurotransmitter initiates or potentiates the action potential of the seizure?*
■ **Glutamate**

Glutamate is an excitatory amino acid neurotransmitter that initiates seizure or initiates depolarization of neurons, causing them to fire rapidly and repeatedly. Glutamate is required for learning and memory, but too much glutamate can lead to seizures and neuronal damage.

> ▶ **HINT:** Inhibiting glutamate can decrease seizure activity and stop a seizure.

■ *What is the inhibitory neurotransmitter that inhibits seizures or depolarization of neurons?*
■ **Gamma-aminobutyric acid (GABA)**

GABA is an inhibitory neurotransmitter that can inhibit seizure or depolarization of the neurons. Animal models have found that the administration of a GABA antagonist can cause a seizure and the administration of a GABA agonist can stop a seizure.

> ▶ **HINT:** Some of the anticonvulsants work by increasing GABA to stop the seizure.

■ *Does the influx of sodium into the cell cause depolarization or repolarization?*
■ **Depolarization**

Depolarization is caused by sodium influx into the cells and potassium leaving the cells. When chloride then enters the cell, the action potential is terminated. Calcium channels then open to allow calcium to enter the cell, resulting in the release of neurotransmitters.

> ▶ **HINT:** Sodium channel blockers and facilitating chloride entry into the cell have been found to decrease a seizure or stop a seizure.

■ *Seizures may or may not have a known underlying cause. If no underlying cause is found, the seizure is considered to be?*
■ **Idiopathic**

Seizures and epilepsy are frequently considered to be idiopathic, without an actual known cause (Box 6.1). Predisposition for epileptic syndromes explains why of two people with similar injury, one may develop seizure, whereas the other one may not.

> ▶ **HINT:** Seizures are managed with anticonvulsants whether there is a known or unknown cause for the seizure.

**Box 6.1** Causes of Seizures

| |
|---|
| Anoxic injury |
| Traumatic brain injury |
| Subarachnoid hemorrhage |
| Intracranial tumors |
| Ischemic or hemorrhagic strokes |
| CNS infections (meningitis, encephalitis) |
| Neurosyphilis |
| Rocky Mountain spotted fever and Lyme disease |
| Electrolyte abnormalities: Hyponatremia, hypocalcemia, hypomagnesemia, hypoglycemia |
| Toxin or drug induced |
| Alcohol withdrawal |

CNS, central nervous system.

- **What is a precipitating factor for patients with epilepsy while being hospitalized to have a seizure?**
- **Sleep deprivation**

Sleep deprivation can lower the seizure threshold and precipitate a seizure (Box 6.2). Sleep deprivation is a common occurrence in hospitalized patients.

> ▶ **HINT:** Sleep deprivation is a technique that can be used in an epilepsy monitoring unit (EMU) to induce a seizure.

**Box 6.2** Situations That May Lower Seizure Thresholds

| |
|---|
| Sleep deprivation |
| Physiological or emotional stress |
| Fever |
| Flashing lights |
| Infection |
| Fatigue |
| Menses |
| Alcohol withdrawal or excessive alcohol intake |

## SYMPTOMS/ASSESSMENT

- **In what type of seizure is the initial neuronal discharge limited to a focal area of the brain?**
- **Partial seizure**

In partial seizures, the initial neuronal discharge is limited to one focal site or cerebral hemisphere. Clinical symptoms usually begin or remain on one side of the body.

> ▶ **HINT:** Partial seizures can progress to a generalized seizure.

■ *Patients with a partial seizure have no recollection of the seizure activity after the event. What type of partial seizure are they experiencing?*
■ **Complex partial seizure**

Partial seizures can be classified into simple partial and complex partial. In simple partial seizure, the person is aware of the seizure activity while the event is occurring and has recollection of the event following the seizure. Patients with complex partial seizures are not aware during the seizure and have no recollection after the seizure event.

> ▶ HINT: People with simple partial seizures can communicate and follow commands during the seizure.

■ *Simple partial seizures can present as hallucinatory events. What are these simple partial seizures called?*
■ **Somatosensory seizures**

Somatosensory seizure is a hallucinatory seizure and includes auditory, gustatory, olfactory, sensory, or visual hallucinations. These are labeled as simple partial seizures and usually originate from the parietal lobe.

> ▶ HINT: An aura is a somatosensory seizure that occurs immediately prior to a generalized seizure.

■ *What is the seizure type called when the motor activity begins with the face and moves down the body but remains on one side of the body?*
■ **Jacksonian march**

Jacksonian march is a simple partial seizure (Box 6.3). The seizure can spread from one muscle area to the next (primary motor cortex in frontal lobe) or from one skin area (sensory cortex in parietal lobe) to the next.

> ▶ HINT: Partial motor seizures usually remain on one side of the body.

**Box 6.3** Types of Simple Partial Seizures

| | |
|---|---|
| Focal motor seizure | Clonic twitching of contralateral muscles, extremities; the face is more often involved |
| Jacksonian march | The spread of seizure from one muscle area to the next remaining on the contralateral side |
| Fencer's position | Contralateral flexion and elevation of arm, contralateral turning of head and eyes, and tonic extension of the ipsilateral arm |
| Postural seizure | Drop seizures |
| Phonatory seizure | Vocalization or arrest of speech |
| Somatosensory seizures | Simple hallucinations |
| Psychic seizures | These include repetitive feelings of déjà vu, jamais vu, and a sense of doom |
| Affective seizures | Uncontrolled bursts of emotion such as anger, tears, laughter |
| Autonomic seizures | Symptoms of the sympathetic autonomic nervous system (tachycardia, dilated pupils, tachypnea, flushing) |

■ **A patient with complex partial seizures experiences repetitive movements. What is this called?**
■ **Automatism**

*Automatism* refers to repetitive movements, picking movements, lip smacking, eye fluttering, excessive swallowing, clapping, buttoning/ unbuttoning, fumbling, grabbing, kicking, hand rubbing, or tapping.

▶ **HINT:** Complex partial seizures can also be focal motor seizures.

■ **What is the classification of a seizure in which the epileptic focus is widespread across both hemispheres at one time?**
■ **Generalized seizure**

Generalized seizures do not have a single area of focus but occur across both hemispheres. They involve generalized activity bilaterally. Patients with generalized seizures lose consciousness and have no recall of the event.

▶ **HINT:** Partial seizures can progress into generalized seizures.

■ **An 8-year-old boy is having difficulty in school, and the teacher tells the parents, "He is frequently staring off into space or daydreaming." What type of seizure is this child most likely experiencing?**
■ **Absence seizure**

Absence seizures are classified as generalized seizures. This seizure presents with brief lapses of awareness and impairment of consciousness lasting 5 to 20 seconds. They can occur frequently throughout the day, and the child appears to be daydreaming. Blank facial expressions and rhythmic eye blinking or other type of automatisms can accompany these lapses. At the end of the seizure, the patient may return to the gesture, sentence, or other activities (retrograde amnesia) in which he was engaged prior to the seizure.

▶ **HINT:** The most common age of onset is 8 to 10 years of age. These used to be called *petite mal seizures*.

■ **What is the generalized seizure called in which the person has an abrupt loss of muscle tone, his or her knees buckle, and the person falls forward?**
■ **Atonic (drop) seizure**

Atonic seizure is a generalized seizure that presents with an abrupt loss of muscle tone, the buckle, and torso/head slumps forward. This results in abrupt falls. It only lasts seconds but can result in injuries.

▶ **HINT:** These have been called *drop seizures* and can cause brain injuries from the falls.

■ **A 3-year-old with a viral infection developed a fever of 104°F and presents in the ED with abnormal motor activity. What is the most likely diagnosis?**
■ **Febrile seizure**

Febrile seizures are more common in younger children and do not typically lead to epilepsy (Box 6.4). They may occur with rectal temperatures greater than 102°F.

> ▶ **HINT:** The child may be prone to experiencing febrile seizures but this does not increase the risk of epilepsy.

**Box 6.4** Types of Generalized Seizures

| |
|---|
| Tonic–clonic |
| Absence |
| Tonic |
| Myoclonic |
| Atonic |
| Febrile |

■ **What is the syndrome called in which a child presents with seizures refractory to anticonvulsants and frequently experiences intellectual impairment?**
■ **Lennox–Gastaut syndrome**

Lennox–Gastaut syndrome has three characteristics: (a) generalized seizures of more than one type, which are difficult to control with anticonvulsants; (b) slowness of intellectual growth and associated personality difficulties; and (c) a specific EEG abnormality called a *slow spike-and-wave pattern*, found when the child is awake, with generalized fast rhythms during sleep.

> ▶ **HINT:** This type of childhood epilepsy continues into adulthood even though the actual type of seizure may change.

■ **What is the type of seizure in which the EEG demonstrates seizure activity, but no activity is seen with the clinical findings?**
■ **Nonconvulsive status epilepticus (NCSE)**

In NCSE, seizure activity is seen on EEG without clinical findings associated with convulsive epileptic seizures. It is frequently underdiagnosed because of the lack of clinical signs of seizure. It may occur after a seizure has been "stopped" with antiepileptic drugs, but the patient continues to have an abnormal mental status. An acutely ill patient with mentally impaired status with or without subtle motor movements may be experiencing nonconvulsant seizures. The diagnosis is with EEG or continuous EEG (cEEG).

> ▶ **HINT:** Subtle motor movement includes rhythmic twitches or tonic eye deviation.

■ **What is the name for an event that clinically appears like a seizure, but there is no activity identified on EEG?**
■ **Nonepileptic event**

These nonepileptic events or seizures may resemble an epileptic seizure, but there are no changes on the EEG. This can be a psychogenic seizure related to the disorder known as *conversion syndrome*. Often the clinical activity resembles seizures but may have longer duration or maintain awareness with bilateral activity.

> ▶ **HINT:** Nonepileptic events used to be called *psychogenic seizures*. Remember, EEGs can be normal in patients with proven epilepsy.

# 6. SEIZURES

▪ *After a seizure, your patient experiences a paralysis of his right arm for a transient period. What is this called?*

▪ **Todd's paralysis**

Todd's paralysis occurs in the period of time immediately following the seizure. It appears as postictal paralysis or focal weakness and usually occurs after a simple partial seizure (Box 6.5). It indicates that seizure activity was from the contralateral hemisphere and is a reversible deficit that rarely lasts longer than 48 hours.

> ▶ **HINT:** Todd's paralysis may also present as blindness if the seizure is in the occipital lobe.

**Box 6.5** Seizure Stages

| | |
|---|---|
| Preictal | Occurs hours to days prior to the seizure; patient experiences general irritability or mood changes |
| Intraictal | Period of the actual seizure; activity depends upon the type of seizure and its location in the brain |
| Postictal | Period after the seizure, which can last hours to days; patient experiences sleepiness and overall muscle soreness |

▪ *A patient is admitted with a history of seizures. What would be important to ask the patient about his or her seizures?*

▪ **Type of seizures**

A good admission history is important when admitting a patient with a history of seizures or epilepsy. There are several aspects about the seizure that are beneficial for healthcare providers to know on admission. The type of seizure, the last time such a seizure was experienced, and what is known to induce the seizure are important questions to ask (Box 6.6).

> ▶ **HINT:** Knowing what has induced the seizure will assist the healthcare providers to prevent a seizure while the patient is hospitalized.

**Box 6.6** Nursing Admission Assessment for Patients With Histories of Seizures or Epilepsy

| |
|---|
| Past seizure description, frequency, pattern, precipitant |
| Current antiepileptic medications and drug levels |
| Compliance with antiepileptic medications |
| Date of last seizure |
| History of status epilepticus |
| Presence of vagal nerve stimulator |

## DIAGNOSTICS

▪ *Which diagnostic study is most commonly used to diagnose a partial or generalized seizure?*

▪ **EEG**

An EEG is the diagnostic study that is used to identify the occurrence of an epileptic seizure (Box 6.7). It has time-limited capabilities following a seizure and should be performed as soon as possible. An EEG may show slowing in the corresponding area of the epileptic activity.

▶ HINT: EEG can be a one-time diagnostic tool or used continuously for a period of time to identify the epileptic activity. The addition of video monitoring can correlate the clinical activity to the EEG findings.

**Box 6.7** Diagnostic Studies for Epilepsy

| | |
|---|---|
| EEG | Used to confirm focal and generalized seizures |
| AED levels | Uses the level of AED in blood to guide medication adjustments |
| Brain MRI | Identifies structural changes and causes of seizure |
| Intraictal PET and SPECT scans | PET and SPECT scans performed during a seizure are used to define specific foci of seizure |
| Wada test | Used to determine language dominance before surgery |

AED, antiepileptic drug; SPECT, single-photon emission computed tomography.

■ *What is the primary goal of an epilepsy-monitoring unit (EMU)?*
■ **To localize epileptic site**

An EMU is used to monitor patients with continuous video EEG in an attempt to localize the epileptic site. This is most commonly used with patients who have intractable seizures and may be candidates for surgical management.

▶ HINT: An EMU can also be used to differentiate an epileptic seizure from a nonepileptic activity.

■ *What is a primary intervention used in an EMU to induce the seizure activity?*
■ **Taper antiepileptic drugs (AEDs)**

Frequently, when a patient is admitted to an EMU, his or her current AEDs are tapered or discontinued to allow the patient to experience seizure while being monitored. Other interventions used to induce seizures include photic stimulation, exercise, hyperventilation, and sleep deprivation.

▶ HINT: EMU patients require close monitoring during the tapering of AEDs to prevent complications of their seizure.

■ *Which of the techniques used to trigger a seizure is most effective with absence seizures?*
■ **Hyperventilation**

Several techniques can be used to lower the threshold or induce a seizure to verify and document the seizure activity. Hyperventilation is one of the most effective triggers to induce absence seizures.

▶ HINT: Hyperventilation may trigger an absence seizure within seconds in an untreated patient.

## 6. SEIZURES

■ *Which antiepileptic drug level can be affected by enteral feeding if the drug is given orally?*
■ **Phenytoin**

Phenytoin drug levels are used to monitor potential efficacy or toxicity of the phenytoin. Enterally feeding a patient on oral phenytoin can cause binding of the drug and lower the phenytoin drug levels.

> ▶ **HINT:** Enteral feed should be held for a time before and after administration of the oral phenytoin to prevent drug binding.

## MEDICAL MANAGEMENT

■ *What is the primary goal of placing someone with a history of seizures on "seizure precautions"?*
■ **Injury prevention**

Seizure precautions are implemented to prevent injury to a patient with a history of seizures or who is currently being evaluated for seizure activity. Seizure precautions are interventions that can be put into place prior to the seizure to protect the patient if a seizure occurs (Box 6.8).

> ▶ **HINT:** Prevention of injury during a seizure involves interventions done during the seizure to prevent injury such as removing objects that can cause injury.

**Box 6.8** Seizure Precautions

| |
|---|
| Bed in the lowest position |
| Padded side rails |
| Pads on floor around bed or chair |
| Suctioning and oxygen equipment available at bedside |

■ *What is the nursing intervention that can be used to decrease the risk of aspiration during or after a seizure?*
■ **Turn the patient on his or her side**

Turning the patient onto his or her side allows the tongue to fall forward and lowers incidence of aspiration of secretions or emesis (Box 6.9).

> ▶ **HINT:** Never put anything in the mouth during a seizure. This can actually cause an airway obstruction.

**Box 6.9** Nursing Care During Seizure

| |
|---|
| If patient is standing, assist him or her to the ground. |
| Do not restrain the patient. |
| If patient is restrained, unrestrain him or her. |

*(continued)*

**Box 6.9** Nursing Care During Seizure *(continued)*

| |
|---|
| Remove furniture or objects that can hurt him or her. |
| Loosen restrictive clothing. |
| Place pillow or soft object under the patient's head. |
| Turn patient on side, if possible. |
| Administer oxygen if needed. |
| Maintain an open airway. |

- **When determining whether the seizure activity was initially a partial seizure progressing to a generalized seizure, what should be noted and documented by the nurse?**
- **Where the activity began**

Observing the seizure activity and noting where it began, the symmetry of movement, progression of the motor activity, and level of awareness can be useful in determining the type of seizure the patient experienced (Box 6.10).

> ▶ **HINT:** When observing the seizure, note the direction of the gaze. Eyes deviate to the contralateral side of the seizure.

**Box 6.10** Nursing Assessment and Observation During Seizure

| |
|---|
| Precipitating factors |
| Presence of an aura or warning |
| Type of seizure (motor, sensory, psychic) |
| Level of consciousness or awareness |
| Length of seizure |
| Direction of eye deviation |
| Note any other eye movement (blinking, eye fluttering, eye rolling, staring, twitching) |
| Note all abnormal motor activities (abnormal posturing, dystonia, head turning, twitching, back arching, bicycling movements, flailing, quivering, speech arrest) |
| Observe for autonomic signs (pupils, heart rate, heart rhythm, respiratory rate and character, GI disturbances, and color of skin—ashen, cyanotic, flushed, pale) |
| Ask about somatosensory disturbances |
| Note facial movements (automatisms, drooling, jerking, or twitching) |
| Note any vocalizations (cursing, barking, gagging, gibberish, groaning, grunting, howling, humming, laughing, moaning, screaming, snorting, talking, whistling) |
| Assess speech if present (neologism—use of novel words; paraphrasia—use of wrong words, repetitive words or sounds, word substitution) |
| Note emotional or behavioral changes |

GI, gastrointestinal.

- **After the seizure, what is the nurse's primary concern for the safety of the patient following a generalized seizure?**
- **Airway obstruction**

# 6. SEIZURES

The patient's level of conscious and ability to maintain an airway is the primary concern following a generalized seizure (Box 6.11). Stimulation of the patient to awaken them may be required to improve breathing. Oxygen saturation should be monitored in the acute period following a seizure.

> ▶ **HINT:** Loss of an airway or difficulty in breathing during or following a seizure is one cause of sudden death in epilepsy patients.

**Box 6.11** Care of Patient in Postictal Stage

| |
|---|
| Assess level of consciousness. |
| Assess airway and breathing. |
| Stimulate patient until responsive (call name, shake, clap loudly). |
| Assess strength for equality. |
| Monitor the length of postictal period. |
| Assess for injury. |
| Note any incontinence. |
| Assess for residual deficits and note duration (behavior changes, confusion, language disturbances, poor coordination, weakness, paralysis, sleep pattern disturbances). |
| Allow patient to rest. |
| Reassure the patient. |
| Reorient the patient to his or her surroundings and recent events. |

■ *Following a seizure, the patient is noted to have developed confusion, irritation, and hallucinations that persist for several days. What is this complication of a seizure called?*

■ **Postictal psychosis**

Postictal aggression or psychosis is a potential complication following a seizure. It consists of symptoms that vary from mood disturbance; confusion; visual, auditory, tactile and olfactory hallucinations; and paranoid ideation with or without delirium to more severe and serious disturbances in behavior, including physical aggression and self-harm.

> ▶ **HINT:** Postictal psychosis can manifest as an episode of psychosis occurring within a week of a seizure or more commonly following a cluster of generalized tonic–clonic seizures.

■ *What is a common side effect found in most AEDs?*

■ **Sedation**

One of the most common side effects of AEDs is sleepiness and drowsiness. AEDs are used to control the frequency of seizures but can adversely affect the patient's quality of life due to the side effects (Box 6.12).

> ▶ **HINT:** Be familiar with the unique side effects of more common AEDs, such as gum hyperplasia in patients taking phenytoin.

**Box 6.12** Common Side Effects of Antiepileptic Drugs

| Sedation |
| Lethargy |
| Dizziness |
| Ataxia |
| Nystagmus |
| Diplopia |

- **When a patient experiences a prolonged seizure, how long before it is considered SE and requires medication to stop the seizure?**
- **5 minutes**

SE is typically defined as a seizure continuing for longer than 5 minutes. A seizure lasting fewer than 5 minutes may not require antiepileptic medications to stop the seizure because it stops on its own in a short period of time.

> ▶ HINT: AEDs used to stop a seizure have the side effect of sedation. A combination of the postictal state and sedative administration can cause respiratory depression.

- **What is the first-line AED of choice during a seizure?**
- **Lorazepam (Ativan)**

Lorazepam (Ativan) is the first-line drug used to manage a seizure or during status epilepticus. It is administered intravenously. If the seizure persists, it can be repeated or a different AED may be used. Benzodiazepines are not used for long-term management and prevention of seizures because of their addicting properties and sedative effects.

> ▶ HINT: The side effects of lorazepam include hypotension, respiratory depression, and sedation.

## SURGICAL MANAGEMENT

- **What is the most common surgical procedure for epilepsy?**
- **Temporal lobectomy**

A temporal lobectomy is the removal of part or all of the anterior temporal lobe. It is indicated for partial seizures that originate in the temporal lobe and are refractory to medical management. Potential complications include visual field cuts and cranial nerve III palsy.

> ▶ HINT: The temporal lobe is the most common foci for partial seizures to originate.

- **What is a surgical procedure that can be used to manage generalized seizures without an identifiable epileptic focus?**
- **Corpus callosotomy**

Most surgical procedures for epilepsy are for partial seizures because an epileptic focus can be identified and removed. In generalized seizures, there is no identifiable focal area so surgical options are more limited. A corpus callosotomy is a surgical procedure that has been used in generalized seizures. It cuts a portion of the corpus collosum, preventing the epileptic activity from crossing to both hemispheres. This maintains the seizure activity on one side of the body, limiting the severity of seizure.

▶ **HINT:** Patients may still have seizure activity and will continue taking their antiepileptic drugs.

■ *What is the "pacemaker-like" device that can be used to control seizures in patients with epilepsy?*
■ **Vagal nerve stimulator (VNS)**

VNSs are implantable pacemaker-like devices with a wire that wraps around the vagal nerve. The generator box is implanted into the chest wall and this emits an electrical stimulus used to decrease the number of seizures in patients refractory to AEDs.

▶ **HINT:** Patients with VNS will have a "wand" that can be placed over the generator box during a seizure to stop the seizure.

## COMPLICATIONS

■ *What is a risk for patients with known history of seizures that should be identified on admission?*
■ **Fall risk**

Falls are a significant risk for most seizures. A patient with a known history of seizures or who is admitted with a current diagnosis of seizure should be placed on a high fall-risk status.

▶ **HINT:** The patient should be placed on fall risk with seizure precautions.

■ *Following a prolonged tonic–clonic seizure, the patient's urine appears to be cola- or tea-colored. What is the most likely cause of the urine color?*
■ **Rhabdomyolysis**

Muscle injury and breakdown occurs following a prolonged tonic–clonic seizure, releasing myoglobin into the blood (myoglobinemia). The myoglobin is filtered by the glomerulonephrons, causing damage to the kidney and acute renal failure. Abnormal lab work includes elevated creatine phosphokinase (CPK) and myoglobin levels.

▶ **HINT:** Rhabdomyolysis is the acute kidney injury that is characterized by the cola- or tea-colored urine.

■ *What does SUDEP refer to in epilepsy patients?*
■ **Sudden unexplained death in epilepsy**

SUDEP is defined as a sudden, unexpected, nontraumatic, nondrowning death in an individual with epilepsy, witnessed or unwitnessed, in which postmortem examination does not reveal an anatomic or toxicologic cause for death (Box 6.13). The risk of SUDEP increases in patients who have a greater number of uncontrolled seizures (Box 6.14).

▶ **HINT:** The risk of SUDEP also increases with nocturnal and unwitnessed seizures.

**Box 6.13** Potential Causes of SUDEP

| |
|---|
| Bradyarrhythmias or lack of sympathetic tone |
| Ventricular arrhythmias |
| Airway obstruction and asphyxiation |
| Central apnea |
| Neurogenic pulmonary edema |

SUDEP, sudden unexplained death in epilepsy.

**Box 6.14** Risks for SUDEP

| |
|---|
| Tonic–clonic seizures |
| Increased frequency uncontrolled seizures |
| Nocturnal seizures |
| Developmental delayed |
| Use of alcohol or recreational drugs |
| Unwitnessed seizure |
| Noncompliance with AEDs |

AEDs, antiepileptic drugs; SUDEP, sudden unexplained death in epilepsy.

■ *The increased circulating catecholamines that occur with a seizure can result in what potentially life-threatening complication?*
■ **Arrhythmia**

During a seizure, catecholamines can elevate and contribute to the development of arrhythmias and heart rate and blood pressure (BP) changes (Box 6.15). The arrhythmias can be lethal ventricular rhythms and are a potential cause of SUDEP.

▶ **HINT:** Patients with seizures should have cardiac monitoring to identify the presence of lethal arrhythmias.

**Box 6.15** Acute Complications of Seizure

| |
|---|
| Falls |
| Skeletal injuries |
| Traumatic brain injury |
| Sudden death |
| Aspiration pneumonia |
| Fever |
| Cardiac arrhythmias (life-threatening) |
| Metabolic changes (metabolic acidosis, hyperkalemia, hyperglycemia, leukocytosis) |
| Rhabdomyolysis (increased CPK, increased myoglobin, acute kidney injury) |
| Drowning |

CPK, creatine phosphokinase.

## What is a potential long-term complication of uncontrolled epilepsy?
## Cognitive changes

Long-term complications increase with the frequency of seizures and uncontrolled epilepsy. Acute hippocampal swelling identified on MRI can be followed by atrophy and mesial temporal sclerosis. The loss of cerebral volume and pyramidal cell loss can lead to generalized cognitive changes.

> ▶ **HINT:** Cognitive changes with epilepsy can affect the younger pediatric patient, and uncontrolled seizures can lead to a lower IQ.

# Sample Exam Questions

1. Which of the following disorders is most commonly associated with Lennox–Gastaut syndrome?
   A. Deafness and visual difficulties
   B. Behavioral and personality disorders
   C. Ataxia
   D. Gastrointestinal disorders

2. Which of the following presentations could indicate nonconvulsive status epilepticus?
   A. Presentation of headaches
   B. Repetitive blinking in an unresponsive patient
   C. Repetitive jerking of an upper extremity
   D. No cerebral blood flow

3. Following presentation with status epilepticus, the patient is noted to have tea-colored urine. Which of the following is the most likely cause?
   A. Glomerulonephritis
   B. Nephritis
   C. Rhabdomyolysis
   D. Contrast-induced nephropathy

4. There are known long-term complications of epilepsy. Which of the following pathological changes contributes to cognitive changes?
   A. Herniation of cerebellum
   B. Ischemic infarction of occipital lobe
   C. Mesial temporal sclerosis
   D. Atrophy of frontal lobe

5. A patient with epilepsy is being evaluated for surgical intervention. A Wada test is ordered. What does the Wada test evaluate?
   A. Motor pathway
   B. Visual acuity
   C. Hemisphere of cerebral dominance for language
   D. Corticospinal tract

6. Which of the following patients would be the best candidate for placement of a vagal nerve stimulator?
   A. Patient who has experienced a fall with seizure
   B. Nonepileptic seizure
   C. Person who experiences longer postictal periods
   D. Patient with drug-resistant seizures

7. A patient with a vagal nerve stimulator (VNS) is admitted into the hospital. He has a magnet "wand" at the bedside. Which of the following statements is the most correct regarding the use of the magnet with the VNS?

   A. The magnet is only used to turn the VNS off when the patient needs an MRI.
   B. Placement over the generator will trigger burst stimulation and is used during a seizure.
   C. Patient's heart rate will increase when placing the magnet over the generator.
   D. Only patients with a history of bradycardia require the use of the magnet.

8. Which of the following injuries is NOT commonly found following seizure or status epilepticus?

   A. Neurogenic pulmonary edema
   B. Dislocation humeral head of shoulder
   C. Rib fractures
   D. Aspiration pneumonia

9. When taking the admission history of a patient with known epilepsy, which of the following would be the most beneficial information to get for the safety of the patient?

   A. Has he or she been diagnosed with any psychiatric issues?
   B. Is there a familial history of epilepsy?
   C. Does the patient have a postictal period?
   D. What are the type and severity of the seizures?

## BIBLIOGRAPHY

Berg, A. T., Berkovic, S. F., Brodie, M. J., Buchhalter, J., Cross, J. H., van Emde Boas, W., … Scheffer, I. E. (2010). Revised terminology and concepts for organization of seizures and epilepsies: Report of the ILAE Commission on Classification and Terminology, 2005-2009. *Epilepsia, 51*(4), 676–685. doi:10.1111/j.1528-1167.2010.02522.x

Birbeck, G. L., French, J. A., Perucca, E., Simpson, D. M., Fraimow, H., George, J. M., … Levy, R. H. (2012). Antiepileptic drug selection for people with HIV/AIDS: Evidence-based guidelines from the ILAE and AAN. *Epilepsia, 53*(1), 207–214. doi:10.1111/j.1528-1167.2011.03335.x

Brophy, G. M., Bell, R., Claassen, J., Alldredge, B., Bleck, T. P., Glauser, T., … Neurocritical Care Society Status Epilepticus Guideline Writing Committee. (2012). Guidelines for the evaluation and management of status epilepticus. *Neurocritical Care, 17*(1), 3–23. doi:10.1007/s12028-012-9695-z

Buelow, J., Miller, W., & Fishman, J. (2018). Development of an epilepsy nursing communication tool: Improving the quality of interactions between nurses and patients with seizures. *Journal of Neuroscience Nursing, 50*(2), 74–80. doi:10.1097/JNN.0000000000000353

Englot, D. J., Chang, E. F., & Auguste, K. I. (2011). Vagus nerve stimulation for epilepsy: A meta-analysis of efficacy and predictors of response. *Journal of Neurosurgery, 115*(6), 1248–1255. doi:10.3171/2011.7.JNS11977

Hirtz, D., Berg, A., Bettis, D., Camfield, C., Camfield, P., Crumrine, P., … Practice Committee of the Child Neurology Society. (2003). Practice parameter: Treatment of the child with a first unprovoked seizure: Report of the Quality Standards Subcommittee of the American Academy of Neurology and the Practice Committee of the Child Neurology Society. *Neurology, 60*(2), 166–175. doi:10.1212/01.wnl.0000033622.27961.b6

Krumholz, A., Wiebe, S., Gronseth, G. S., Gloss, D. S., Sanchez, A. M., Kabir, A. A., … French, J. A. (2015). Evidence-based guideline: Management of an unprovoked first seizure in adults. Report of the Guideline Development Subcommittee of the American Academy of Neurology and the American Epilepsy Society. *Neurology, 84*, 1705–1713. doi:10.1212/WNL.0000000000001487

Kwan, P., Arzimanoglou, A., Berg, A. T., Brodie, M. J., Allen Hauser, W., Mathern, G., ... French, J. (2010). Definition of drug resistant epilepsy: Consensus proposal by the ad hoc Task Force of the ILAE Commission on Therapeutic Strategies. *Epilepsia, 51*(6), 1069–1077. doi:10.1111/j.1528-1167.2009.02397.x

Ma, L., & McCauley, S. (2017). Management of pediatric febrile seizures. *Journal for Nurse Practitioners, 14*(2), 74–80. doi:10.1016/j.nurpra.2017.09.021

Ng, Y. T., Conry, J. A., Drummond, R., Stolle, J., & Weinberg, M. A. (2011). Randomized, phase III study results of clobazam in Lennox-Gastaut syndrome. *Neurology, 77*(15), 1473–1481. doi:10.1212/WNL.0b013e318232de76

Shorvon, S., & Tomson, T. (2011). Sudden unexpected death in epilepsy. *Lancet, 378*(9808), 2028–2038. doi:10.1016/S0140-6736(11)60176-1

Smith, G., Wagner, J., & Edwards, J. (2015). Epilepsy update part 2: Nursing care and evidence based treatment. *American Journal of Nursing, 115*(6), 34–44. doi:10.1097/01.NAJ.0000466314.46508.00

Steering Committee on Quality Improvement and Management, Subcommittee on Febrile Seizures American Academy of Pediatrics. (2008). Febrile seizures: Clinical practice guideline for the long-term management of the child with simple febrile seizures. *Pediatrics, 121*(6), 1281–1286. doi:10.1542/Peds.2008-0939

# 7

# Pediatric and Developmental Disorders

## INTRODUCTION

■ *Where is the Chiari malformation located in the brain?*
■ **Cerebellum**

A Chiari malformation is a developmental anomaly at the base of the skull, which results in downward displacement of the cerebellum and brainstem structures into the spinal canal.

▶ **HINT:** It is the herniation of the cerebellum through the foramen magnum.

■ *What structures are displaced into the spinal canal in a type I Chiari malformation?*
■ **Cerebellar tonsils**

Type I Chiari malformation is a downward displacement of cerebellar tonsils by greater than 4 mm (Box 7.1). The malformation typically occurs during fetal development.

▶ **HINT:** Chiari malformations type I and type II are typically found in adolescents and young adults. Type III and IV are recognized at birth.

**Box 7.1** Types of Chiari Malformations

| Type | Degree of Injury |
| --- | --- |
| I | Downward displacement of cerebellar tonsils |
| II | Downward displacement of cerebellar tonsils, vermis, fourth ventricles, choroid plexus, and medulla |
| III | Associated with a herniation of fluid sac (spinal bifida in the neck region) in which the lower structures of the brainstem are herniated into this sac |
| IV | Refers to a hypoplasia (incomplete development) or aplasia (lack of development) of a portion of the cerebellum (not an actual herniation) |

■ *What is the term used to describe fluid accumulation within the central portion of the cord?*
■ **Syringomyelia**

During the downward displacement of the cerebellar and brainstem structures, pressure increases and "pushes" cerebrospinal fluid (CSF) into the central portion of the cord.

▶ **HINT:** Terminology: A *hydromyelia* is the widening of the central portion of cord.

■ *What is the motor disorder that appears in infancy and early childhood that can permanently affect motor movement and coordination?*
■ **Cerebral palsy (CP)**

CP is a neurological disorder that permanently affects motor movement and coordination. CP has multiple etiologies and abnormal motor presentations.

▶ **HINT:** CP causes a permanent, nonprogressive abnormal motor movement.

■ *When can an injury occur to the brain resulting in abnormal motor pathways and cerebral palsy (before, during, or after birth)?*
■ **All are correct answers**

Damage is the result of an injury to fetal/infant brain either during the brain development before birth, during delivery of the infant, or after birth within the first several years of life.

▶ **HINT:** CP can result due to damage of the motor cortex before it is completely developed.

■ *What is the childhood disorder that is a result of incomplete closure of the neural tube during development?*
■ **Spina bifida (SB)**

SB is a result of the incomplete closure of the neural tube that develops into the spinal cord. This occurs during fetal development. There are varying degrees of severity with SB.

▶ **HINT:** SB is the most common birth defect in the United States and means *split spine*.

■ *Which type of SB is the least severe?*
■ **SB occulta**

SB occulta is the mildest form of SB. SB occulta presents as a small gap or separation in one or more vertebral bodies in the spine. It does not involve any external exposure of the spine or nerve roots.

▶ **HINT:** It may not be diagnosed unless identified with an MRI.

■ *What is the name of the form of spina bifida in which the meninges and spinal cord protrude through an opening of the back at birth?*
■ **Myelomeningocele**

A myelomeningocele is the most severe form of spina bifida (Box 7.2). It involves an opening of the spinal column with protrusion of the meningeal sac containing the spinal cord and spinal nerve roots.

▶ **HINT:** In some cases of myelomeningoceles, the meningeal sac is covered with skin.

**Box 7.2** Forms of Spina Bifida

| Spina bifida occulta | Abnormal separation or gap between two or more vertebral bodies in the spine |
| Meningocele | Opening of the vertebral laminae with the protrusion of the meningeal sac without spinal cord or nerve roots |
| Myelomeningocele | Opening of the vertebral laminae with the protrusion of a meningeal sac with spinal cord and spinal nerve roots present within the sac |

## PATHOPHYSIOLOGY

■ *What is the tissue that hangs off the inferior surface of the cerebellum?*
■ **Tonsils**

Cerebellar tonsils consist of two pieces of tissue that hang off the inferior surface of the cerebellum. Type I Chiari malformations involve the herniation of the cerebellar tonsils.

▶ **HINT:** The vermis is a bundle of tissue connecting the two halves of the cerebellum and is a part of the structures that herniate in type II Chiari malformations.

■ *What is considered to be the underlying pathologic change that allows for the herniation of the cerebellum?*
■ **Small posterior fossa**

The posterior fossa, which houses the cerebellum, is too small for the cerebellum. During brain growth, it causes the brain to be pushed down through the foramen magnum.

▶ **HINT:** Genetics may play a role in the development of Chiari malformations.

■ *What is the physiological cause of the development of hydrocephalus in a type II Chiari malformation?*
■ **Herniation of the fourth ventricle**

The displacement or herniation of the fourth ventricle results in the obstruction of CSF flow. This causes a noncommunicating hydrocephalus. Both Chiari I and II malformations can develop hydrocephalus. Tonsillar herniation in Chiari malformation leads to obstruction of outflow of CSF.

▶ **HINT:** The hydrocephalus caused by a blockage is called *noncommunicating hydrocephalus*.

■ *What causes the development of type III Chiari malformation?*
■ **Bony defect**

The Chiari malformation type III is characterized by a portion of the cerebellum and brainstem pushing out through an occipital encephalocele (abnormal opening in the base of the skull). It is a bony defect similar to spina bifida but located in the cervical region. It is very rare and has a high, early mortality rate.

▶ **HINT:** Chiari malformation type III and IV are identified at birth.

■ **What is the most common etiology of CP that is caused during the birthing process?**
■ **Hypoxic/anoxic injury**

A complication of delivery can be hypoxic or anoxic injuries. This injury is one of the etiologies of CP. Ischemia and/or anoxia can also occur during the pregnancy. There are several causes or underlying etiologies that can result in CP (Box 7.3).

▶ **HINT:** The causes of CP can be divided into injuries that occur during the pregnancy, during delivery, and after birth.

**Box 7.3** Etiology of Cerebral Palsy

| During Pregnancy | During Delivery | After Delivery (First Few Years of Life) |
| --- | --- | --- |
| Fetal stroke | Hypoxia | Bacterial or viral meningitis |
|   Maternal hypertension | | |
|   Blood clotting abnormalities | | |
| Maternal infections | Rh incompatibility | Brain trauma |
| Maternal exposure to toxic substances | Fetal stroke | |
| Methylmercury | | |
| Maternal seizure | | |
| Maternal hyperthyroidism | | |
| Maternal trauma | | |

■ **What is considered a high-risk delivery for hypoxic or anoxic injury?**
■ **Breech presentation**

There are some "red flags" when evaluating a newborn's risk for development of CP (Box 7.4). This includes situations that increase the newborn's risk for hypoxia, including breech position.

▶ **HINT:** Asphyxiation during complicated delivery is a significant cause of hypoxic/anoxic-induced CP.

**Box 7.4** Red Flags for Newborns at Risk for Developing Cerebral Palsy

| |
| --- |
| Breech position |
| Complicated labor and/or delivery |
| Small for gestational age |
| Premature or low birth weight |
| Multiple births (twins, triplets, etc.) |
| Low Apgar score |

*(continued)*

**Box 7.4** Red Flags for Newborns at Risk for Developing Cerebral Palsy *(continued)*

| |
|---|
| Pathological jaundice |
| Seizures |

- **Cerebral palsy caused by damage to the white matter of the fetus's brain resulting in tiny holes is called?**
- **Periventricular leukomalacia (PVL)**

PVL is a pathological change in the white matter of the brain and is described as damage that looks like tiny holes in the brain. The white matter of the brain is responsible for transmitting motor impulses, and the holes cause gaps in this transmission. PVL can be caused by maternal or fetal exposure to infections or trauma (Box 7.5).

> ▶ **HINT:** Fetal brains are susceptible to motor cortex injury during the first 20 weeks of pregnancy.

**Box 7.5** Maternal Infections That Increase Risk of Cerebral Palsy

| |
|---|
| Rubella (German measles) |
| Cytomegalovirus |
| Herpes simplex |

- **When does the neural tube close during the development of the fetus?**
- **28th day after conception**

The neural tube closes early in the pregnancy and fetal development. As the neural tube is closing, a section does not close appropriately or reopens later during fetal development, resulting in the incomplete closure of the spinal cord or herniation of the spinal nerves and cord. Later in development, the top of the neural tube forms the brain and the remainder of the tube becomes the fetus' spinal cord (Box 7.6).

> ▶ **HINT:** Frequently, the woman may not even be aware of the pregnancy during the first 28 days after conception. Exposure to certain elements, such as high temperatures, during this time can cause spina bifida.

**Box 7.6** Neural Tube Malformations

| |
|---|
| Craniorachischisis |
| Iniencephaly |
| Anencephaly |
| Encephalocele |
| Spina bifida |

- **What dietary deficiency is most often associated with SB?**
- **Folic acid deficiency**

Folic acid is an important vitamin in the development of the fetus. Folic acid (vitamin B9) deficiency is a primary cause of SB and other neural tube defects (Box 7.7).

> ▶ **HINT:** The anticonvulsant medication valproic acid (Depakene) can cause SB when taken during pregnancy because it interferes with the ability to utilize folic acid.

**Box 7.7** Risks for Development of Spina Bifida

| |
|---|
| Genetics |
| Folic acid deficiency |
| Certain medications |
| Maternal diabetes |
| Obesity |
| Exposure to high body temperatures |

## SYMPTOMS/ASSESSMENT

- *What is the main determinant of the severity of the symptoms caused by Chiari malformations type I and type II?*
- **Degree of displacement**

The degree of displacement of the cerebellum and brainstem structures into the spine determines the severity of symptoms. Displacement of the cerebellar tonsils only is classified as a Chiari type I. The displacement of more structures, such as the vermis, fourth ventricle, and medulla, is more severe and is called a *Chiari type II malformation*.

> ▶ **HINT:** Symptoms progressively worsen with a greater degree of displacement and the development of a syringomyelia.

- *What are the primary symptoms of pediatric patients presenting with a Chiari malformation?*
- **Nystagmus and spastic paralysis**

Infants and young children can present with Chiari malformations. Common symptoms in this age group are nystagmus, spastic paralysis, bulbar dysfunctions (dysphagia, dysarthria), and apnea (predominantly in infants; Box 7.8).

> ▶ **HINT:** Signs and symptoms may vary among people even within the same age groups.

**Box 7.8** Symptoms of Chiari Malformations Based on Age Group

| Infants | Children | Adolescents |
|---|---|---|
| Apnea | Nystagmus | Progressive spasticity |
| Decreased gag reflex | Spastic paralysis | Pain and temperature losses in upper extremities |
| Nystagmus | Bulbar dysfunction | |
| Spasticity | | |

- *What is the most common presenting symptom in adults with Chiari malformations?*
- **Headache**

The most common symptom in adults is headache. The headache is frequently described as dull, chronic pain located at the base of the skull (Box 7.9).

▶ **HINT:** Headaches commonly radiate into the neck and shoulders and worsen with coughing or sneezing.

**Box 7.9** Common Characteristics of Headache in Adults With Chiari Malformations

| |
|---|
| Located at the base of the skull/upper neck |
| Dull and chronic |
| Paroxysmal, severe headache with Valsalva maneuver |
| Postural headaches |

- *What spinal deformity is commonly associated with Chiari malformations in adolescents and young adults?*
- **Scoliosis**

Progressive scoliosis is commonly associated with Chiari malformations and can be corrected with decompressive surgery in the majority of patients (Box 7.10).

▶ **HINT:** Anomalies of the base of the skull occur in 30% to 50% of patients with Chiari malformations.

**Box 7.10** Spine Deformities Associated With Chiari Malformations

| |
|---|
| Basilar impressions |
| Atlantooccipital fusion |
| Atlantoaxial assimilation |
| Cervical spina bifida occulta |

- *A patient with a Chiari malformation presents with disequilibrium and a history of falling. Which of the following structures is most likely involved?*
- **Cerebellum**

The downward displacement of cerebellar structures occurs in Chiari malformations type I and type II. Cerebellar symptoms include ataxia, disequilibrium, uncoordination, and low muscle tone.

▶ **HINT:** Symptoms of cerebellar injury make the patient appear to be drunk.

- *What is a bulbar symptom that may be found in Chiari malformations?*
- **Dysphagia, dysarthria, or dysphonia**

Bulbar symptoms are a result of injury to cranial nerves (CNs) IX, X, XI, and XII, located in the brainstem. In patients with Chiari malformations, herniation of brainstem structures causes compression to the CNs located in the medulla (IX, X, XI, XII).

▶ **HINT:** Know the CN origin. Think about dividing the 12 CNs into three groups of four CNs. CNs I through IV originate in the cerebral cortex and midbrain. CNs V to VIII originate in the pons and CNs IV to VII originate in the medulla.

**Box 7.11** Symptoms of Chiari Malformations

| Cerebellar Symptoms | Base of Skull Anomalies | Brainstem Compression/ CN Deficits |
|---|---|---|
| Balance | Scoliosis | Drop attacks |
| Equilibrium | Atlantooccipital fusion | Headaches |
| Coordination | Atlantoaxial fusion | Nystagmus |
| Low muscle tone | Cervical spina bifida | Diplopia |
| Tremor | | Dysarthria |
| | | Dysphagia |
| | | Sensorimotor deficits |
| | | Transient visual losses |

CN, cranial nerve.

- **What is the most common symptom of CP?**
- **Abnormal motor movement**

CP can present with a wide variety of abnormal movement and severity (Box 7.12). For example, the movement can be a spasticity or ataxic gait. The symptoms and severity vary between children and adults with CP.

▶ **HINT:** CP may also involve one limb or all four limbs.

**Box 7.12** Common Motor Abnormalities of Cerebral Palsy

| |
|---|
| Ataxia |
| Spasticity |
| Dragging a foot or leg with ambulation |
| "Scissoring" gait, crossing one leg over the other |
| Walking on toes in crouched position |
| Difficulties with precise movements |
| Athetoid movement (writhing movement) |
| Tremors |
| Muscle weakness or flaccidity |
| One side of body is favored |

- **What is the most common motor presentation of an infant under the age of 2 years with CP?**
- **Flaccidity**

Infants under the age of 1 year with CP tend to initially present with motor weakness (hypotonia) or flaccidity. In some cases, an early period of hypotonia will progress to hypertonia after the first 2 to 3 months of life.

▶ **HINT:** Not meeting the developmental milestones for motor development in the early ages is a sign of CP (Box 7.13).

**Box 7.13** Developmental Milestones for Motor Development in the Early Ages

| |
|---|
| Rolling over |
| Sitting up |
| Crawling |
| Smiling |
| Pulling oneself up |
| Walking |

- **CP can be associated with other medical conditions. Name one of the most common presentations of CP other than motor disturbances?**
- **Sensory abnormalities**

CP is primarily a motor disorder, but sensory abnormalities can occur as well. The sensory component commonly presents as hyperalgesia (increased pain sensation) or allodynia (pain sensation with an innocuous stimuli).

> ▶ **HINT:** The other conditions listed in Box 7.14 are not found consistently in all patients with CP and can vary widely.

**Box 7.14** Medical Conditions Associated With Cerebral Palsy

| |
|---|
| Mental impairment |
| Seizures |
| Impaired vision |
| Impaired hearing |
| Abnormal physical sensations or perception |
| Sleep abnormalities |
| Excessive drooling |
| Dysphagia |
| Dysarthria to nonverbal |

- **What is the primary external sign of a child with spina bifida occulta?**
- **Dimple with tuft of hair**

An abnormal tuft of hair, a collection of fat, a small dimple, or a birthmark on the child's skin in the area of the spinal defect may be the only visible indication of the condition.

> ▶ **HINT:** An MRI may identify the gap between the vertebral bodies as a sign of spina bifida occulta.

- **What is the clinical sign of hydrocephalus in neonates with myelomeningocele and Chiari malformations?**
- **Increase head circumference**

Head circumference measurements can be used in neonates to determine the presence or increase in hydrocephalus. This is due to the skull not being closed so it expands as CSF increases.

> **HINT:** After the closure of fontanels, the head circumference will not increase with hydrocephalus.

## DIAGNOSIS

- **What is the most accurate diagnostic radiographic examination used to diagnose Chiari malformations?**
- **MRI**

An MRI is used to identify small posterior fossa, herniated tonsils, the cerebellum, fourth ventricle, and brainstem structures.

> **HINT:** Both brain and cervical spine scans should be obtained.

- **What should be used during scanning that will identify a syrinx?**
- **Contrast**

Contrast can be used to assist with diagnosing abnormal pathology. It is especially useful in identifying a syrinx and obstruction of CSF.

> **HINT:** Skull and cervical spine radiographs have very little diagnostic value in Chiari malformations.

- **What is the issue during the first year of life that can result in a clinical diagnosis of CP?**
- **Not reaching developmental milestones**

Typically, the diagnosis of CP is made within the first 2 to 3 years of life. The initial issue in most cases is the lack of motor skill development such as rolling over, crawling, ability to pulling themselves up, and walking. This is usually a clinical diagnosis but requires other causes be ruled out.

> **HINT:** If symptoms are mild, the diagnosis may be delayed.

- **Which of the pathophysiological changes in CP can be seen on MRI?**
- **PVL**

An MRI is superior to CT scan for identifying changes in the motor cortex, which assists with the clinical diagnosis of CP. Not all children with CP will have identifiable changes on the MRI. The physiology of PVL yields the greatest changes, which are identified by MRI.

> **HINT:** A negative MRI does not rule out CP. CP is predominantly a clinical diagnosis.

- **What is the primary maternal blood test used to screen for spina bifida during pregnancy?**
- **Maternal serum alpha-fetoprotein (AFP) test**

AFP is a protein that is produced by the fetus. It is normal for a small amount of AFP to cross the placenta and enter the maternal bloodstream. But abnormally high levels of AFP may indicate the fetus has a neural tube defect. False positives can occur with this test.

> ▶ HINT: Twins or multiple gestations will produce a higher level of AFP.

- *What two tests can be used to verify the maternal serum alpha-fetoprotein (MSAFP) test for spina bifida?*
- Human chorionic gonadotropin (HCG) and estriol

HCG and estriol are two maternal blood tests that can be used to verify the accuracy of the MSAFP test. These are hormones produced in the placenta. Amniocentesis may also be used to identify higher-than-normal levels of alpha fetoprotein levels.

> ▶ HINT: MSAFP is a screening test that can have false positives.

- *Which diagnostic exam can be used to identify the presence and severity of SB in the fetus?*
- Ultrasound

Ultrasonography is used to determine the gestational age of the fetus. An advanced ultrasound study can visualize the open spine and assist with determining the severity of the SB.

> ▶ HINT: Ultrasound for gestational age can improve the accuracy of the MSAFP test.

## MEDICAL MANAGEMENT

- *A Chiari malformation is found incidentally on MRI. The patient is asymptomatic. What is the recommended plan of care?*
- Observation

Patients with few or no symptoms may be observed and followed regularly using MRI to monitor the progression of the condition.

> ▶ HINT: Minimal herniation in Chiari I malformations may not be symptomatic but can progress to type II and become symptomatic.

- *Which class of medications is commonly prescribed to people with CP?*
- Antispasmodics

Antispasmodics are used to correct stiff, contracted, or overactive muscle (Box 7.15). Spasticity can interfere with activities of daily living and quality of life. Botulinum toxin (BOTOX, BT-A) injected locally has become a standard treatment for overactive muscles with spastic movement disorders. It relaxes contracted muscles by keeping nerve cells from overactivating muscle. Baclofen can be administered continuously into the intrathecal space by pump.

> ▶ HINT: Anticholinergics can be used to decrease the amount of saliva and drooling.

**Box 7.15** Examples of Antispasmodics

| |
|---|
| Benzodiazepines |
| Baclofen (Lioresal) |
| Tizanidine (Zanaflex) |

- **What is the primary goal of the nurse when caring for a neonate with a myelomeningocele prior to surgery?**
- **Maintain sterility**

The first and primary goal of the nurse caring for a neonate with a myelomeningocele is to maintain sterility of the defect (Box 7.16). This is an open area for direct transmission of pathogens to enter the central nervous system (CNS).

▶ **HINT:** Leaking of CSF is associated with an increased risk of CNS infection.

**Box 7.16** Nursing Care for Neonates With Open Spines

| Nursing Goal | Physiology | Intervention |
|---|---|---|
| Prevention of CNS infection | Open track for pathogens to CNS | Use of sterile technique when caring for the defect |
| Prevention of hypothermia | Open defect causes increased heat loss | Active management to maintain heat (e.g., plastic wrap) |
| Maintain infant in prone position | Supine position causes damage to the exposed neural tissue | Nursing care of the patient in the prone position to avoid mechanical injury |
| Protect neural tissue to prevent further injury | Exposed neural tissue is potentially salvageable | Cover the defect in a saline-moistened dressing |
| Decrease risk of developing latex sensitivities | Altered neuroimmune interactions and frequent exposure to latex can cause latex sensitivities | Avoid use of latex when caring for the neonate |

CNS, central nervous system.

## SURGICAL MANAGEMENT

- **What is the surgical management for a symptomatic Chiari malformation?**
- **Decompressive surgery**

Posterior fossa decompression is the surgery of choice to prevent further herniation of brainstem structures through the foramen magnum. It creates more room in the base of the skull to restore CSF flow between the brain and spinal cord.

▶ **HINT:** A laminectomy may be performed with the craniectomy to provide room for the cerebellum.

- **What is the recommended surgery in cases of severe spasticity with cerebral palsy?**
- **Selective dorsal rhizotomy (SDR)**

This surgical procedure is recommended only in cases of severe spasticity when all of the more conservative treatments have failed to reduce spasticity or chronic pain.

This procedure selectively severs overactivated nerves at the spinal nerve roots.

> ▶ **HINT:** This procedure may need to be repeated after the nerves begin to regenerate.

- **What is the surgical management of the hydrocephalus associated with Chiari II malformations and myelomeningocele?**
- **Ventriculoperitoneal (VP) shunt**

Hydrocephalus or ventriculomegaly can be managed with the placement of a VP shunt. The hydrocephalus is typically a result of obstruction of outflow from the aqueduct of Sylvius into the fourth ventricle.

> ▶ **HINT:** VP shunt complications include obstruction and infections.

## COMPLICATIONS

- **A fluid-containing cyst in the spinal cord is called?**
- **Syrinx**

Syringomyelia (syrinx) is a complication of Chiari type II malformations. It is a cavity filled with CSF within the central portion of the cord.

> ▶ **HINT:** Syringomyelia can enlarge over a period of time. Hydromyelia are benign fluid collections that do not expand.

- **CP is frequently associated with visual abnormalities. What is the name for a visual abnormality in which the child is "cross-eyed"?**
- **Strabismus**

Some of the medical conditions associated with CP include strabismus, visual field cuts, and abnormally poor visual acuity (Box 7.17). Strabismus is the appearance of being "cross-eyed," which affects visual acuity. Losses of visual fields include homonymous hemianopsia (loss of the same-side visual field bilaterally).

> ▶ **HINT:** Associated medical conditions may also be considered complications of CP.

**Box 7.17** Symptoms Associated With Strabismus and Cerebral Palsy

| |
|---|
| Seizures |
| Impaired intellectual development |
| Scoliosis |
| Delayed growth and development |

*(continued)*

**Box 7.17** Symptoms Associated with Strabismus and Cerebral Palsy *(continued)*

| |
|---|
| Drooling |
| Visual changes and loss |
| Hearing loss |
| Abnormal sensations and perceptions |

- *What is the major complication of a myelomeningocele?*
- **Paralysis**

Myelomeningocele is the most severe form of spina bifida and frequently results in paralysis due to the spinal cord involvement (Box 7.18).

▶ **HINT:** The anatomical level of the myelomeningocele sac can correlate with the patient's neurological, motor, and sensory deficits.

**Box 7.18** Complications of Spina Bifida

| |
|---|
| Paralysis of lower extremities |
| Bowel incontinence |
| Neurogenic bladder |
| Seizures |
| Meningitis |
| Hydrocephalus |
| Learning disabilities |
| Latex allergies |
| Urinary tract infections |
| Gastrointestinal disorders |
| Emotional abnormalities |
| Poor cognition |
| Brain malformations |
| Scoliosis and kyphosis |

- *Which brain malformation is most commonly associated with myelomeningocele?*
- **Chiari II malformation**

Of the spina bifida types, myelomeningoceles have a greater association with brain malformations. One of the most common malformations is Chiari II malformation.

▶ **HINT:** Corpus callosum is another area of the brain that is found to be abnormal in patients with spina bifida.

- *A 5-year-old child with the history of surgical repair for a meningocele at birth begins to develop a new weakening in his lower extremities. What is the potential cause of this motor weakness?*
- **Tethered cord syndrome**

The surgical repair of the meningocele can cause scarring of the spinal cord region in the lower back. As the child grows, the spinal cord becomes tethered with the scarring, compressing the spinal cord. Symptoms can include lower-extremity weakness or paralysis and loss of bowel and bladder.

> ▶ **HINT:** New onset symptoms or worsening of motor symptoms are signs of tethered cord syndrome.

# Sample Exam Questions

1. Myelomeningocele children may have cognitive involvement as well as orthopedic. Which of the following brain abnormalities is commonly associated with myelomeningocele?
   A. Ischemic strokes
   B. Chiari II malformations
   C. Glioblastoma multiforme
   D. Normal-pressure hydrocephalus

2. A Chiari malformation, type I and II, can result in hydrocephalus. Which of the following is the most likely etiology of the hydrocephalus?
   A. Vermis herniation
   B. Increased production of cerebrospinal fluid (CSF)
   C. Obstruction of CSF flow
   D. Hypoplasia of the cerebellum

3. Which of the following is NOT considered to be a pathophysiological reason for presenting symptoms of Chiari malformation type II?
   A. Compression of medulla and upper spine
   B. Increased intracranial pressure
   C. Compression of the cerebellum
   D. Disruption of cerebrospinal fluid through the foramen magnum

4. Which of the following neurological injuries would indicate need for a decompressive foramen magnum craniectomy?
   A. Pons hemorrhagic stroke
   B. Cerebrospinal fluid hypotensive syndrome
   C. Cerebellar brain tumor
   D. Chiari malformation

5. Which of the following is a potential risk of neonates born with myelomeningocele that should be monitored closely?
   A. Dehydration
   B. Hypothermia
   C. Acidosis
   D. Hypokalemia

6. Which of the following is NOT a complication of myelomeningocele spina bifida in a neonate?
   A. Cerebrospinal fluid leak
   B. Latex allergies
   C. Developmental delay
   D. Neurogenic bladder

## BIBLIOGRAPHY

Abd-El-Barr, M. M., Strong, C. I., & Groff, M. W. (2014). Chiari malformations: Diagnosis, treatments and failures. *Journal of Neurosurgical Sciences, 58*(4), 215–221.

Copp, A., Adzick, S., Chitty, L., Fletcher, J., Holmbeck, G., & Shaw, G. (2015). Spina bifida. *Nature Reviews. Disease Primers, 1*, 15007. doi:10.1038/nrdp.2015.7

Handley, J. (2016). Spina bifida: A case study. *Journal of Nursing, 2*(1), 6–10.

Jensen, A. (2012). Nursing care and surgical correction of neonatal myelomeningocele. *Infant, 8*(5), 142–146.

Labuda, R., Loth, F., & Slavin, K. (2011). National Institutes of Health Chiari Research Conference: State of the research and new directions. *Neurological Research, 33*(3), 227–231. doi:10.1179/016164111X12962202723689

Mukherjee, S., & Pasulka, J. (2017). Care for adults with spina bifida: Current state and future directions. *Topics in Spinal Cord Injury Rehabilitation, 23*(2), 155–167. doi:10.1310/sci2302-155

Novak, I. (2014). Evidence-based diagnosis, health care, and rehabilitation for children with cerebral palsy. *Journal of Child Neurology, 29*(8), 1141–1156.

Nurse, S. (2010). Nursing babies at risk of cerebral palsy in the neonatal period. *Journal of Neonatal Nursing, 16*(5), 215–220.

Radcliff, E., Cassell, C. H., Laditka, S. B., Thibadeau, J. K., Correia, J., Grosse, S. D., & Kirby, R. S. (2016). Factors associated with the timeliness of postnatal surgical repair of spina bifida. *Child's Nervous System, 32*(8), 1479–1487. doi:10.1007/s00381-016-3105-3

Savage, K., & Pierce, L. (2012). The puzzle of Chiari malformation. *Nursing Made Incredibly Easy, 10*(4), 14–16. doi:10.1097/01.NME.0000413353.05812.73

Schuster, J. M., Zhang, F., Norvell, D. C., & Hermsmeyer, J. T. (2013). Persistent/recurrent syringomyelia after Chiari decompression—natural history and management strategies: A systematic review. *Evidence Based Spine Care Journal, 4*(2), 116–125. doi:10.1055/s-0033-1357362

Siasios, J., Kapsalaki, E. Z., & Fountas, K. N. (2012). Surgical management of patients with Chiari I malformation. *International Journal of Pediatrics, 2012*, 640127. doi:10.1155/2012/640127

Torpy, J. M., Lynm, C., & Glass, R. M. (2010). JAMA patient page. Cerebral Palsy. *JAMA, 304*(9), 1028. doi:10.1001/jama.304.9.1028

Wilkinson, D. A., Johnson, K., Garton, H. J., Muraszko, K. M., & Maher, C. O. (2017). Trends in surgical treatment of Chiari malformation Type I in the United States. *Journal of Neurosurgery Pediatrics, 19*(2), 208–216. doi:10.3171/2016.8.PEDS16273

# 8

# Neurological Trauma: Traumatic Brain Injury

## MECHANISM OF INJURY

- **What is the most common blunt mechanism of injury that causes traumatic brain injury (TBI)?**
- **Motor vehicle collision (MVC)**

MVC is one of the most common mechanisms of injury that results in TBI (Box 8.1). The TBI can range from mild to severe. Falls are the most common mechanism of TBI in pediatric patients under the age of 12 years. Adolescents experience MVC, sports injuries, and assaults more often.

> ▶ **HINT:** A major component of prevention of TBI in MVC is the proper use of seatbelts and car seats for the pediatric population.

**Box 8.1** Common Causes of Blunt TBI

| |
|---|
| MVC |
| Motor/pedestrian injury |
| Falls |
| Sports-related injury |
| War injury |
| Domestic violence |

MVC, motor vehicle collision; TBI, traumatic brain injury.

- **What is it called when a moving object impacts a stationary head?**
- **Acceleration injury**

Blunt trauma to the head is described based on the mechanism of injury. The term *acceleration injury* indicates a moving object, such as a baseball bat, impacted the head. Deceleration injury occurs when the head is moving and impacts a stationary object, such as in MVC when the head impacts the windshield.

▶ **HINT:** When you accelerate, you put something into motion. So, when an object hits the head, it causes the head to accelerate or move. This is an acceleration injury.

■ *What is it called when a brain injury occurs without any impact to the head itself?*
■ **Indirect injury**

An indirect injury occurs when the brain moves in the cranial vault following an acceleration–deceleration movement without the head impacting an object. A direct injury is an impact to the head, either through an acceleration, deceleration, or acceleration–deceleration mechanism.

▶ **HINT:** There are bony protrusions in the skull, and when the brain moves against these rough edges, it causes injury, even without a direct impact to the head.

■ *Following a gunshot to the head, the bullet is found within the cranial vault. What type of injury is this?*
■ **Penetrating injury**

Penetrating injury resulting from a gunshot wound indicates that the bullet entered the cranial vault but did not exit it. The bullet remains in the skull. Perforating injury occurs when the bullet enters and exits the cranium. Penetrating injuries to the brain also include stab wounds through the cranium or penetrating stab wounds to the face, which can enter the cranium. Tangential injury occurs when the bullet glances off the skull and may have a lower mortality rate.

▶ **HINT:** In some penetrating injuries to the skull, the bullet is left in the cranium and not retrieved because of the location bullet being in an eloquent area of the brain. Retained bullet or skull fragments have not been found to significantly increase infection risk.

■ *Following an impact to the head, an injury to the brain occurs on the opposite side of the impact. What is this injury called?*
■ **Contrecoup injury**

A coup injury occurs under the area of impact, and a contrecoup injury is brain injury that occurs on the opposite side of the impact. Coup–contrecoup injuries are commonly associated with epidural and subdural hematomas.

▶ **HINT:** The mechanism of injury that most commonly causes a coup–contrecoup injury is an impact to the lateral side of the skull.

■ *What type of injury results in diffuse axonal injury (DAI) to the brain?*
■ **Rotational injury**

Rotational injury, such as vehicle rollover, can result in shearing of the brain tissue. This injury is called a *DAI*. Presence of DAI indicates a poorer functional outcome for the TBI patient.

▶ **HINT:** A decreased level of consciousness (LOC) that is out of proportion to CT scan findings is indicative of DAI.

## 8. NEUROLOGICAL TRAUMA: TRAUMATIC BRAIN INJURY

▪ *What type of injury causes chronic traumatic encephalopathy (CTE)?*
▪ **Repetitive injuries**

Repetitive TBIs that trigger progressive degeneration of brain tissue result in CTE. The injuries frequently are mild TBIs related to contact sports injuries.

> ▶ HINT: CTE may also be found in veterans of war and victims of domestic violence.

▪ *What patient population is most likely to present with a chronic subdural hematoma (SDH)?*
▪ **Elderly**

Elderly patients are likely to present with chronic SDH. Other SDH patient populations include alcoholics and dementia patients. Chronic SDHs tend to be slower to hemorrhage, and these patient groups have cortical atrophy, which allows for more blood volume to accumulate before an increase in intracranial pressure occurs (Box 8.2).

> ▶ HINT: Chronic SDH patients are frequently misdiagnosed initially with "old age" or stroke.

**Box 8.2** Classifications of SDH

| Acute SDH | Onset within 24 hours |
|---|---|
| Subacute SDH | Onset within 24 to 48 hours |
| Chronic SDH | Onset days to weeks after injury |

SDH, subdural hematoma.

▪ *Secondary injuries include cerebral edema. Cerebral edema caused by ischemic or hypoxic insult following a TBI is called?*
▪ **Cytotoxic edema**

Cytotoxic edema causes intracellular swelling and is a result of hypoxic or anoxic injuries. Vasogenic cerebral edema is swelling or extra fluid in the interstitial space and is a result of trauma to the tissue. TBI will have a combination of both cytotoxic and vasogenic edema. Following brain trauma, there is a loss of autoregulation in areas of injury. Cerebral blood flow is shunted away from uninjured areas of the brain to areas of injury. This causes a "steal phenomenon" and results in hypoxia in uninjured areas of the brain.

> ▶ HINT: Mannitol is used to treat cerebral edema and is more effective with vasogenic cerebral edema because the fluid is in the interstitial space.

▪ *What is the anatomical difference in pediatric patients that makes them more likely to experience a brain injury with a trauma?*
▪ **Head is larger in proportion to body**

The head of pediatric patients is larger in proportion to the rest of the body, and the stability of the neck through ligaments is not fully developed. This makes the child susceptible to TBI in MVC.

> ▶ HINT: Once the child is no longer in a car seat, the child typically places the shoulder harness behind him or her because it no longer fits appropriately. This increases the likelihood of TBI.

■ *What is the triad of symptoms typically seen in shaken baby syndrome (SBS)?*
■ **Subdural hematoma, retinal hemorrhage, and cerebral edema**

SBS is a result of violent shaking of the child. This is also called *abusive head trauma* (Box 8.3). The head may or may not have contacted an object, but the movement of the brain contents causes a shearing effect. The result is typically bilateral SDH and diffuse axonal injury. The injury is often fatal and can cause lifelong severe, neurological disabilities.

▶ **HINT:** Retinal hemorrhages have a characteristic pattern for SBS and are used frequently to assist with the diagnosis of SBS.

**Box 8.3** Signs of TBI Caused by Child Abuse

| |
|---|
| Injuries cannot be explained by reported trauma |
| Associated long bone fractures |
| Associated cervical injuries |
| Poor hygiene |
| Bruises at varying stages of healing |
| Multiple complex skull fractures with reported single-impact history |

TBI, traumatic brain injury.

## TRAUMATIC INJURIES

■ *A displaced comminuted fracture of the skull is what type of fracture?*
■ **Depressed skull fracture**

A depressed skull fracture is a comminuted fracture that is displaced into the meninges and brain tissue. This injury is commonly associated with epidural, subdural, and parenchymal hematomas. A linear skull fracture involves a nondisplaced fracture line.

▶ **HINT:** The displacement of bony pieces into the meninges causes the tearing of meningeal vessels and development of epidural and subdural hematomas.

■ *A patient develops a cerebrospinal fluid (CSF) leak following a blow to the side of the head. What type of fracture does this patient have?*
■ **Basilar skull fracture**

Basilar skull fractures may result in CSF leaks from ears (otorrhea) or from the nose (rhinorrhea). The base of the skull is divided into the anterior, middle, and posterior skull base or fossa. Fractures may occur anywhere throughout the skull bases, but the anterior fossa is the most common area for basilar skull fractures.

▶ **HINT:** A blow to the side of the head causes the basilar skull to buckle, resulting in fracture lines along the basilar skull.

■ *An area of the brain parenchyma that hemorrhages following TBI is called?*
■ **Contusion**

Contusions are areas of parenchymal hemorrhage due to acceleration/deceleration injury and blunt impact. Contusions may initially appear as several areas of small hemorrhages, but these can increase and combine into larger hematoma. Approximately, one third of the patients with contusion will experience contusion expansion within 24 hours.

> ▶ **HINT:** Initial CT scan following TBI may not show the contusion. Frequently, follow-up CT scans obtained 24 hours later are used to identify the contusion or to determine the increased size of the contusion.

- **Is an epidural hematoma (EDH) most commonly caused by laceration of an artery or bridging veins?**
- **Artery**

Laceration of an artery is the most common cause of EDH. The most common artery involved in EDH is the middle meningeal artery. Laceration of veins may also result in bleeding in the epidural space, but is less common than arterial involvement. Tearing of bridging veins will hemorrhage into the subdural space (venous sinuses are located in subdural space) causing SDH.

> ▶ **HINT:** An EDH typically expands rapidly due to its being an arterial hemorrhage, and SDH may be slower to hemorrhage due to venous involvement.

- **Tearing of pial veins will cause bleeding following a trauma. Where is the hemorrhage located?**
- **Subarachnoid space**

Tearing of small pial veins causes bleeding into the subarachnoid space and is called *subarachnoid hemorrhage (SAH)*. SAH may also involve blood in the ventricles, but isolated ventricular hemorrhage following trauma is unusual.

> ▶ **HINT:** SAH following trauma does not usually result in vasospasms as does SAH following aneurysm rupture.

- **What are the two secondary injuries that have the greatest effect on neurological outcomes following TBI?**
- **Hypotension and hypoxia**

Secondary injuries are those neurological injuries that occur to the brain after the initial trauma (Box 8.4). It has been found that hypotension and hypoxia are the two most important determinants of neurological outcomes.

> ▶ **HINT:** Priority of care for managing TBI patients is airway/breathing to improve oxygenation and resuscitation to reestablish perfusion to prevent further neurological injury.

**Box 8.4** Secondary Injuries: Neurological Injuries Occurring to the Brain After an Initial Trauma

| Systemic Secondary Injuries | Intracranial Secondary Injuries |
|---|---|
| Hypotension | Increased intracranial pressure |
| Hypoxia | Cerebral edema |
| Anemia | Expanding mass lesions (hematomas) |

*(continued)*

**Box 8.4** Secondary Injuries: Neurological Injuries Occurring to the Brain After an Initial Trauma *(continued)*

| Systemic Secondary Injuries | Intracranial Secondary Injuries |
|---|---|
| Hypercapnia | Hydrocephalus |
| Hypocapnia | CNS infections |
| Hyperthermia | Seizures |
| Hyperglycemia | Brain ischemia |
| Electrolyte abnormalities | |
| Acid–base abnormalities | |

CNS, central nervous system.

## ASSESSMENT/DIAGNOSIS

- *A patient develops bilateral periorbital ecchymosis following traumatic injury to the head. What is the cause of the ecchymosis?*
- **Basilar skull fracture**

Patients with basilar skull fracture may develop periorbital ecchymosis (raccoon eyes) and bruising on the mastoid process called the *Battle sign*.

> ▶ **HINT:** Raccoon eyes and Battle sign may not appear immediately following a trauma and typically develop later following injury.

- *What is the best method to use to test drainage from the nose for the presence of CSF?*
- **Halo test**

Halo test is used to determine the presence of CSF in drainage from the nose (rhinorrhea) or from the ears (otorrhea). To perform the halo test, dab the drainage onto gauze and look for a yellow ring surrounding the drainage. This is a positive halo sign and indicates the presence of CSF.

> ▶ **HINT:** Halo test is more reliable than testing the drainage for glucose as drainage may contain blood, which also has glucose. Glucose test for CSF yields more false positives.

- *To improve accuracy of the diagnosis for CSF in drainage, which lab test may be used?*
- **Beta-2 transferrin**

The halo ring test can cause false positives so the gold standard (most diagnostic) is lab testing of the drainage for CSF. Beta-2 transferrin is a variant of transferrin and is used as an endogenous marker for CSF in other body fluids.

> ▶ **HINT:** Beta-2 transferrin has been called *CSF-specific transferrin* because it is highly specific for CSF.

- *What diagnostic study is considered the gold standard for identifying skull base fractures?*
- **CT scan**

High-resolution CT scan of the head is considered the gold standard in identifying skull base fractures. Differentiation between suture lines and fracture is required to ensure an accurate diagnosis.

> ▶ **HINT:** Clinical findings may be used to assist with diagnosis of basilar skull fracture if unable to visualize the fracture on head CT scan.

- *Diagnostic CT scan of the brain found air present in the cranium and basilar skull fracture. What is the air in the cranium called?*
- **Pneumocephalus**

Pneumocephalus is a complication of basilar skull fracture and may be identified on brain CT scan. Air enters the cranium through the fracture. Management of pneumocephalus may be achieved with oxygen administration.

> ▶ **HINT:** Pneumocephalus can become a tension pneumocephalus with a resulting elevation of intracranial pressure.

- *A mild traumatic brain injury (MTBI) may be defined using Glasgow Coma Scale (GCS). What GCS score would indicate minor brain injury?*
- **GCS 13–15**

MTBI (used to be called a *concussion*; see Box 8.5) is often classified as a GCS score between 13 and 15 (Box 8.6). The patient does not have to experience a loss of consciousness to have a TBI. MTBI can be graded on its severity.

**Box 8.5** Diagnosis of Mild TBI

| |
|---|
| GCS between 13 and 15 |
| Temporary loss of consciousness |
| Posttraumatic amnesia for <24 hours |
| Transient neurological abnormalities |
| Transient confusion |

GCS, Glasgow Coma Scale; TBI, traumatic brain injury.

> ▶ **HINT:** Neurological abnormalities must not be due to alcohol or drugs or caused by other injuries to qualify as an MTBI.

**Box 8.6** GCS Classification Severity and TBI

| | |
|---|---|
| GCS 13–15 | Mild traumatic brain injury |
| GCS 9–12 | Moderate traumatic brain injury |
| GCS 3–8 | Severe traumatic brain injury |

GCS, Glasgow Coma Scale; TBI traumatic brain injury.

> ▶ **HINT:** Limitations of using GCS to determine severity of neurological injury exist in intubated and aphasic patients.

■ **A patient presents with an altered LOC following a head trauma. What is the best diagnostic procedure used initially to identify skull and brain injuries?**
■ **Noncontrast CT scan**

Noncontrast CT scan is useful during the immediate posttraumatic period to identify intracranial pathology that would indicate the need for immediate surgical management (Box 8.7). Noncontrast CT scan is used to identify skull fractures, hematomas, contusions, mass effects, presence of foreign objects, and presence of cerebral edema.

▶ **HINT:** Pediatric patients with GCS <15 may be an indication for noncontrast CT scan.

**Box 8.7** Indications for Noncontrast CT Scan of TBI

| |
|---|
| Loss of consciousness or posttraumatic amnesia is possible; if one of the following is present:<br>  Vomiting, age >60 years, headache, drug or alcohol intoxication, deficits in short-term memory, GCS <15, focal neurological deficit |
| Signs of basilar skull fracture |
| Posttraumatic seizures |
| Presence of coagulopathy |
| Dangerous mechanism of injury (e.g., ejection from vehicle) |

GCS, Glasgow Coma Scale.

■ **What is the most sensitive indicator of an increased intracranial pressure (ICP)?**
■ **Change in LOC**

A change in LOC is a sensitive indicator for neurological deterioration and an increased ICP (Box 8.8). When performing neurological assessments, it is very important to assess for LOC.

▶ **HINT:** A change in LOC can include both a change in alertness and a change in orientation.

**Box 8.8** Symptoms of Neurological Deterioration

| |
|---|
| Decreased level of consciousness |
| Development of confusion or disorientation |
| Unequal pupils and change in pupillary response |
| Dilated pupil(s) or constricted pupils |
| Vision changes |
| Vomiting |
| Seizures |
| Worsening headache |
| Changes in respiratory patterns |
| Cushing's triad |

▶ **HINT:** Cushing's triad (increased systolic pressure, widened pulse pressure, and bradycardia) are signs of impending herniation but are late signs of an increased ICP.

■ *What is the most commonly used diagnosis of diffuse axonal injury (DAI)?*
■ **Clinical diagnosis**

Clinical diagnosis is poor neurological status and decreased LOC that is out of proportion to injury observed on CT scan. DAI involves microscopic injuries so it is not seen as large changes on diagnostic studies such as CT scan. CT imaging may demonstrate small punctate foci of hemorrhage, but is not found in all cases of DAI.

> ▶ **HINT:** It may be several days before the diagnosis of DAI due to delay of contusions in CT presentation.

■ *A patient presents to the ED following a fall off a ladder. The family reports some altered LOC after the fall. What should be included in the nurse's admission history?*
■ **Duration and severity of altered LOC**

A report of altered LOC requires more information from those who observed the injury. This includes the duration of the altered mentation, degree of altered LOC, other neurological symptoms experienced, and mechanism of injury.

> ▶ **HINT:** The observer of the traumatic event is a better historian than the person who experienced the altered LOC. Patients typically cannot recall the event, deny the LOC, or are not really aware of how long they were unconscious.

■ *The trauma nurse, to evaluate presence of retrograde amnesia following a traumatic brain injury, may use what question?*
■ **"What was the last event you remember before your injury?"**

*Retrograde amnesia* refers to the loss of memory before the traumatic event. It is commonly determined by asking what the last thing the patient remembers before the traumatic event. *Posttraumatic amnesia* is the loss of memory from the time of unconsciousness until the first memory after the event. *Antegrade amnesia* is the inability to create new memory after the event. An example of antegrade amnesia is when a person is unable to remember anything that happened during the remainder of the day, but was conscious.

> ▶ **HINT:** "What is the first thing you remember after the event" is a question used to evaluate for posttraumatic amnesia.

■ *A rapidly expanding epidural hematoma following a severe TBI can result in an uncal herniation. Which pupil will dilate following uncal herniation?*
■ **Ipsilateral**

Uncal herniation is a lateral displacement and herniation of brain tissue due to a unilateral expanding mass. The pupil affected by the herniation is the ipsilateral pupil. It will dilate and become nonreactive. Subdural hematoma may also be a rapidly expanding mass and can cause uncal herniation in a dilated ipsilateral pupil.

> ▶ **HINT:** Dilated pupil is caused by injury or stretch of cranial nerve (CN) III (oculomotor nerve). CNs do not cross in the brainstem like motor and sensory tracts (except CN IV), so symptoms are ipsilateral.

■ *Which of the hematomas following TBI has the classic presentation of a lucid period?*
■ **EDH**

EDH classically presents with a period of lucidity. The patient may have been unconscious initially, experiences a period of being awake, and then loses consciousness again.

> ▶ HINT: Not all EDHs will have this classical presentation, but of all the hematomas, EDH is the most likely cause of the presentation.

■ **What complication of abdominal trauma can increase ICP and worsen neurological outcomes?**
■ **Abdominal compartment syndrome (ACS)**

ACS is a complication of abdominal trauma. It causes an increase in abdominal pressure that results in a decrease in venous drainage from the brain. This elevates the intracerebral blood volume and ICP. Increased pressure in the thoracic cavity can have the same effect as ACS. Multisystem trauma patients with the combination of abdominal or thoracic trauma with brain injury should be assessed for the presence of ACS, and treatment should be initiated to lower abdominal and thoracic pressures.

> ▶ HINT: ACS can be measured and monitored with bladder pressure readings.

■ **What is a commonly used assessment tool to measure the deficit in cognitive functioning following a TBI?**
■ **Ranchos Los Amigos Scale**

The Ranchos Los Amigos Scale is used to measure deficits in cognitive functioning. The tool is frequently used to determine the patient's level of cognitive functioning for rehabilitation capabilities and prognosis following TBI. The scale is divided into eight stages (or 10 stages with revised version) ranging from appropriate to coma.

> ▶ HINT: Level VI on the revised score is the point at which the patient requires moderate assistance (versus maximal assistance) and is the point when he or she will have a greater benefit from rehabilitation.

## MEDICAL/SURGICAL INTERVENTION

■ **What is the primary management of a depressed skull fracture?**
■ **Surgical debridement**

Following a depressed skull fracture, surgical debridement is used to remove the bony pieces that cause damage to the meninges and brain tissue. This is followed later by cranioplasty to replace the portion of the skull that was debrided.

> ▶ HINT: The use of cranioplasty to repair the skull defect is also done for cosmetic purposes.

■ **What is the priority of prehospital and ED care when treating severe TBI patients?**
■ **Check airway and breathing.**

Hypoxia and hypotension are secondary injuries that will worsen neurological outcomes. The prehospital goals are to initiate treatment to prevent secondary injuries. This includes obtaining and maintaining airway and breathing to prevent hypoxia and initiating fluid resuscitation to prevent hypotension and hypoperfusion. Care should also be taken to secure the cervical spine because cervical spine injuries are commonly associated with head trauma.

> ▶ **HINT:** Intubation is considered in patients with GCS score of less than or equal to 8.

### What is the mean arterial pressure (MAP) and the PaO$_2$ goal for TBI?
### MAP >80 mmHg and PaO$_2$ >80 mmHg

Systemic hypoxia is an independent predictor of increased morbidity and mortality. A single episode of hypotension (BP <90 mmHg) is associated with worsening of outcomes. Maintaining a MAP >80 in severe TBI patients (GCS <8) will improve brain perfusion. If GCS is >8, then MAP is maintained at >70 mmHg. The oxygenation goal is to maintain PaO$_2$ between 80 and 120 mmHg and arterial saturation greater than 92% to prevent secondary hypoxic injuries.

> ▶ **HINT:** Goal in managing severe TBI is to optimize cerebral blood flow while minimizing cerebral edema and intracranial pressure.

### An ICP monitor was placed in the trauma ICU to monitor patients with severe TBI. What should be the goal for the cerebral perfusion pressure (CPP)?
### Maintain >60 mmHg

CPP is a measurement used at the bedside to estimate cerebral blood flow (CBF) (Box 8.9). The CPP is calculated when the patient has an ICP monitor (Box 8.10), and the goal is to maintain CPP greater than 60 mmHg to improve CBF. An ICP should be maintained less than 20 mmHg. If CPP is less than 60 mmHg following adequate fluid resuscitation, a vasoconstrictor may be administered to increase MAP. CPP higher than 70 mmHg is not recommended due to risk of volume overload, cerebral edema, and acute respiratory distress syndrome (ARDS).

> ▶ **HINT:** To improve CPP, increase MAP and reduce the ICP. Focus of interventions is on both sides: the driving force (MAP) and the opposing force (ICP).

**Box 8.9** Calculation of Cerebral Perfusion Pressure

| |
|---|
| Mean arterial pressure − intracranial pressure = cerebral perfusion pressure |

**Box 8.10** Indications for Intracranial Pressure Monitor

| |
|---|
| GCS <8 |
| Abnormal brain CT scan includes:<br>  Hemorrhage<br>  Contusions<br>  Swelling<br>  Herniation<br>  Compressed basal cisterns |
| Normal brain CT scan and two or more of the following:<br>  Age >40<br>  Unilateral or bilateral motor posturing<br>  Systemic hypotension |
| Patient will not be examined for a prolonged period of time |

GCS, Glasgow Coma Scale.

▶ **HINT:** Infants and young children may tolerate increased intracranial pressures better because of open sutures and fontanelles, but they can still experience increase ICP and may require ICP monitoring similar to adults.

■ **What osmotic diuretic is used to treat cerebral edema and lower ICP?**
■ **Mannitol**

Mannitol is an osmotic diuretic that is used to increase serum osmolality, creating a pull of fluid from extravascular to intravascular space. This lowers cerebral edema and ICP. While administering mannitol, care should be taken to avoid hypovolemia (due to the diuresis) and hypotension. Fluid resuscitation may be required to prevent hypovolemia. Serum osmolality and sodium levels need to be obtained at least every 6 hours with hyperosmolar therapy.

▶ **HINT:** Hold mannitol if serum osmolality is greater than 320 Osm/L.

■ **What is the potential adverse effect of administering hypertonic saline to lower cerebral edema?**
■ **Central pontine myelinolysis (CPM)**

Hypertonic saline (3%, 7.5%, 23%) may also be used to increase serum osmolality instead of mannitol (Box 8.11). The highest risk for causing CPM occurs in hyponatremic patients. If the patient has a normal serum $Na^+$ level, the chance of causing CPM when using 3% saline in appropriate dosages is rare. Monitor serum $Na^+$ levels while administering hypertonic saline, and hold if $Na^+$ levels are greater than 155 mEq/L.

▶ **HINT:** Avoid administering hypertonic saline in patients who are hyponatremic. Mannitol would be the better answer in that situation (Box 8.12).

**Box 8.11** Types of Hyperosmolar Therapy

| 3% saline | 100 mL IV q2h PRN |
|---|---|
| Mannitol | 0.25–1 gm/kg IV q6h PRN |

IV, intravenous.

**Box 8.12** Adverse Effects of Hyperosmolar Therapy

| Mannitol | Hypertonic Saline |
|---|---|
| Rebound phenomenon | Rebound phenomenon |
| Hyperosmolar state | Central pontine myelinolysis |
| Dehydration | Hypernatremia |
| Acute renal failure | Worsening pulmonary edema |

■ **Sustained hyperventilation with hypocarbia and respiratory alkalosis can cause what harmful effects in a TBI patient?**
■ **Reduced cerebral blood flow (CBF)**

$PaCO_2$ is a potent cerebral vasodilator. If the $PaCO_2$ is decreased due to hyperventilation and hypocarbia occurs, this causes cerebral vasoconstriction, reduced CBF, and a decrease in ICP. Sustained or aggressive hyperventilation is not recommended due to the effect on

CBF, even though it can lower an ICP. The PaCO$_2$ goal is 35 to 45 mmHg (maintaining on the low side of normal if ICP is elevated).

▶ **HINT:** A patient suddenly loses consciousness due to a rapidly elevating ICP; the trauma nurse may hyperventilate for a short period to lower the ICP until definitive management of the patient can occur.

▪ *Patient is admitted to ICU after craniotomy to remove acute SDH. The bone is left out and will be replaced at a later date. What is this bone called?*
▪ **Bone flap**

A bone flap is removed during the craniotomy and is not replaced to allow for more room for the brain to swell. This is called *decompressive surgery*. Patients still can herniate through the bone flap causing strangulation of brain tissue and will still need to be treated for an increase in iICP.

A hemicraniectomy may also be performed to allow for a greater amount of decompression.

▶ **HINT:** The trauma nurse assesses the bone flap for tension or bulging, which indicate an increase in ICP.

▪ *What is the temperature goal when caring for a severe TBI patient?*
▪ **Between 36 and 37°C**

Elevated body temperatures have adverse effects on TBI patients, and normothermia should be maintained. Even though fever in non–brain-injured patients is allowed to increase body temperatures to 38.3–38.5°C, the brain may begin to experience greater injury at temperatures above 37°C. Fever increases brain metabolism, elevates levels of proinflammatory cytokines, and may increase ICP. Hypothermia has also been found to worsen outcomes in TBI patients and should be avoided unless patient has refractory elevated ICP.

▶ **HINT:** Remember that neurological patients are also at risk for central neurogenic fever and body temperatures can elevate rapidly and severely.

▪ *Which type of intravenous (IV) fluid is most commonly used to maintain fluid volume in a TBI patient?*
▪ **Normal saline (NS)**

NS is an isotonic crystalloid commonly used to resuscitate and maintain fluid volume in a TBI patient. NS may also be used initially to correct hyponatremia (Na$^+$ <140 mEq/L).

▶ **HINT:** Avoid dextrose in the IV fluids because hyperglycemia is considered a secondary injury and can worsen neurological outcomes.

▪ *Sedation and analgesia may be provided to control agitation and pain following TBI. What adverse effect should be monitored closely to prevent secondary brain injuries?*
▪ **Hypotension**

Analgesia and sedation can lower the intracranial pressure and facilitate mechanical ventilation but may cause vasodilation with hypotension and decreased CBF. Hypotension is a secondary injury that may worsen neurological outcomes. Close monitoring of blood pressure is required when administering analgesics and sedatives. Analgesia and sedation may also affect respiratory rate and should be used cautiously to prevent respiratory depression and hypoxia unless mechanically ventilated.

▶ **HINT:** Sedation also involves a potential loss of accurate neurological assessment.

■ *How long should seizure prophylaxis be continued following a severe TBI?*
■ **7 days**

Seizure prophylaxis is recommended for 7 days following a severe TBI. If the patient has not had a seizure within 7 days following the trauma, antiepileptic drugs may be discontinued. Seizure prophylaxis is not recommended in mild to moderate TBI patients.

▶ **HINT:** Continuous EEG monitoring may be used to identify nonconvulsive seizures in TBI patients who do not regain consciousness following the trauma.

■ *When would a barbiturate coma be considered following a severe TBI?*
■ **In cases with persistent elevation of ICP**

Inducing a barbiturate coma is not a first-line treatment to manage an increased ICP but may be used if the ICP is refractory despite tier 1 interventions (i.e., osmolar therapy; Box 8.13). Continuous EEG monitoring is frequently used to titrate the barbiturate therapy by burst suppression.

▶ **HINT:** Monitor hemodynamics of patient in a barbiturate coma due to the adverse effect of myocardial depression.

**Box 8.13** Potential Treatments for Refractory Increased ICP

| |
|---|
| Barbiturate coma |
| Decompressive craniotomy |
| Mild hyperventilation (PaCO$_2$ 30–34 mmHg) |
| Mild hypothermia (33–35°C) |
| Neuromuscular blocking agents |

ICP, intracranial pressure.

▶ **HINT:** Corticosteroids are not recommended in managing cerebral edema or increased ICP in TBI patients.

## NURSING INTERVENTIONS

■ *A gastric tube is required for a patient with TBI. What type of gastric tube should be placed?*
■ **Orogastric tube (OGT)**

OGT is the preferred gastric tube in patients with TBI at risk of having basilar skull fracture. Nasogastric tube placement can result in the tube entering the brain through the cribriform fracture in basilar skull fractures. The cribriform plate is located in the anterior fossa or skull base.

> ▶ **HINT:** Never place any nasal tube following facial or head injury due to risk of brain cannulation.

- *What is the placement of gauze in patients with rhinorrhea?*
- **Taped under the nose**

Frequently, gauze is taped under the nose to absorb the drainage. This allows for the estimation of the amount of drainage or CSF leak that is occurring.

> ▶ **HINT:** Never pack the nose with gauze in patients with rhinorrhea. This can increase risk of meningitis.

- *Following a basilar skull fracture with a known CSF leak, at what level should the head of the bed (HOB) be placed?*
- **Greater than 30 degrees**

HOB should be elevated greater than 30 degrees in patients with a known CSF leak. Conservative treatment is usually recommended for basilar fractures and CSF leaks, which include strict bedrest, elevated HOB, no coughing, sneezing, or straining. Antibiotic prophylaxis is not recommended following a basilar skull fracture and CSF leak.

> ▶ **HINT:** Instruct the patients with CSF not to forcefully blow their nose.

- *Patient is being discharged home from ED following a mild TBI from playing football. What is the most appropriate recommendation on when the patient can return to play?*
- **When symptom free**

Current guidelines recommend a graduated increase in the level of activity of the athlete progressing from the initial stage of "light exercise" toward "full contact" activity once the athlete is completely symptom free at rest. This is to prevent a secondary impact event syndrome, which can result in death and repetitive injuries.

> ▶ **HINT:** Secondary impact syndrome can occur with a second impact within hours to weeks after the initial TBI.

- *A patient with a TBI should be placed in what position to lower the ICP?*
- **Elevated HOB**

Elevating the HOB by 30 degrees facilitates venous drainage and lowers blood volume in the cranium, thus lowering the ICP. Laying the HOB flat will increase the ICP. Also maintain the neck in a neutral position to avoid jugular vein constriction.

> ▶ **HINT:** Maintain an elevated HOB in TBI patients unless contraindicated due to their other injuries.

- **A patient in the ICU with severe TBI develops a temperature of 39°C. What nursing intervention should be done to lower the body temperature?**
- **Apply cooling blanket**

Elevated body temperatures should be managed quickly in brain-injured patients to prevent secondary brain injury. Applying a cooling blanket to lower the body temperature is a nursing intervention that may be used. Other methods to lower the body temperature may include administering antipyretic medications, controlling room temperature, and intravascular cooling. The goal is a normothermic body temperature. See Box 8.14 for additional nursing interventions for TBI patients.

> ▶ **HINT:** Shivering can also increase metabolism and should be treated if it occurs during cooling of the patient.

**Box 8.14** Nursing Interventions for TBI Patients

| |
|---|
| Appropriate and early nutrition |
| Venous thrombosis prophylaxis |
| Stress ulcer prophylaxis |
| Early mobility |
| Prevent infections |
| Treat hyperglycemia (>180 mg/dL) |
| Prevent skin breakdown |
| Maintain normothermic body temperature |

## COMPLICATIONS

- **Following a depressed skull fracture, the patient develops fever and elevated white blood cell (WBC) counts. What would be the potential complication of the depressed skull fracture?**
- **Meningitis**

Central nervous system (CNS) infections, such as meningitis, are potential complications following a depressed and basilar skull fracture.

> ▶ **HINT:** Signs of an infection are elevated fever and WBC count so the infection associated with depressed skull fracture is meningitis.

- **Which CN may be injured due to basilar skull fracture if patient presents with asymmetrical facial expressions?**
- **CN VII (facial nerve)**

CN injuries can be associated with basilar skull fractures. CN I (olfactory nerve/sense of smell) can be affected if the cribriform plate is fractured. CN II (optic nerve) injury can result in unilateral blindness and dilated pupil. Facial nerve (CN VII) is more commonly damaged in middle fossa and temporal bone fractures.

> ▶ **HINT:** CN injuries can occur with skull fractures and facial fractures.

## 8. NEUROLOGICAL TRAUMA: TRAUMATIC BRAIN INJURY

■ *Brain CT scan of a trauma patient finds intracerebral hemorrhage. What medication therapy would the trauma nurse suspect the patient to be taking?*

■ **Anticoagulation and/or antiplatelet therapy**

Anticoagulation and antiplatelet therapy are common therapies that result in intracerebral hemorrhage and may occur following any trauma. Reversal of the bleeding complications is considered a priority and may include administering a reversal agent if there is an antidote for the medication. Correct the coagulopathy with prothrombin complex concentrates (PCCs) in life-threatening bleeds. Other blood products may include fresh frozen plasma (FFP) and cryoprecipitate.

▶ **HINT:** If the patient is on antiplatelet therapy, administer platelets.

■ *Repetitive mild TBIs in contact sports can result in what complication?*

■ **Chronic traumatic encephalopathy (CTE)**

CTE is a complication of repetitive brain trauma frequently seen in players of contact sports. This used to be called *punch drunk* in boxing. These repetitive injuries result in the deposit of tau proteins in the cortex, resulting in degeneration and atrophy of the brain similar to that of cortical dementia (Box 8.15).

▶ **HINT:** CTE is similar to Alzheimer's disease and Parkinson's disease in its pathophysiology, but is a preventable dementia.

**Box 8.15** Symptoms of CTE

| |
|---|
| Memory loss |
| Depression |
| Suicidal thoughts and suicides |
| Aggressive behavior |
| Tremors |
| Ataxia (gait abnormality) |
| Slowed movements |
| Speech abnormalities |
| Confusion |

CTE, chronic traumatic encephalopathy.

■ *A patient presents to the clinic with frequent headaches and states that he had a concussion about 2 months ago. What is the cause of the headaches?*

■ **Posttraumatic headache**

Posttraumatic headaches develop in about 30% to 40% of patients following mild TBI (Box 8.16). The headaches may increase during periods of stress, tension, or activity.

▶ **HINT:** Management of posttraumatic headache is similar to benign headaches and includes abortive treatments with triptans.

**Box 8.16** Complications of Mild TBI

| |
|---|
| Headache |
| Posttraumatic stress disorder |
| Fatigue, exhaustion |
| Sleep disturbances |
| Posture and balance issues |
| Memory problems |
| Seizures |

TBI, traumatic brain injury.

## REHABILITATION

- *The brain's ability to reorganize neural pathways is called?*
- **Plasticity**

Plasticity is the ability of the neural pathways to reorganize based on stimulation, new experiences, and new learning. Pediatric brains have greater plasticity, but adult brains can reorganize neural pathways to learn and improve recovery. Engaging in activities helps the brain develop new pathways.

> ▶ **HINT:** Brain is most susceptible to plasticity soon after the trauma, so rehabilitation begins on admission.

- *How many months after the TBI will the neurological improvement begin to slow down?*
- **6 months**

The greatest improvements following TBI occur within the first 6 months and then begin to slow down with minimal improvements after 1 year.

> ▶ **HINT:** It is usual to inform family that it may take up to 1 year after injury to have an understanding of the degree of physical recovery needed; however, psychological recovery may take even longer.

# Sample Exam Questions

1. Which of the following statements is most correct regarding surgical management of subdural hematomas (SDHs)?
   A. Lateral shift of 2 cm is present
   B. Clinical symptoms are compatible with the CT scan findings
   C. Presence of bilateral SDH
   D. Acute on chronic SDH

2. Which of the following is a nursing intervention used to facilitate venous drainage and lower the intracranial pressure?
   A. Maintain head of the bed greater than 30 degrees
   B. Secure cervical collar snugly for head alignment
   C. Elevate the foot of the bed
   D. Place ventriculostomy to drain cerebrospinal fluid

3. Which of the following does NOT increase the intracranial pressure of a patient with severe traumatic brain injury?
   A. Coughing
   B. Sneezing
   C. Pain
   D. Upright position

4. Which of the following would be considered the highest priority prehospital event when transporting a traumatic brain-injured patient?
   A. Provide hyperventilation.
   B. Administer an osmotic diuretic.
   C. Prevent hypotension.
   D. Maintain the stretcher in reverse Trendelenburg.

5. Which of the following scales is the most widely accepted scale in traumatic brain-injured patients?
   A. National Institutes of Health Stroke Scale
   B. Injury Severity Score
   C. Glasgow Coma Scale
   D. Apache score

6. Following a traumatic brain injury, the patient is hypotensive in the ED. Which of the following intravenous fluids is the best option for this patient?
   A. Normal saline
   B. Lactated Ringers
   C. Dextrose 5% normal saline
   D. Dextrose

7. A trauma patient with a gunshot to the head is being evaluated neurologically in the ED. Which of the following diagnostic studies would be contraindicated in this patient?
   A. CT scan
   B. Skull radiograph
   C. MRI
   D. Doppler flow study

8. Which of the following arteries is commonly involved with epidural hematoma?
   A. Middle cerebral artery
   B. Anterior cerebral artery
   C. Posterior inferior cerebellar artery
   D. Middle meningeal artery

9. Which of the following outcome scales is most commonly used to evaluate cognition in traumatic brain-injured patients for rehabilitation purposes?
   A. Rancho Los Amigos Scale
   B. Glasgow Coma Scale
   C. Apache score
   D. Hunt and Hess Scale

## BIBLIOGRAPHY

Barbosa, R. R., Jawa, R., Watters, J. M., Knight, J. C., Kerwin, A. J., Winston, E. S., ... Eastern Association for the Surgery of Trauma. (2012). Evaluation and management of mild traumatic brain injury: An Eastern Association for the Surgery of Trauma practice management guideline. *Journal of Trauma and Acute Care Surgery, 73*(5, Suppl. 4), S307–S314. doi:10.1097/TA.0b013e3182701885

Bohman, L. E., & Schuster, J. M. (2013). Decompressive craniectomy for management of traumatic brain injury: An update. *Current Neurology and Neuroscience Reports, 13*(11), 392. doi:10.1007/s11910-013-0392-x

Bullock, M. R., & Povlishock, J. T. (2007). Guidelines for management of severe traumatic brain injury. Editor's Commentary. *Journal of Neurotrauma, 24*(Suppl. 1), 2 p preceding S1. doi:10.1089/neu.2007.9998

Carney, N., Totten, A. M., O'Reilly, C., Ullman, J. S., Hawryluk, G. W., Bell, M. J., ... Ghajar, J. (2017). Guidelines for the management of severe traumatic brain injury, fourth edition. *Neurosurgery, 80*(1), 6–15. doi:10.1227/NEU.0000000000001432

Cecil, S., Chen, P., Callaway, S., Rowland, S., Adler, D., & Chen, J. (2010). Traumatic brain injury: Advanced multimodal neuromonitoring from theory to clinical practice. *Critical Care Nurse, 31*(2), 25–36. doi:10.4037/ccn2010226

Geyer, K., Meller, K., Kulpan, C., & Mowery, B. (2013). Traumatic brain injury in children: Acute care management. *Pediatric Nursing, 39*(6), 283–289.

Thompson, H., & Mauk, K. (2011). Care of the mild traumatic brain injured patient. *AANN and ARN Clinical Practice Guideline Series*. Retrieved from www.AANN.org

# 9

# Neurological Trauma: Spinal Cord Injury

## MECHANISM OF INJURY

- *A hyperflexion injury may result in rupture of which ligament?*
- Posterior longitudinal

Hyperflexion injury occurs when the spine is flexed beyond its normal range of motion. An example is a head-on motor vehicle collision (MVC). The head continues forward with sufficient speed and force for the chin to touch the chest. The stretch occurs posteriorly, causing the rupture or tearing of the posterior ligaments. The anterior vertebral body may be involved as a compression or wedge fracture. This injury may result in subluxation and/or disc herniation. Pediatric patients are at high risk for this mechanism of injury due to laxity of longitudinal ligaments.

▶ **HINT:** A *lipstick sign* refers to a lipstick smear on the trauma patient's shirt, which can indicate a hyperflexion injury.

- *A patient is diagnosed with cervical injury following a rear-end MVC. What is the most likely mechanism for the spinal injury?*
- Hyperextension

Hyperextension injuries occur when the spine is moved into an extreme hyperextension position. The stretch of the spine occursanteriorly, so the anterior longitudinal ligament would be the most likely ligament to be injured. The posterior vertebral body is at highest risk for fracture. Subluxation and herniated discs may also occur with this mechanism of injury. Extreme hyperextension can cause compression injury form the ligamentum flavum, resulting in cord contusion and hypoxia.

▶ **HINT:** Whiplash is commonly caused by a hyperextension mechanism of injury.

- *Axial loading or vertical compression mechanisms result in what type of vertebral fracture?*
- Burst fractures

Axial loading is the force applied vertically through the spine, causing increased pressure and vertebral burst fractures. Bone and disc matter are sent in all directions, including inward into the spinal canal, causing cord injury. This is commonly seen with diving injuries.

> ▶ **HINT:** Burst fractures are considered unstable even if ligaments are intact due to risk of bony pieces impinging or penetrating the spinal cord.

- *Side-impact MVC can result in which type of mechanism of injury to the spinal column?*
- **Rotational**

Rotational injuries occur with a twisting motion of the spine. Lateral flexion of the spine along with axial rotation is the mechanism of injury that causes rupture of the posterior longitudinal ligament, dislocation of facets, and vertebral compression fractures.

> ▶ **HINT:** The most common cause for rotational injury is side-impact MVC with an unrestrained occupant.

- *What type of trauma is most likely to result in a distraction injury to the cervical spine?*
- **Hanging**

Distraction injuries occur when the spine comes to a sudden stop while weight and momentum of the body continues to pull, causing tearing and laceration of the spinal cord.

> ▶ **HINT:** Another trauma that has been associated with distraction mechanism of injury is bungee cord jumping.

- *Following a gunshot wound, the bullet is found to have traveled near the spinal cord but did not transverse the cord. The injury to the spinal cord would be due to what mechanism?*
- **Concussion**

Concussive forces from the velocity of the bullet can cause injury to tissue without direct contact with the tissue. Penetrating cord injuries are caused by gunshot wounds and stab wounds. Gunshot injuries can penetrate the spinal cord and may be of high velocity or low velocity. Low-velocity injuries may not be associated with bony fractures.

> ▶ **HINT:** Avoid MRI if bullet fragments are present within the spinal cord or cord canal because of the effects of the magnet.

- *Trauma to spinal column resulting in burst fractures may cause cord injury through which mechanism of injury?*
- **Direct compression**

Primary injuries are injuries that occur due to the initial traumatic injury. This includes tissue destruction (lacerations, avulsions), compression (bony fragments, hematomas), and ischemia (damage or impingement spinal arteries). Spinal cord injuries can occur without radiographic evidence of vertebral fractures or dislocations. Secondary injuries are those injuries to the spinal cord that result in further injury and neurological deficits that occur after the initial trauma (Box 9.1).

> **HINT:** Level of function may be one to two levels above the level of injury due to secondary injuries worsening effect on neurological function.

**Box 9.1** Secondary Injuries to Spinal Cord

| |
|---|
| Ischemia/hypoperfusion |
| Vasogenic edema |
| Release of oxygen-free radicals |
| Acid–base imbalances |
| Inflammation |
| Hemorrhage/hematomas |
| Obstruction of CSF flow |

CSF, cerebrospinal fluid.

## TRAUMATIC INJURIES

- *Which type of odontoid fracture is considered to be a stable fracture?*
- **Type I**

Odontoid (also called *the dens*) is the bony structure of C2 that comes up anteriorly into the ring of C1 and allows for rotational movement of the neck. Fractures of the odontoid are classified as type I, II, and III, based on where the odontoid fracture occurred (Box 9.2). This grading system is also used to describe stability and guide treatment of the fracture. Type I is considered the most stable of the odontoid fractures. Instability of odontoid fractures is due to either cord compression or penetration of a bony fragment or ligament disruption between the odontoid process and the anterior aspect of C1.

> **HINT:** Type II odontoid fractures are the most common and are considered most unstable of the odontoid fractures.

**Box 9.2** Types of Odontoid Fractures

| | |
|---|---|
| Type I | Tip of odontoid bone above transverse ligament |
| Type II | Base of odontoid bone<br>Between transverse ligament and body of axis |
| Type III | Extends into the vertebral body |

> **HINT:** Another less common odontoid fracture is a vertical fracture through the odontoid and axis body.

- *The bilateral fracture of the ring of C2 with or without subluxation is called?*
- **Hangman's fracture**

Hangman's fracture (also called *traumatic spondylolisthesis*) is a bilateral fracture through the neural arch of C2. This injury may or may not be associated with anterior subluxation. Even though it is called *Hangman's fracture*, it is less likely to be seen in hangings. It is most commonly associated with falls and MVCs. Hangings typically cause fracture dislocation of C2 and complete disruption of ligaments between C2 and C3. The burst fracture of the ring of C1 is called *Jefferson's fracture*.

> **HINT:** Hangman's fracture is often associated with other spine pathologies including osteoarthritis and may be seen in elderly patients.

■ **Which type of cervical injury commonly results in death at the scene of an MVC?**
■ **Atlantooccipital dislocation**

Atlantodislocation (also called *internal decapitation*) is the avulsion of the atlas (C1) from the occiput and is usually fatal or results in prehospital cardiopulmonary arrest. The severe disruption of ligaments allows the cranium to move out of alignment of the spine. There are cases of patients presenting without neurological injury who commonly complain of the sensation of their "head falling off."

> **HINT:** Atlantooccipital dislocation is more common in pediatric patients than adults.

■ **Instability between C1 and C2 resulting in excessive movement between these two joints is called?**
■ **Atlantoaxial instability**

Atlas (C1) and axis (C2) instability may result from a cervical trauma and commonly involves injury to the transverse ligament or odontoid process. Injury severity varies from subluxation to dislocation.

> **HINT:** Congenital disorders may increase risk of atlantoaxial instability due to ligament laxity. An example is Down syndrome.

■ **A patient with total loss of motor and sensory function below the level of injury is called?**
■ **Complete cord injury**

There is some degree of correlation between the level of function and level of radiographic injury but this is not always consistent. The neurological level of injury (NLI) is the most caudal spinal cord level at which the normal motor/sensory function persists following spinal cord injury.

> **HINT:** An incomplete cord injury may initially appear functionally as a complete cord injury due to inflammation and edema in the cord.

■ **Following a traumatic injury, a football player presents with motor impairment greater in the upper extremities than the lower extremities. What is this incomplete injury called?**
■ **Central cord syndrome**

This spinal cord injury occurs in the central portion of the cord and is characterized by greater upper-extremity involvement of the upper extremities and especially the hands. The upper-extremity axons are located in the central portion of the spinal cord, and the axons that control the lower-extremity movement are located laterally in the cord. This incomplete cord syndrome is frequently caused by hyperextension injury or a fall. There is often a gradual return to function with the lower extremities first, followed by the upper, with finger movement returning last, with the hand being the most common site of residual motor weakness. Urinary retention and sensory abnormalities vary with severity of injury.

▶ **HINT:** Key to recognizing this syndrome is upper-extremity weakness greater than less lower-extremity weakness.

■ *What is typically spared in a patient with an anterior cord syndrome following a traumatic injury?*
■ **Vibratory sensation and proprioception**

Anterior cord syndrome is characterized by immediate onset of complete motor paralysis, loss of pain and temperature, with preservation of sensation in the posterior columns (includes vibration sense, position sense, deep pressure, two-point discrimination, and light touch). The anterior horn of the spinal cord contains the lower motor neurons (LMNs), and signs of LMN injuries include flaccid paralysis, atrophy of muscles, and areflexia. These symptoms are frequently associated with anterior cord syndromes and are caused by occlusion/compression mechanism of injury (e.g., traumatic herniated or dislocated disc, bone fragments, or epidural hematoma) or infarcted spinal cord in the areas supplied by the anterior spinal artery.

▶ **HINT:** This is the worst prognosis of the incomplete injuries, with 10% to 20% recovery of motor function.

■ *In Brown–Sequard syndrome, there is an ipsilateral loss of what function?*
■ **Motor function**

Brown–Sequard syndrome involves a hemisection of the spinal cord, which results in the ipsilateral loss of motor function and contralateral loss of pain and temperature. It is often seen with penetrating injuries, but may also be seen with epidural hematomas and a traumatically herniated cervical disc.

▶ **HINT:** This syndrome has the best prognosis with a 90% recovery of ambulation, regaining of sensation, and bowel/bladder function if caused by compression.

■ *When the lumbosacral spinal nerve roots are damaged at the level of L1 to L5, the syndrome is called?*
■ **Cauda equina syndrome (CES)**

CES is the result of damage to the lumbosacral nerve roots within the spinal canal at the level of L1 to L5. The cauda equina (CE) is a bundle of nerves distal to the conus medullaris. *Cauda equina* is Latin for *horse's tail*, and the nerve roots are called this because of the resemblance. CES results in areflexic bladder and bowel and lower-extremity paralysis. It is a peripheral nerve injury so it is considered to be a lower motor neuron injury. The syndrome result in variable motor and sensory losses. The prognosis of the recovery of motor function is good, however.

▶ **HINT:** A common sensory abnormality is called *saddle anesthesia* in which there is a paresthesia in the perineal region.

## ASSESSMENT/DIAGNOSIS

■ *A lateral plain radiograph can be used to diagnose what type of injury?*
■ **Bony or vertebral fractures**

A lateral x-ray is used to visualize bony abnormalities and fractures. Ligament injuries are not identified on plain radiographs unless the spinal column is out of alignment.

Flexion/extension x-rays may be obtained in an awake, cooperative patient without distracting injuries. MRI is the more definitive radiographic study used to identify ligament injuries.

> ▶ **HINT:** A patient with normal lateral cervical spine x-rays but complaints of pain in neck region should remain in cervical immobilization until flexion/extension views or MRI is obtained.

■ *While obtaining lateral radiographs of the cervical spine, what is most likely to interfere with visualization of the lower cervical vertebrae?*

■ **Shoulders**

Visualization from the occiput to T1 is required on lateral cervical x-ray to clear the presence of bony fractures. The shoulders frequently interfere with the ability to visualize C7 and the top of T1 in lateral cervical-spine radiographs. Obtaining a lateral x-ray using the swimmer's view can assist in identifying C7 and T1 vertebral bodies. Swimmer's view with a lateral x-ray involves downward traction on one arm and upward traction on the other with the x-ray beam aimed through the axilla of the abducted arm.

> ▶ **HINT:** The trauma nurse can retract downward on both arms equally to pull the shoulders out of the way to improve visualization of the cervical spine.

■ *Which radiographic view is used to determine the height and alignment of vertebral bodies?*

■ **Anterior–posterior (AP) view**

AP view allows the visualization of the vertebral bodies and determination of the height and alignment of the vertebral bodies.

> ▶ **HINT:** *AP view with open-mouth techniques* refers to the odontoid view and is used to recognize odontoid fractures.

■ *Which radiographic study can distinguish between spinal cord hemorrhage and vasogenic edema?*

■ **MRI**

An MRI is the gold standard radiographic study for the spinal cord. It is able to distinguish among ischemic injury, edema, and hemorrhage within the cord.

> ▶ **HINT:** MRI is also considered the gold standard for recognizing spinal ligament injuries.

■ *What is the purpose of magnetic resonance angiography (MRA) following a blunt trauma to the cervical region?*

■ **To evaluate vertebral arteries**

A complication of a blunt trauma or flexion/extension injury to the neck may result in vertebral or carotid artery injuries. Arterial dissections are associated with cervical fractures and spinal cord injuries.

> ▶ **HINT:** Altered mentation or neurological changes may indicate vertebral or carotid injury.

- *The presence of sacral sparing following a traumatic spinal cord injury (SCI) indicates what type of injury?*
- Incomplete injury

Anal contraction with stimulation or ability to feel pinprick or touch around the anus is called *anal sparing* and indicates incomplete injury. This is a phenomenon of sensation in the sacral region even though sensation is absent in the thoracic and lumbar areas. Sacral fibers may be protected more from compression injury, thus sparing the sacral dermatomes.

> ▶ HINT: Assessing for sacral sparing assists with determining an incomplete from complete injury.

- *How many cervical levels has sensory assessment tested?*
- C8

There are seven cervical vertebrae and eight paired cervical nerve roots. Sensory assessment of the cervical region is tested through C8. The cervical region is the only portion of the spinal column that has a greater number of paired nerve roots than vertebrae.

> ▶ HINT: Sensory assessment is performed using dermatome levels in spinal cord–injured patients, whereas motor assessment is performed using myotome levels.

- *Motor evaluation of the patient assesses which spinal cord tract?*
- Corticospinal

The corticospinal tract controls voluntary movement assessed with motor evaluation. The spinothalamic tract controls pain and temperature and is assessed by pinprick, light touch, and temperature. The posterior column of the spinal cord is responsible for proprioception and stereognosis. Proprioception is the ability to know where the body and extremities are in space. Stereognosis is the ability to perceive or understand an object by sense of touch.

> ▶ HINT: To determine spinal tract function; the first part of the word identifies where the spinal tract originates and the second part identifies where it terminates.

- *What does the Modified Barthel Index (MBI) tool measure?*
- Functional outcomes

The MBI is a functional outcome tool that may be used to assess the deficits associated with SCIs. The Functional Independence Measure (FIM) is another tool recommended to assess the deficits associated with SCIs.

> ▶ HINT: Acute spinal cord assessment may be done with American Spinal Injury Association (ASIA) scores, which use a motor index score, sensory index score, and functional outcome score.

## MEDICAL/SURGICAL MANAGEMENT

- *What is the primary prehospital intervention used to prevent further injury to the spinal cord?*
- Immobilization

The initial goal when caring for a trauma patient at the scene is to limit motion of a potentially injured spine and prevent further neurological involvement. A combination of a rigid cervical collar and supportive blocks on a backboard with straps is commonly used to stabilize the spine in the prehospital setting. The "neutral" position with the chin in midline position without hyperextension is recommended for spine immobilization.

▶ HINT: The use of rigid collars and spinal stabilization can increase intracranial pressure (ICP) and increase the risk of skin breakdown as well as aspiration.

- **What is the primary management of a patient with burst fractures of cervical vertebrae?**
- **Surgical cord decompression**

Burst fractures may require surgical removal of bone to achieve cord decompression. Bony pieces may compress the spinal cord and cause neurological injury. This injury requires surgical management, and closed reduction with cervical traction is not recommended for burst fractures.

▶ HINT: Immobilization of the spinal column is important to prevent further injury to the spinal cord from bony pieces.

- **What nonsurgical treatment is used on a patient with cervical subluxation and significant narrowing of the spinal column?**
- **Cervical traction**

Cervical facet dislocation or subluxation can cause cord compression and may require closed reduction with cervical traction. Early closed reduction of traumatic cervical fractures with subluxation or a narrowing spinal canal improves neurological outcomes. A halo vest may be used to stabilize cervical fractures externally, especially odontoid fractures.

▶ HINT: An inability to reduce a subluxation with external traction and weights may indicate a locked facet.

- **What is the primary treatment for neurogenic shock?**
- **Fluid administration**

The complication of neurogenic shock causes systemic vasodilation with hypotension. Fluid resuscitation is the treatment of choice to correct the hypotension. If fluids do not improve the blood pressure and perfusion, vasopressors may be initiated. A goal is to maintain the mean arterial pressure (MAP) between 85 and 90 mmHg to increase perfusion and improve neurological outcomes. The bradycardia associated with neurogenic shock does not typically require treatment, but, if symptomatic, an external pacemaker may be placed.

▶ HINT: Neurogenic shock is classified as a distributive shock.

## NURSING INTERVENTIONS

- **What respiratory parameter should be closely monitored in a spontaneously breathing acute SCI patient?**
- **Forced vital capacity (FVC) and/or negative inspiratory force (NIF)**

To determine the ability to ventilate, the respiratory parameters to monitor in a patient with an SCI to determine the ability to ventilate include FVC and NIF. The FVC is the forced maximal breath in followed by the maximal breath out. NIF is the ability to generate enough negative pressure in the chest to allow for inspiration. The FVC and NIF are used to evaluate the respiratory muscles and ability to generate an adequate breath.

> ▶ **HINT:** These parameters are commonly used to evaluate a person's ability to breathe spontaneously effectively.

- *When should a bowel regimen begin following an acute SCI?*
- **Upon admission**

When an acute SCI patient is admitted, the bowel regimen should be ordered and initiated. A bowel regimen includes adminstration of a suppository with finger stimulation timed appropriately for a once-a-day bowel movement. Timing of daily suppository for bowel training should be scheduled in acute care to facilitate rehabilitation and daily routines once the patient is discharged. An SCI above T12 may have reflex or spastic bowel, whereas an SCI below T12 level may be hyporeflexic with a flaccid bowel.

> ▶ **HINT:** The bowel regimen should only be discontinued with severe diarrhea.

- *A patient is able to void spontaneously following an acute SCI. What should the nurse assess for following the void?*
- **Postvoid residuals**

If a patient with an SCI is able to void spontaneously, use a bladder scan to assess for residual postvoiding. If greater than 200–300 mL, straight catheterization is recommended even if patient is spontaneously voiding. *Bladder training* refers to the removal of the indwelling bladder catheter with intermittent catheterization used in the presence of urinary retention.

> ▶ **HINT:** Bladder training is initiated as soon as patient is on maintenance fluids or oral intake.

- *What may be used to prevent postural hypotension in an SCI patient when getting the patient out of bed?*
- **Abdominal binder**

Postural hypotension is a common complication following an SCI. Position changing should be performed slowly to avoid syncope or near-syncope. Applying compression hose or leg wraps and abdominal binders to patients with SCI prior to getting them out of bed can help prevent orthostatic hypotension.

> ▶ **HINT:** Maintain adequate fluid volume to assist with management of orthostatic hypotension.

- *A patient is readmitted from rehabilitation following a cervical SCI. The patient suddenly develops hypertension with a blood pressure of 210/120 mmHg. What is the nurse's priority of care?*
- **Find the source of stimulation and remove it**

Priority of care with a hypertensive SCI patient due to autonomic hyperreflexia is to find the source of obnoxious stimulation and remove it (Box 9.3). The trauma nurse should elevate the head of the bed to lower the pressure and assess the patient for the cause of the autonomic hyperreflexia. Once the source is identified and removed, the patient's hypertension should resolve.

> ▶ HINT: Administration of an antihypertensive should not be the priority or first choice to manage the hypertension associated with autonomic hyperreflexia because once the source is removed, the patient will become hypotensive.

**Box 9.3** Nursing Interventions for Potential Sources of Autonomic Hyperreflexia

| Potential Sources of AH | Nursing Interventions |
| --- | --- |
| Urinary retention | Bladder scan and intermittent catheterization |
| Restrictive clothing | Loosen or remove clothing |
| Pressure sores | Reposition off of pressure scores |
| Fecal impaction | Remove fecal impaction |

AH, autonomic hyperreflexia.

## COMPLICATIONS

- *If a complete injury, at what level of spinal injury is the diaphragm affected and requires ventilatory support if a complete injury?*
- **Fourth cervical level**

The C4 level innervates the diaphragm. A patient with a cervical injury to the spinal cord at C4 level or above loses innervation to the diaphragm and usually requires intubation and mechanical ventilation. Cervical injuries at the six or seventh cervical level (C6 and C7) may still require intubation and ventilation at least in the acute period due to cord edema.

> ▶ HINT: Airway and breathing are the priorities of care in cervical spinal injuries.

- *What is the term for the lack of ability to regulate internal temperature following an SCI?*
- **Poikilothermia**

Loss of thermoregulatory function occurs in cord injuries above the thoracolumbar outflow due to loss of sympathetic nervous system (SNS) stimulation. Poikilothermia is the lack of internal regulation of the body temperature that occurs after an SCI. SCI patients are unable to vasoconstrict and shiver to conserve heat or sweat to dissipate heat.

> ▶ HINT: Nursing interventions for SCI patients include controlling the body temperature through external interventions.

- *What is the loss of motor function and reflexes below the level of injury called?*
- **Spinal shock**

Spinal shock is the loss of reflexes and motor function below the level of injury. Spinal shock occurs immediately after the injury and typically resolves within 2 to 16 weeks.

## 9. NEUROLOGICAL TRAUMA: SPINAL CORD INJURY

▶ **HINT:** Two of the reflexes routinely assessed in SCI patients include the ano-cutaneous and bulbocavernosus reflexes.

- *During neurogenic shock, what is the most common dysrhythmia?*
- **Sinus bradycardia**

Neurogenic shock is caused by the interruption of descending sympathetic fibers in the thoracic and cervical cord, producing vasodilation below the level of injury and hypotension. At the cervical level, complete injury interrupts sympathetic outflow to the heart, whereas the parasympathetic outflow remains intact via the vagus nerve, causing bradycardia in neurogenic shock.

▶ **HINT:** Neurogenic shock is associated with symptoms of hypotension and bradycardia, whereas spinal shock involves loss of motor function and reflexes.

- *What is the hypertensive crisis that can occur with patients following an SCI?*
- **Autonomic hyperreflexia (AH)**

An SCI with lesions above T6 may exhibit signs of AH. AH occurs with an obnoxious stimulation below the level of injury followed by life-threatening hypertension. Some of the potential causes of AH include bladder distension, catheterization, urinary tract infection, testicular torsion, pressure sores, and fecal impaction.

▶ **HINT:** AH is not an early complication and only occurs after spinal shock has resolved.

- *What electrolyte abnormality may commonly occur in a paraplegic patient due to prolonged inability to bear weight?*
- **Hypercalcemia**

Having a non–weight-bearing status for a prolonged period of time allows calcium to move from bone to serum, thus increasing calcium levels. This is a long-term complication and may require administration of calcitonin.

▶ **HINT:** Hypercalcemia can cause vasoconstriction and hypertension.

## REHABILITATION

- *What is the level of innervation required for the SCI patients to be able to feed themselves independently?*
- **C5 through C7**

The fifth cervical level innervates the biceps, allowing for flexion of the elbow, whereas the seventh cervical level innervates the triceps, allowing the elbow to extend. The flexion and extension of the arm allow patients to be able to feed themselves, even if they require utensils to be strapped to the hands.

> **HINT:** Flexing the wrist and spreading the fingers occurs at the C8 and T1 level of innervation and enables fine motor control. This allows the patient to perform greater independent activities of daily living (ADL).

■ *What is the level of innervation in which a paraplegic is able to push himself or herself in a wheelchair?*

■ **Level of C6**

The level of C6 innervation is considered to be the level that SCI patients require to perform ADL such as feeding, grooming, dressing, and pushing a wheelchair.

> **HINT:** This is the level of function not necessarily the actual level of injury.

# Sample Exam Questions

1. Which of the following is the BEST recommendation for bladder training of a spinal cord–injured patient in the acute care setting following a trauma?

    A. Perform an intermittent straight cath procedure following bladder scanning.
    B. Maintain an indwelling urinary catheter until able to void.
    C. Surgically place a suprapubic catheter.
    D. Allow patient to void spontaneously when the bladder becomes overfilled.

2. When a spinal cord–injured patient has greater weakness in the upper extremities than the lower extremities, which of the following incomplete cord injuries should be suspected?

    A. Posterior cord syndrome
    B. Brown–Sequard cord syndrome
    C. Anterior cord syndrome
    D. Central cord syndrome

3. What is the American Spinal Injury Association impairment scale used to assess in a trauma patient?

    A. Level of consciousness
    B. Risk for anticoagulation therapy
    C. Spinal cord function
    D. Gait analysis

4. Which of the following would be the most appropriate goal in a patient with a penetrating incomplete injury to the spinal cord within the first 24 hours of injury?

    A. Initiate bowel and bladder training.
    B. Administer high-dose steroids.
    C. Maintain mean arterial pressure ≥80 mmHg.
    D. Administer low-dose unfractionated heparin to prevent venous thromboembolism.

5. A nonintubated patient with cervical fractures and cord compression is admitted to the ICU for close monitoring of respiratory status. Which of the following respiratory function tests is NOT routinely used to evaluate the respiratory function of a nonintubated patient with a spinal cord injury?

    A. Forced vital capacity
    B. Tidal volume
    C. Forced expiratory volume in 1 second
    D. Negative inspiratory force

6. Upon getting a spinal cord–injured (SCI) patient out of bed, the nurse notes the patient's blood pressure has decreased significantly. Which of the following should be used to prevent orthostatic hypotension in an SCI patient?

    A. Utilization of spine brace when out of bed
    B. Administration of a vasopressor
    C. Maintain foot elevation
    D. Abdominal binder

7. Which of the following conditions is best described as a temporary areflexic state with the loss of autonomic control and muscle tone below the level of injury?
   A. Neurogenic shock
   B. Autonomic hyperreflexia
   C. Brachial plexus syndrome
   D. Spinal shock

8. Which of the following best describes the physiology of neurogenic shock?
   A. Loss of thoracic sympathetic innervation
   B. Spinal cord concussion
   C. Ischemic and reperfusion injuries to the spinal cord
   D. Compression of the spinal nerve roots

9. Urinary bladder function may be affected by spinal cord injury (SCI). Which of the following is NOT a physiological effect of SCI on bladder control?
   A. Incontinence due to reflexive bladder
   B. Bladder retention due to loss of reflexive bladder
   C. Obstruction to outflow
   D. Combination of reflexive and flaccid bladder

10. Which of the following is a TRUE statement regarding autonomic hyperreflexia (AH) following a spinal cord injury (SCI)?
    A. AH is common during the acute period following an SCI.
    B. AH occurs in patients with SCI at the level of T11 or higher.
    C. Hypotension is the most common presenting symptom of AH.
    D. Noxious stimulus below the level of injury can trigger AH.

11. Which of the following would be the BEST nursing intervention to prevent the incidence of autonomic hyperreflexia in rehabilitation centers?
    A. Bladder education program with the patient and family
    B. Administration of antihypertensive agents
    C. Initiation of a bowel program
    D. Use of alternatives to indwelling catheters such as condom catheters for males

## BIBLIOGRAPHY

Coggrave, M., Mills, P., Willms, R., & Eng, J. J. (2014). Bowel dysfunction and management following spinal cord injury. In J. J. Eng, R. W. Teasell, W. C. Miller, D. L. Wolfe, A. F. Townson, J. T. C. Hsieh, … A. McIntyre (Eds.), *Spinal cord injury rehabilitation evidence* (pp. 1–48). Vancouver, BC: SCIRE Project. Retrieved from https://scireproject.com/wp-content/uploads/bowel_management-1.pdf

Evans, L. T., Lollis, S. S., & Ball, P. A. (2013). Management of acute spinal cord injury in the neurocritical care unit. *Neurosurgery Clinics of North America*, 24(3), 339–347. doi:10.1016/j.nec.2013.02.007

Fehlings, M., Tetreuit, L., Wilson, J., Kwon, B., Burns, A., Martin, A., … Harrop, J. (2017). A clinical practice guideline for the management of acute spinal cord injury: Introduction, rationale, and scope. *Global Spine Journal*, 7(3, Suppl.), 84S–94S. doi:10.1177/2192568217703387

Hadley, M., & Walters, B. (2003). Guidelines for the management of acute cervical spine and spinal cord injuries. *American Association of Neurological Surgeons, 72*(Suppl. 2), 1–259.

Hadley, M. N., & Walters, B. C. (2013). Introduction to the guidelines for the management of acute cervical spine and spinal cord injuries. *Neurosurgery, 72*(Suppl. 2), 5–16. doi:10.1227/NEU.0b013e3182773549

Phillips, A. A., & Krassioukov, A. V. (2015). Contemporary cardiovascular concerns after spinal cord injury: Mechanisms, maladaptations, and management. *Journal of Neurotrauma, 32*(24), 1927–1942. doi:10.1089/neu.2015.3903

Rundquist, J., Gassaway, J., Bailey, J., Lingefelt, P., Reyes, I., & Thomas, J. (2011). Nursing bedside education and care management time during inpatient spinal cord injury rehabilitation. *Journal of Spinal Cord Medicine, 34*(2), 205–215. doi:10.1179/107902611X12971826988255

Stein, D. M., & Sheth, K. N. (2015). Management of acute spinal cord injury. *Continuum (Minneap Minn), 21*(1), 159–187. doi:10.1212/01.CON.0000461091.09736.0c

# 10

# Practice Exam

1. Which of the following tumor types will have a higher incidence in pediatric populations and have a decreased incidence with age?

   A. Glioblastoma
   B. Pilocytic astrocytoma
   C. Central nervous system lymphoma
   D. Metastatic brain tumor

2. A patient presents with progressive neurological deficits and has a recent history of transient neurological attack. This patient is most likely experiencing which of the following types of stroke?

   A. Thrombotic stroke
   B. Embolic stroke
   C. Subarachnoid hemorrhage
   D. Vasospasms

3. Which of the following best describes a coup injury?

   A. Injury occurs at the point of impact.
   B. Injury occurs on the contralateral side of impact.
   C. It is an acceleration injury.
   D. It is a deceleration injury.

4. A patient is admitted to the ICU with persistent epileptic seizures lasting beyond 90 minutes. Which of the following best describes the seizure activity?

   A. Epileptic seizure
   B. Epilepsy
   C. Refractory seizure
   D. Nonepileptic seizure

5. Which of the following would be the best technique to use to assess for cerebrospinal fluid in bloody drainage from the nose following a traumatic brain injury?

   A. Glucose test
   B. Halo test

C. Send to lab for hemoglobin level
D. Litmus test

6. Which of the following is the most common cause of an embolic stroke?
   A. Atrial septal defect
   B. Atrial fibrillation
   C. Calcified lesion
   D. Angioplasty

7. Cranial nerve (CN) VII (facial nerve) is commonly involved with Bell's palsy. Where does this CN originate?
   A. Pons
   B. Medulla
   C. Midbrain
   D. Basal ganglia

8. Which of the following electrolyte abnormalities is LESS likely to result in a seizure?
   A. Hyponatremia
   B. Hyperkalemia
   C. Hypocalcemia
   D. Hypomagnesemia

9. A patient in the ICU following a severe traumatic brain injury suddenly demonstrates profuse sweating, sustained tachycardia, hypertension, and fever. Which of the following is the most likely cause?
   A. Neurogenic fever
   B. Diencephalic seizure
   C. Paroxysmal sympathetic hyperactivity
   D. Cerebral salt wasting syndrome

10. In severe cases of cerebral palsy, there may be a delay in growth and development. Which of the following conditions can occur in these cases?
    A. Coagulopathy
    B. Immunocompromise
    C. Failure to thrive
    D. Locked-in syndrome

11. Which of the following best describes the penumbra in an ischemic stroke?
    A. Irreversibly damaged tissue
    B. Normal healthy tissue
    C. Presence of vasogenic cerebral edema
    D. Reversible ischemic tissue

12. A patient is admitted to the trauma ICU following a traumatic brain injury due to vehicle rollover. The patient is hypotensive and tachycardic. Which of the following is the most accurate statement?
    A. Hypotension following traumatic brain injury (TBI) indicates presence of epidural hematoma.

B. Hypotension is sign of blood loss but is not considered a sign of TBI.
C. Scalp lacerations can be easily controlled with direct compression.
D. Neurogenic shock following TBI results in hypotension.

13. Which of the following has been found to be the most effective in preventing embolic strokes due to atrial fibrillation?

    A. Aspirin
    B. Low-molecular-weight heparin
    C. Warfarin (Coumadin)
    D. Clopidogrel (Plavix)

14. Which of the following scales are used to determine the overall prognosis in patients with a brain tumor?

    A. PedsQL
    B. Functional Iindependence Measure
    C. CHADS2 score
    D. Karnofsky Performance Status Scale

15. Which of the following best describes a radiculopathy?

    A. Compression of the cord with central stenosis
    B. Inflammation of bone and cartilage of joint
    C. Compression of nerve roots with foraminal stenosis
    D. Symptomatic degenerative changes of osteoarthritis

16. Your patient presents with left upper extremity weakness and facial droop. Which of the following vessels is most likely involved in this stroke?

    A. Anterior cerebral artery
    B. Middle cerebral artery
    C. Posterior cerebral artery
    D. Basilar artery

17. Your patient has sustained a traumatic brain injury and a basilar skull fracture. The physician has ordered a nasogastric tube (NG) be placed. Which of the following is your best response?

    A. Place the NG according to the physician's order.
    B. Discuss with the physician the need to place an enteral feeding tube.
    C. Insert the gastric tube orally.
    D. Ask the physician to place the NG.

18. During a stroke assessment, the patient has been found to have a deviated gaze. Which of the following would be the most correct statement regarding the gaze?

    A. Dysconjugate gaze
    B. Upward gaze
    C. Gaze toward the affected side
    D. Gaze away from affected side

19. What type of seizure is an aura classified as?
    A. Simple partial
    B. Complex partial
    C. Generalized
    D. Nonconvulsive

20. Your patient presents with the diagnosis of Guillain–Barré syndrome. Which of the following is the priority of care for this patient?
    A. Assessment of vital capacity
    B. Reassurance of the patient
    C. Preparing for electromyography testing
    D. Obtaining CT scan of the spine

21. A patient sustained cervical fractures at the C4 and C5 level from a motor vehicle collision. In the ED, initially he was moving all extremities equally. He suddenly became hemiplegic on the left side. Which of the following is the most likely cause for this neurological change?
    A. Carotid artery dissection
    B. Spinal cord injury
    C. Spinal epidural hematoma
    D. Cerebral edema

22. Which of the following therapeutic interventions is frequently recommended to manage a cerebrospinal fluid (CSF) leak?
    A. Drain CSF with a lumbar drain.
    B. Administer mannitol.
    C. Limit fluid intake.
    D. Maintain head-of-the-bed elevation greater than 30 degrees.

23. The mother of a 6-year-old girl just diagnosed with pilocytic astrocytoma asks the nurse what her child's prognosis is. Which of the following would be the best response by the nurse?
    A. This type of tumor has a good prognosis and can usually be managed with surgery.
    B. The tumor is malignant and frequently metastasizes to the spine.
    C. This tumor is associated with poor prognosis. I would encourage you to speak with a palliative care physician.
    D. The prognosis is not well known. She will probably require long-term chemotherapy.

24. Which of the following cerebral arteries is most likely involved in the presentation of "locked-in" syndrome during a stroke?
    A. Anterior cerebral artery
    B. Posterior communicating artery
    C. Internal carotid artery
    D. Basilar artery

25. Following a minor brain injury (concussion), the patient may experience which of the following symptoms over the next 6 months?
    A. Periods of aphasia
    B. Swallowing deficits
    C. Difficulty concentrating
    D. Ataxia

26. A patient presents with signs of occipital headache and abnormal motor strength. The MRI found herniation of the cerebellar tonsils, vermis, and fourth ventricle. How would this Chiari malformation be classified?
    A. Type I
    B. Type II
    C. Type III
    D. Type IV

27. The patient presents in the ED with expressive aphasia and paralysis of the right arm and leg. He has a decreased level of consciousness and rapid respiration. Which of the following is your priority of care?
    A. Obtain a STAT CT scan.
    B. Administer alteplase immediately.
    C. Perform a baseline National Institutes of Health Stroke Scale (NIHSS).
    D. Secure an airway and ensure ventilation.

28. A patient presents with low-back pain. Upon review of the spinal radiographs, multiple levels of osteophytes are noted. Which of the following best describes an osteophyte?
    A. Inflammation of synovial joints
    B. Degeneration of vertebral body with increased bone formation
    C. Stenosis of the nerve root as exits lateral foramen
    D. Compression of lumbar disc

29. Anticholinesterase agents are used to improve myasthenia gravis muscle function through which of the following actions?
    A. Increase secretion of acetylcholine.
    B. Prevent breakdown of acetylcholine.
    C. Increase sensitization postsynaptic receptors.
    D. Increase number of postsynaptic muscle receptors.

30. Which of the following diagnostic studies is considered the most reliable to identify spinal cord and soft-tissue injuries?
    A. Lateral cervical spine radiographs
    B. CT scan
    C. MRI
    D. Flexion/extension radiographs

31. A patient reports he or she experiences irritability and mood changes days prior to a seizure. What is this period called?
    A. Preictal
    B. Aura
    C. Intraictal
    D. Postictal

32. Which of the following secondary injuries would be the most important determinants of outcomes in patients following traumatic brain injuries?
    A. Hyponatremia and tachycardia
    B. Hypoxia and hypotension
    C. Hyperglycemia and hypothermia
    D. Hyperthermia and metabolic acidosis

33. Which of the following would be a contraindication for administering a thrombolytic?
    A. Patient's home medications include Eliquis
    B. National Institutes of Health Stroke Scale score of 10
    C. Patient on a daily aspirin
    D. Negative CT scan

34. Your patient has a sudden loss of consciousness. An emergency CT is obtained and an intracerebral hemorrhage (ICH) is seen. Which of the following would be the LEAST common cause of an ICH?
    A. Anticoagulation therapy
    B. Hypertensive crisis
    C. Aneurysm rupture
    D. Vascular tumor

35. Which of the following statements is a true regarding cerebral palsy (CP)?
    A. CP is not preventable.
    B. CP is a disease found in children but can be cured.
    C. Most children with CP will die by the age of 10 years.
    D. CP has no cure.

36. Plasmapheresis is treatment commonly used in managing Guillain–Barré. It involves the:
    A. Complete exchange of red blood cells
    B. Removal of antibodies with plasma exchange
    C. Washing of the white blood cells to clear allergens
    D. Filtering of the immunoglobulins

37. Which of the following best describes Moyamoya disease?
    A. Small, multiple aneurysms in the microcirculation
    B. Arteriovenous malformations
    C. Hyperlipidemia deposits of fat in the cerebral vessel wall
    D. Progressive occlusion of the intracranial internal carotid artery with collateral flow

38. When clearing a cervical spine injury in the acute period following a traumatic event, which of the following is NOT required?
    A. Maintain cervical immobilization until cleared of ligament injury
    B. Flexion/extension evaluation in an awake, asymptomatic patient
    C. Visualization of C1 through T1 on lateral cervical radiographs
    D. MRI of cervical spine

39. Which of the following is a known risk factor for a brain tumor?
    A. Use of cellular phones
    B. Exposure to ionized radiation
    C. Consumption of fish with high mercury levels
    D. Use of microwaves

40. Lobar intracerebral hemorrhage frequently presents with which neurological symptom?
    A. Cranial nerve deficits
    B. Decreased level of consciousness
    C. Pinpoint pupils
    D. Horner's syndrome

41. Patients with Mèniére's disease often complain of feelings of aural fullness accompanied by which of the following other symptoms?
    A. Worst headache of their lives
    B. Urinary incontinence
    C. Roaring sound in ears
    D. Frequent ear infections

42. A patient is experiencing a tonic–clonic seizure on the floor next to the bed. To prevent injury during the seizure, which of the following is the most appropriate intervention by the nurse?
    A. Move the bed and any other objects away from the patient to prevent injury.
    B. Just monitor the patient and do not attempt to make any interventions during the seizure.
    C. Move the patient away from the bed and to the middle of the floor.
    D. Restrain the patient to prevent injury.

43. Which of the following is NOT considered a cholinergic side effect of anticholinesterase medications used in managing myasthenia gravis?
    A. Diarrhea
    B. Nausea and vomiting
    C. Increased salivation
    D. Urinary retention

44. Intracellular swelling in the brain occurred following an anoxic brain injury. What is this called?
    A. "Steal" phenomenon
    B. Neurogenic cerebral edema

C. Vasogenic cerebral edema
D. Cytotoxic cerebral edema

45. Which of the following frequently presents with nausea, vomiting, and ataxia?

    A. Cerebellar hemorrhage
    B. Thalamic hemorrhage
    C. Pituitary hemorrhage
    D. Frontal lobe hemorrhage

46. Which of the following radiographs is best used to identify spinal segmental instability in an awake, nontraumatic patient?

    A. Cervical CT scan
    B. Diffusion-weighted imagery
    C. Myelogram
    D. Flexion extension x-rays

47. Which of the following is a TRUE statement about rehabilitation with spinal cord–injured (SCI) patients?

    A. Rehabilitation begins after the patient is stabilized in the acute period.
    B. The goal of rehabilitation in SCI patients is to return the patient to his or her prior level of functioning.
    C. Preventing secondary injuries in SCI patients is a component of rehabilitation.
    D. It provides long-term assistance to patients with SCI.

48. The cardinal feature of Guillain–Barré includes which of the following?

    A. Unilateral ascending paralysis
    B. Descending bilateral paresthesia
    C. Bilateral ascending paralysis
    D. Bilateral spasticity in upper extremities

49. Which of the following has been associated with a genetic increase in risk of brain tumor?

    A. Down syndrome
    B. Autoimmune disorders
    C. Glioblastoma gene
    D. Neurofibromatosis

50. Which of the following is the priority of care of a patient following a seizure?

    A. Reorient the patient to place and time.
    B. Determine whether the patient has a recollection of the seizure.
    C. Maintain the patient's airway and breathing.
    D. Assess for the presence of Todd's paralysis.

51. When assessing a patient with meningitis, you passively flex the patient's neck and his or her knees automatically flex upward. What is this called?

    A. Brudzinski's sign
    B. Romberg sign

C. Kernig's sign
D. Kehr's sign

52. A patient presents to your unit with the diagnosis of an intracerebral hemorrhage. Which of the following blood pressure (BP) parameters orders would be expected?

    A. Keep systolic BP >220 mmHg.
    B. Maintain systolic BP <100 mmHg.
    C. Maintain systolic BP between 130 and 150 mmHg.
    D. Treat BP only if patient rebleeds.

53. Postoperative management of carotid endarterectomy (CE) includes monitoring of neurological assessment. Which of the following physiological changes is NOT considered a common cause for the neurological deterioration following the CE?

    A. Reperfusion injury with cerebral edema
    B. Embolic showers
    C. Cerebral ischemia
    D. Subdural hematoma

54. Which of the following patients is LEAST likely to experience a chronic subdural hematoma?

    A. An 85-year-old male patient
    B. A patient with severe dementia
    C. Patient on anticoagulation therapy
    D. An alcoholic patient

55. Which of the following types of headache may be accompanied by an aura?

    A. Cluster headaches
    B. Migraine headaches
    C. Stress headaches
    D. Daily headaches

56. Which of the following is LESS meaningful when talking to the patient about the brain tumor pathology and prognosis?

    A. Malignant or benign
    B. Tumor growth
    C. Location of tumor
    D. Patient's comorbidities

57. Aneurysms can be classified based on the shape, size, and origin of the aneurysm. Which of the following terms best describes an aneurysm with a neck?

    A. Saccular aneurysm
    B. Fusiform aneurysm
    C. Giant aneurysm
    D. Mycotic aneurysm

58. A patient is diagnosed with disc protrusion (propulsion). Which of the following best describes disc herniation?
    A. Occurs when nucleus ruptures through innermost fibers of the annulus fibrosus with no disruption to outer annular fibers.
    B. Rupture of nucleus distorts the outermost fibers of the annulus and causes bulge outward.
    C. Complete split of annulus allows nuclear material to leak out of surrounding spaces.
    D. Extruded nuclear substance is no longer attached to material remaining within the disc and fragments may float around the spinal canal.

59. A paraplegic patient is being taught in rehabilitation to prevent pressure ulcers while sitting in the wheelchair. Which of the following strategies is the MOST important to preventi pressure ulcers?
    A. Use air cushion pad at all times.
    B. Perform frequent shifts in the chair.
    C. Use a Hoyer lift to move in the chair.
    D. Massage skin frequently to improve skin circulation.

60. Hydrocephalus present in Chiari type II malformations is classified as which of the following?
    A. Communicating hydrocephalus
    B. Noncommunicating hydrocephalus
    C. Degenerative hydrocephalus
    D. Productive hydrocephalus

61. Which of the following autoimmune disorders is most commonly associated with trigeminal neuralgia?
    A. Lupus
    B. Multiple sclerosis
    C. Myasthenia gravis
    D. CREST syndrome

62. Which of the following aneurysms is caused by septic emboli associated with bacterial endocarditis?
    A. Charcot–Bouchard
    B. Giant aneurysm
    C. Ehler's aneurysm
    D. Mycotic aneurysm

63. Hyperventilation with the lowering of $PaCO_2$ causes which of the following physiological effects in the cerebral circulation?
    A. Cerebral vasodilation
    B. Cerebral vasoconstriction
    C. Increased intracranial pressure
    D. Cerebral edema

64. Which of the following best describes the pain syndrome associated with trigeminal neuralgia?
    A. Dull, constant aching pain along the jaw line
    B. Constant, severe, knifelike facial pain occurs bilaterally
    C. Muscle spasms along the V1 and V2 branches, which result in cramping-like pain
    D. Shock-like sensations, intermittent or episodic facial pain that occurs unilaterally

65. Which of the following is the most common result of an intracranial aneurysm rupture?
    A. Subarachnoid hemorrhage
    B. Epidural hematoma
    C. Subdural hematoma
    D. Intracerebral hemorrhage

66. A vaccine has been developed for which of the following types of meningitis?
    A. Tuberculosis meningitis
    B. Meningococcal meningitis
    C. *Haemophilus influenzae* meningitis
    D. *Listeria*

67. Which of the following neurotransmitters will inhibit seizure activity?
    A. Glutamine
    B. Dopamine
    C. Acetylcholine
    D. Gamma-aminobutyric acid

68. Which of the following types of tremor occur due to a fixed posture against gravity?
    A. Kinetic intentional tremor
    B. Postural tremor
    C. Magnetic gait tremor
    D. Ataxic tremor

69. When administering an osmotic diuretic, such as mannitol, which of the following laboratory values should be closely monitored?
    A. Calcium
    B. Creatinine
    C. Potassium
    D. Serum osmolality

70. Which of the following is the least severe or mildest form of spina bifida (SB)?
    A. Myelomeningocele
    B. SB occulta
    C. Syrinx
    D. Meningocele

71. Cerebral aneurysms can occur throughout the cerebral circulation. Which of the following is the most common location of a cerebral aneurysm?
    A. Anterior circulation
    B. Extracranial internal carotid artery
    C. Basilar artery
    D. Vertebral artery

72. Which of the following brain tumors is classified as an extraaxial tumor?
    A. Oligodendrioglioma
    B. Astrocytoma
    C. Pituitary adenoma
    D. Ependymoma

73. Trigeminal neuralgia is a type of neuropathic pain. The best treatment for neuropathic pain includes which of the following?
    A. An antiepileptic
    B. Opioid
    C. Nonsteroidal anti-inflammatory drug
    D. Benzodiazepine

74. The most common presentation for a subarachnoid hemorrhage is which of the following?
    A. Sudden development of paralysis
    B. Ascending bilateral paralysis
    C. Complaints of "worst headache" of one's life
    D. Expressive aphasia

75. Which of the following cranial nerves (CNs) is most commonly involved in long-term complications of bacterial meningitis?
    A. CN V (trigeminal nerve)
    B. CN I (olfactory nerve)
    C. CN IX (glossopharyngeal nerve)
    D. CN VIII (acoustic nerve)

76. Which of the following would be the most appropriate method used to lower intracranial pressure?
    A. Elevate the head of the bed.
    B. Elevate the foot of the bed.
    C. Perform carotid massage.
    D. Place rolled towels on either side of the neck.

77. A patient has a seizure that is localized to the right upper extremity without impairment of consciousness. What is the classification of the seizure?
    A. Simple partial
    B. Complex partial
    C. Generalized seizure
    D. Nonepileptic seizure

78. A patient is admitted with an acute ischemic stroke with a current history of sleep apnea. Which of the following would be the most appropriate intervention to improve outcomes?

    A. Continuous positive airway pressure
    B. Monitor end-tidal carbon dioxide levels
    C. Intubation and mechanical ventilation
    D. Place patient on ketogenic diet

79. Neuroleptic agents are most commonly used to suppress symptoms of Tourette's syndrome. Which of the following is the most common neurological side effect of neuroleptic agents?

    A. Dystonic movements
    B. Weight loss
    C. Acute renal failure
    D. Angioedema

80. Which of the following pituitary adenomas is most amendable to medical management?

    A. Adrenocorticotropic-secreting adenoma
    B. Nonsecreting adenoma
    C. Growth hormone-secreting adenoma
    D. Prolactinoma

81. Mechanism of hyperflexion of the neck during a trauma can result in which of the following patterns of injury?

    A. Disruption of anterior ligament with posterior vertebral fracture
    B. Central cord syndrome
    C. Brown–Sequard cord syndrome
    D. Disruption of the posterior ligament and fractures of the anterior vertebral body

82. Which of the following forms of spina bifida has the highest risk for experiencing complications from the time of birth?

    A. Meningocele
    B. Chiari malformation type I
    C. Spina bifida occulta
    D. Myelomeningocele

83. A patient is admitted with the diagnosis of a Hunt and Hess scale grade III subarachnoid hemorrhage. You would expect the patient to have which of the following symptoms on neurological examination?

    A. Asymptomatic presentation
    B. Unresponsive with Glasgow Coma Scale score of 5
    C. Abnormal posturing
    D. Drowsy or confused

84. In benign essential tremor (BET), the tremor occurs when?

    A. During rest
    B. At night

C. During intentional activity
D. Only during stress

85. A burst fracture of the vertebral body is most commonly associated with which mechanism of injury?

    A. Hyperflexion
    B. Hyperextension
    C. Torsion injury
    D. Axial loading

86. Which of the following radiographic studies is considered the gold standard used to identify the location and characteristic of a central nervous system tumor?

    A. CT without contrast
    B. CT with contrast
    C. MRI
    D. Magnetic resonance arteriogram

87. Following an injury to the spinal cord, your patient exhibits the following symptoms: bilateral loss of motor function, pain, and temperature, but the patient maintains proprioception and light touch. Which of the following spinal cord syndromes does he or she exhibit?

    A. Anterior cord syndrome
    B. Central cord syndrome
    C. Brown–Sequard cord syndrome
    D. Complete cord injury

88. Creutzfeldt–Jakob disease is a spongiform encephalopathy, which is considered a prion disease. Which of the following is a prion disease?

    A. Abnormal version of infectious protein
    B. Protozoa infection found in stagnant water
    C. Bovine tapeworm that invades brain tissue
    D. Tick-borne disease that infects meninges

89. Which of the following is NOT classified as a simple partial seizure?

    A. Somatosensory seizure
    B. Psychogenic seizure
    C. Autonomic seizure
    D. Atonic seizure

90. Which of the following may be a complication of a lumbar puncture in a patient with a subarachnoid hemorrhage?

    A. Herniation syndrome
    B. Development of aphasia
    C. Kernig's sign
    D. Brudizinski's sign

91. A patient requiring a posterior cervical fusion is placed in the prone position for a prolonged period of time and experiences significant blood loss and hypotension. Which of the following is the most likely complication of this scenario?
    A. Visual losses
    B. Mesenteric ischemia
    C. Acute kidney injury
    D. Intracerebral hemorrhage

92. Vasospasm is the focal narrowing of cerebral vessels. This is most likely to appear during which of the following time periods after the subarachnoid hemorrhage (SAH)?
    A. 2 to 3 days post SAH
    B. 14 days post SAH
    C. 7 to 10 days post SAH
    D. 3 months post SAH

93. Which of the following is most commonly used to manage the vasogenic cerebral edema surrounding a brain tumor?
    A. Corticosteroids
    B. Mannitol
    C. Hypertonic saline
    D. Hypothermia

94. Which of the following is a recognized management of vasospasm following subarachnoid hemorrhage?
    A. Hypervolemia
    B. Hypertension
    C. Hypothermia
    D. Hemodilution

95. The goal of medical treatment for benign essential tremor is best described as which of the following?
    A. Cessation of all tremor activity
    B. Decreasing the frequency of the tremors
    C. Decreasing the amplitude of the tremors
    D. Treating the emotional effects of the tremors

96. A cerebrospinal fluid analysis of bacterial meningitis includes all of the following except?
    A. Elevated protein
    B. Elevated glucose
    C. Increased lactate
    D. Elevated neutrophils

97. Which of the following can increase the risk of spina bifida during fetal development?
    A. Exercise
    B. Maternal trauma

C. Vitamin C deficiency
D. Exposure to high temperatures

98. Which of the following electrolyte abnormality most commonly follows subarachnoid hemorrhage?

    A. Hyperphosphatemia
    B. Hyponatremia
    C. Hyperkalemia
    D. Hypocalcemia

99. A patient presents with neurological deficits lasting 20 minutes followed by complete resolution of symptoms. During the transient ischemic attack workup, the intracranial internal carotid artery was found to be 70% obstructed. Which of the following is NOT recommended at this time?

    A. Dual antiplatelet with clopidogrel (Plavix) and aspirin
    B. Maintain systolic blood pressure less than 140 mmHg
    C. Immediate angioplasty and stenting
    D. High intensity statins

100. Which of the following has been identified as a precipitating factor that can trigger the onset of Guillain–Barré syndrome?

    A. Hyperthyroidism
    B. Vaccinations
    C. Urinary tract infection
    D. Bacteremia

101. A patient with Brown–Sequard cord syndrome would present with which of the following patterns of symptoms?

    A. Ipsilateral motor loss and contralateral pain and temperature loss
    B. Loss of both motor and sensory function below the level of injury
    C. Greater upper-extremity weakness verus lower-extremity weakness
    D. Loss of sensory function but maintains motor function bilaterally

102. The larval stage of the pig tapeworm eventually enters through the gastrointestinal tract and moves into brain tissue. This larvae is acquired by which of the following?

    A. Swimming in stagnant water
    B. Tick bites
    C. Eating undercooked pork
    D. Mosquito bite

103. Which of the following brain tumor types is amendable to surgical gross resection and tumor biopsy?

    A. Frontal lobe glioblastoma
    B. Brainstem glioma
    C. Tumor located in Broca's area
    D. Vascular tumor

104. Which of the following best describes cerebral palsy (CP)?

    A. CP is a progressive motor movement disorder.
    B. CP is always caused by hypoxic injuries during delivery.
    C. CP is a permanent injury that is nonprogressive.
    D. CP is a reversible ischemic injury.

105. Complementary medicine has been used to manage pain in trigeminal neuralgia. Which of the following would be the most appropriate treatment?

    A. Spinal manipulation
    B. Acupuncture
    C. Meditation
    D. Herbal supplements

106. Following spinal cord injury, the nurse needs to know complications that can occur at the different levels of spinal cord injury. At which level is the diaphragm innervated?

    A. C2
    B. C4
    C. C6
    D. T1

107. A long-term complication of a subarachnoid hemorrhage includes which of the following:

    A. Vasospasm
    B. Cerebral edema
    C. Hydrocephalus
    D. Nausea and vomiting

108. Which of the following types of encephalopathy is described as an acute process, resulting in cerebral edema induced by rapid changes in serum osmolality?

    A. Septic encephalopathy
    B. Drug-induced delirium
    C. Hepatic encephalopathy
    D. Dialysis disequilibrium syndrome

109. Your patient is experiencing a seizure. Upon recovery of the seizure, it was noted he had left arm paralysis. This is phenomenon is called?

    A. Postictal period
    B. Aura
    C. Todd's paralysis
    D. Electromechanical dissociation (EMD)

110. Normal-pressure hydrocephalus (NPH) typically presents with all of the following except:

    A. Nausea and vomiting
    B. Gait disturbances

C. Urinary symptoms
D. Dementia

111. Which of the following tests is most commonly used to screen for fetal spina bifida during pregnancy?

    A. Maternal serum alpha-feto protein test
    B. Amniocentesis
    C. Estriol
    D. Human chorionic gonadotropin

112. The cervical region contains seven vertebral bodies. How many paired cervical nerve roots are found in the cervical region?

    A. Six
    B. Seven
    C. Eight
    D. Nine

113. A fusiform aneurysm is best described as which of the following?

    A. Aneurysm with a neck
    B. Aneurysm measuring greater than 2.5 cm in diameter
    C. Tiny aneurysm in the microcirculation
    D. Aneurysm forms an outpouching of the vessel wall

114. Which of the following statements best describes multiple sclerosis (MS)?

    A. MS is a demyelinating disorder characterized by relapses and remissions.
    B. MS affects the postsynaptic junction of the muscle.
    C. MS is a motor neuron disorder.
    D. MS presents as an ascending bilateral paralysis.

115. Which of the following commonly presents with visual changes, headaches, and depression?

    A. Viral encephalitis
    B. Meningioma
    C. Pseudotumor cerebri
    D. Normal-pressure hydrocephalus

116. Which of the following statements is most correct regarding the goal of brain tumor resection?

    A. The goal in all brain tumors is to resect the entire tumor to prevent reoccurrence.
    B. Resection of the tumor should only include enough brain tissue to send to pathology for tumor recognition.
    C. The goal is to resect to the greatest extent possible with the least amount of damage of eloquent areas.
    D. Chemotherapy and radiation are always preferred methods before surgical resection.

117. Which of the following is NOT a common side effect of antiepileptic medications?
    A. Drowsiness
    B. Dizziness
    C. Nausea and vomiting
    D. Diplopia

118. Which of the following is the most accurate statement regarding strokes caused by central venous thrombosis (CVT)?
    A. CVT is due to a hypercoagulable state.
    B. Obstruction of a dural artery is the underlying cause of CVT.
    C. CVT presents as an ischemic stroke only.
    D. Thrombosis of the external jugular vein is the most commonly affected area of CVT.

119. Which of the following statements is most correct about normal-pressure hydrocephalus (NPH)?
    A. To determine whether the hydrocephalus is of normal pressure, a ventriculostomy is inserted and the intracranial pressure is measured.
    B. All patients with NPH will improve with a ventriculoperitoneal (VP) shunt.
    C. Placement of a VP shunt will not improve symptoms but can slow the progression of the disease.
    D. Draining cerebrospinal fluid with lumbar drain trials may be used to evaluate patients for VP shunt placement.

120. Lhermitte's sign may be present in multiple sclerosis. Which of the following best describes Llhermitte's sign?
    A. Paresthesia of arms
    B. Head tremors
    C. Electric-shock sensations
    D. Word-finding abnormalities

121. Which of the following signs would be an indication of the presence of spinal shock following a spinal cord injury?
    A. Hyperspasticity
    B. Positive Babinski's reflex
    C. Loss of anal tone
    D. Hypertension

122. A tumor in which of the following lobes of the brain is most likely to present with seizures?
    A. Frontal lobe
    B. Parietal lobe
    C. Temporal lobe
    D. Occipital lobe

123. Which of the following is NOT considered a cause of central venous thrombosis?
    A. Malignancy
    B. Eye infections

C. Factor VIII deficiency
D. Pregnancy

124. Which of the following time intervals for presentation of a stroke patient with a central venous thrombosis is most common?
    A. Acute (within 48 hours)
    B. Subacute (48 hours to 30 days)
    C. Chronic (greater than 30 days)
    D. Ultraacute (within 12 hours)

125. Which of the following diagnostic exams can be used to assist in determining the severity of spina bifida in a fetus?
    A. Amniocentesis
    B. Maternal serum alpha-fetal protein test
    C. Ultrasonography
    D. CT

126. Which of the following is NOT an appropriate instruction for a patient with cerebrospinal fluid leak following a transphenoidal approach to resect a pituitary tumor?
    A. Place packing in the nose.
    B. Avoid Valsalva maneuvers.
    C. Perform an open-mouth cough.
    D. Avoid nose blowing.

127. A patient presents in the ED following a witnessed seizure at home. She is awake and states she has been having headaches for the past 2 weeks. A CT scan identified a subacute ischemic stroke with some hemorrhagic components. Upon further diagnostic workup, she is diagnosed with a central venous thrombosis. Which of the following would most likely be the recommended treatment?
    A. Anticoagulation therapy
    B. Steroid therapy
    C. Decompressive craniotomy
    D. Statin therapy

128. Management of multiple sclerosis includes all of the following except?
    A. Steroid
    B. Acetylcholinesterase inhibitor
    C. Immunosuppressive
    D. Interferon

129. Pseudotumor cerebri is most commonly linked with which of the following?
    A. Hyperlipidemia
    B. Obesity
    C. Hispanic population
    D. Pet dandruff

130. A 35-year-old patient is admitted for new-onset right-sided weakness. He reports that playing football about 2 weeks ago, he developed a sore neck. He went to a chiropractor this morning, and the weakness started about 2 hours after his appointment. Which of the following would be the most likely cause of the patient's stroke?
    A. Basilar artery occlusion
    B. Extracranial vertebral dissection
    C. Intracranial internal carotid dissection
    D. Central venous thrombosis

131. Ativan (lorazepam) is administered as a primary antiepileptic medication during an active seizure. What is the action of benzodiazepines in stopping a seizure?
    A. Blocks the $Na^+$ channels.
    B. Enhances the inhibitory effects of gamma-aminobutyric acid (GABA).
    C. Overpaces the neurons.
    D. Induces a medical coma.

132. Which of the following statements best describes trigeminal neuralgia (TN)?
    A. TN most commonly occurs bilaterally.
    B. TN most commonly affects the mandibular and maxillary divisions of the trigeminal nerve.
    C. Brain MRI is used to diagnose TN and rule out other causes of facial pain.
    D. Pain is constant and increases in intensity with progression.

133. GS has a complete spinal cord injury at the level of C6. The patient complains of a headache and stuffy nose. Blood pressure (BP) is 210/120 mmHg. Which of the following is your first response in managing the patient?
    A. Immediately call the physician for a STAT CT scan.
    B. Elevate the head of the bed and remove the source of pain stimulus.
    C. Administer an antihypertensive.
    D. Continue to monitor the patient's BP.

134. Which of the following is an incorrect statement regarding radiation treatment of a brain tumor?
    A. It affects tumor cells only.
    B. It causes brain tissue necrosis within area of radiation.
    C. Certain brain structures are more radiosensitive than others.
    D. Radiation effects are irreversible.

135. A patient presents with unilateral ptosis, miosis, and anhydrosis on the ipsilateral face. Which of the following syndromes is the most likely cause of this patient's symptoms?
    A. Chagall's syndrome
    B. Duvet's syndrome
    C. Locked-in syndrome
    D. Horner's syndrome

136. A 1-year-old infant sustains a brain injury in a motor vehicle collision. The child develops abnormal motor movements. Which of the following is the most accurate statement?
    A. The abnormal movement is not considered to be cerebral palsy because the injury occurred after birth.
    B. This injury will always progress to mental retardation.
    C. The presentation of a motor movement abnormality caused by trauma during an early age can be classified as CP.
    D. Traumatic brain injuries do not cause abnormal motor movements.

137. A patient with a spinal cord injury that occurred 10 years ago presents with hypertension and diaphoresis above the level of injury. Which of the following is the patient most likely experiencing?
    A. Spinal shock
    B. Neurogenic shock
    C. Autonomic hyperreflexia
    D. Lacunar stroke

138. Surgical instruments that have been used to biopsy brain tissue of a patient suspected of Creutzfeldt–Jakob disease should be:
    A. Autoclaved
    B. Destroyed
    C. Disinfected
    D. Washing

139. Which of the following chemotherapy medications is most commonly used as first-line medical management of a glioblastoma?
    A. Doxorubicin (Adriamycin)
    B. Temozolomide (Temodar)
    C. Paclitaxel (Taxol)
    D. Bevacizumab (Avastin)

140. Which of the following does NOT require surgical management?
    A. Myelomeningocele
    B. Chiari malformation type II
    C. Myelomeningocele
    D. Spina bifida occulta

141. Myasthenia gravis is a chronic autoimmune disorder that is commonly associated with which of the following disorders?
    A. Vaccinations
    B. Lyme disease
    C. Thyroid disorder
    D. Renal disease

142. Which of the following neurological complications is NOT associated with Ehlers–Danlos syndrome?
    A. Cerebral aneurysm
    B. Carotid dissection

C. Arteriovenous malformation
D. Vertebral dissection

143. Which of the following diagnostic tests is considered the gold standard for diagnosing leptomeningeal tumor?

    A. CT scan
    B. PET scan
    C. Tumor biopsy
    D. Cerebrospinal fluid analysis

144. A spinal cord–injured patient commonly experiences orthostatic hypotension when changing positions. Which of the following interventions may help prevent the hypotension?

    A. Abdominal binder
    B. Halo vest
    C. "Quad" cough
    D. Bowel stimulation

145. Which of the following diagnostic radiographic tests is considered the gold standard for identifying cavernous malformations?

    A. Transcranial Doppler
    B. Cerebral angiogram
    C. Noncontrast CT scan
    D. Gradient echo MRI

146. Which of the following is the most common presenting symptom of Mèniére's disease?

    A. Dementia
    B. Vertigo
    C. Neuropathic pain syndrome of the face
    D. Facial numbness

147. Your patient had a tonic–clonic seizure. The physician has ordered you to load the patient on intravenous (IV) phenytoin (Dilantin). Which of the following is the most accurate statement regarding administering Dilantin via IV?

    A. Rapid intravenous push (IVP)
    B. Administer no faster than 50 mg/min
    C. Administer over 4 hours only
    D. Cannot be administered using the IV route

148. A patient presents with nonlocalized symptoms of muscle weakness and confusion. The EEG indicates encephalopathy. Which of the following studies is recommended to diagnose primary central nervous system vasculitis?

    A. Transcranial Doppler
    B. Cerebrospinal fluid drainage over 3 days
    C. Temporal artery biopsy
    D. MRI

149. Which of the following statements is most accurate regarding the presentation of myasthenia gravis?
    A. Causes hyperalgesia of lower extremities
    B. Bilateral ascending muscle weakness
    C. Progressive muscle weakness occurs with repetitive muscle activity
    D. Upper-extremity weakness greater than lower extremity

150. Which of the following types of central nervous system (CNS) tumor is most likely to benefit from intrathecal administration of chemotherapy medication?
    A. CNS lymphoma
    B. Pituitary tumor
    C. Glioma
    D. Leptomeningeal tumor

151. Following a stroke, the patient undergoes a cerebral angiogram. It is noted that the patient has "haze-like smoke puffs" bilaterally around the internal carotids. Which of the following would be the most likely diagnosis?
    A. Leptomeningeal fibrosis
    B. Neurofibromatosis
    C. Ehlers–Danlos disease
    D. Moyamoya disease

152. A patient presents with unilateral facial droop and paralysis. When assessing the patient, it is noted that the paralysis also involves the forehead. Which of the following would be the most likely cause?
    A. Lyme disease
    B. Bell's palsy
    C. Trigeminal neuralgia
    D. Ischemic stroke

153. Following administration of alteplase in an acute stroke, the patient is placed in the ICU. According to the American Heart Association/American Stroke Association guidelines, the systolic blood pressure be kept below what?
    A. 220 mmHg
    B. 180 mmHg
    C. 160 mmHg
    D. 140 mmHg

154. Which of the following is the best intervention to prevent spina bifida?
    A. Genetic testing
    B. Dietary supplement
    C. Maternal vaccinations
    D. Use of seatbelts

155. Which of the following treatment plan would be indicated in a patient with one unprovoked seizure?
    A. Admit for video EEG monitoring.
    B. Initiate an antiepileptic agent.

C. Avoid typical precipitants.
D. Send home with no further follow-up.

156. Which of the following is an indication for a decompressive craniectomy following a traumatic brain injury?

   A. Contusion in frontal lobe
   B. Organ donor following brain death determination
   C. Impending herniation
   D. Pediatric patient only

157. Following an ischemic stroke, the patient is in the progressive care unit (PCU). The following vital signs and laboratory data are obtained: blood pressure (BP) 190/92 mmHg, heart rate (HR) 84 beats/minute, respiratory rate (RR) 16 breaths/minute, temperature = 38.5°C, glucose = 130 mg/dL, Na$^+$ 142 mEq/L. Which of the following interventions is recommended at this time based upon the patient's above findings?

   A. Administer antihypertensive.
   B. Administer acetaminophen for fever.
   C. Place patient on sliding scale insulin and administer insulin subcutaneous (SQ).
   D. Obtain a urine osmolality and urine specific gravity.

158. A common side effect of the anticholinergic drugs used to manage Mèniére's disease includes which of the following?

   A. Tachycardia
   B. Excessive drooling
   C. Blurred vision
   D. Nausea

159. A patient is recently diagnosed with a grade II astrocytoma. The biopsy report was discussed with the patient, including that the tumor is considered to be benign. Which of the following statements would be most appropriate at this time?

   A. You are really lucky this is a benign tumor and easily managed.
   B. Even though the results are benign, this can be an invasive, progressive tumor.
   C. *Benign* means this is not cancer and will not require radiation or chemotherapy after surgical resection.
   D. An astrocytoma typically metastasizes to the lungs. You will need a routine chest x-ray to monitor for tumors.

160. Which of the following statements regarding the care of a patient after an ischemic stroke is most correct?

   A. Place all patients on supplemental oxygen to improve tissue oxygenation levels.
   B. Administer prophylactic antiepileptic medications to all patients.
   C. Antihypertensives should be administered to keep the systolic blood pressure less than 160 mmHg.
   D. A bedside swallow test should be obtained prior to administration of oral medications or oral intake on all patients.

161. Which of the following best describes the allodynia patients with cerebral palsy can experience?
    A. Inability to differentiate temperature changes
    B. Loss of pain sensation
    C. Inability to control body temperature
    D. Light touch can become painful

162. Following an unprovoked first seizure, which of the following findings would NOT increase the risk for a second seizure?
    A. Epileptiform abnormalities on EEG
    B. Partial-onset seizure
    C. Presence of hydrocephalus
    D. Generalized seizure

163. An ischemic stroke patient had passed a bedside swallow test prior to admission to the progressive care unit. While the nurse is administering an oral medication with a sip of water, she notes the patient coughs. Which of the following would be the most appropriate response?
    A. Continue to administer medications, the patient has passed the bedside swallow test.
    B. Hold oral medications, put the patient on nothing per os status, and consult speech therapy.
    C. Place a STAT order for a video endoscopic evaluation.
    D. Obtain a STAT chest x-ray and place the patient on supplemental oxygen.

164. A neurological patient develops polyuria with a urine output of 450 mL/hr. Which of the following would NOT be found in diabetes insipidus?
    A. Urine specific gravity <1.005
    B. Serum osmolality <275 mOsm/L
    C. Urine osmolality <200 mOsm/L
    D. $Na^+$ levels >145 dg/L

165. Which of the following treatments for cerebral edema and increased intracranial pressure is NOT recommended following severe traumatic brain injury?
    A. Hypertonic saline
    B. Mannitol
    C. Therapeutic hypothermia
    D. Cerebrospinal fluid drainage

166. A stroke patient on warfarin (Coumadin) is being bridged with heparin infusion until the international normalized ratio (INR) meets goal. On day 7, the patient's platelet count decreased from 120,000 to 50,000. Which of the following is the most likely cause?
    A. Immune-mediated thrombocytopenia purpura
    B. Elevated INR affected the platelet count
    C. Heparin-induced thrombocytopenia
    D. Suppression of bone marrow production of platelets

167. Which of the following is NOT a known cause of trigeminal neuralgia?

    A. Aneurysm
    B. Tumor
    C. Multiple sclerosis
    D. Traumatic brain injury

168. A brainstem glioma in the pons commonly presents with cranial nerve (CN) deficits. Which of the following CNs are most likely involved?

    A. CN I (olfactory nerve) and II (optic nerve)
    B. CN III (oculomotor nerve) and IV (trochlear nerve)
    C. CN V (trigeminal nerve), VI (abducens nerve), VII (facial nerve), and VIII (acoustic nerve)
    D. CN IX (glossopharyngeal) nerve, X (vagus nerve), and XII (hypoglossal nerve)

169. A patient with an acute ischemic stroke states he is allergic to aspirin (acetylsalicylic acid [ASA]). Which of the following would be the most appropriate response?

    A. Call the pharmacy to check out ASA allergies.
    B. Explain to the patient that he needs the ASA and encourage him or her to take the ASA.
    C. Document the patient is refusing the ASA.
    D. Discuss with the physician changing the order to clopidogrel (Plavix)

170. Upper motor neuron injury presents with which of the following symptoms?

    A. Flaccidity of muscles
    B. Significant muscle atrophy
    C. Hypertonicity of muscles
    D. Depressed deep tendon reflexes

171. Which of the following terms best describes motor activity of sustained focal stiffening?

    A. Atonic
    B. Tonic
    C. Myoclonic
    D. Clonic

172. An 8-year-old, previously diagnosed with attention deficit hyperactivity disorder, now presents to the neurologist with repetitive involuntary movements and vocalizations. Which of the following is the most likely cause?

    A. Tourette's syndrome
    B. Miller Fisher syndrome
    C. Absence seizures
    D. Dravet syndrome

173. A patient is admitted to the trauma ICU following severe traumatic brain injury. An intracranial pressure (ICP) monitor is placed, and the patient is noted to have increased ICP. The following are the patient's data:

$$K^+ \ 4.2 \ mEq/L$$
$$Na^+ \ 130 \ mEq/L$$
$$Serum \ osmolality = 280 \ mOsm/L$$

Which of the following international normalized ratio results would be considered appropriate for a patient with an acute embolic stroke and atrial fibrillation?

A. 1.8
B. 2.4
C. 3.1
D. 3.8

174. Which of the following would be the most likely ordered hyperosmolar agent to manage this patient's increased intracranial pressure?

A. 3% saline
B. Mannitol
C. 7.5% saline
D. Glycerol

175. Which of the following cranial nerves (CNs) is commonly affected by an acoustic neuroma?

A. CN III (oculomotor nerve)
B. CN VII (facial nerve)
C. CN II (optic nerve)
D. CN XII (hypoglossal nerve)

176. Focal seizures may demonstrate automatism. Which of the following best describes automatism behaviors?

A. Motor arrest
B. Hyperkinetic activity
C. Irregular, brief focal jerking movement
D. Purposeless repetitive motor activity

177. The neurologist ordered a statin for your acute ischemic stroke patient. Which of the following statements would be the most appropriate for patient education regarding the statin?

A. If your urine turns "reddish, or cola colored," come to the ED.
B. It is recommended to take the statin with grapefruit juice to improve absorption.
C. This medication is ordered because diet alone will not lower your cholesterol.
D. You will need to have your kidney function monitored closely while taking the statin.

178. Which of the following complications of mannitol should be monitored closely in multisystem trauma patients with severe traumatic brain injury?

A. Hypokalemia
B. Hypernatremia

C. Increased serum osmolality
D. Diuresis

179. Which of the following is a postoperative complication following a vestibular nerve resection?

    A. Cerebrospinal fluid leak
    B. Epidural hematoma
    C. Cushing's triad
    D. Cerebellar herniation

180. A patient is 24 hours postoperative following pituitary tumor removal by the transphenoidal route. The nurse taking care of the patient noted the urine output to have increased from to 400 mL/hr. Which of the following is the most likely cause for the increase in urine output?

    A. Shifting of fluids postoperatively
    B. Cerebral salt wasting syndrome
    C. Diabetes insipidus
    D. Syndrome of inappropriate antidiuretic hormone

181. While providing education to a stroke patient, which of the following is considered to be the most important concept to ensure understanding?

    A. Document all education provided to the patient and family.
    B. Perform "teach back" by asking the patient to repeat the information in his or her own words.
    C. Use a variety of teaching methods.
    D. Provide a large amount of information during the short period of time the patient is hospitalized.

182. Which of the following is the most powerful determinant of cerebral blood flow?

    A. $PaO_2$
    B. $PaCO_2$
    C. Arterial pH
    D. Bicarbonate

183. A patient presents to the ED with altered mentation. The patient then stiffens bilaterally followed by rhythmic movement and is not responding to external stimuli. Which of the following is the most correct description of the seizure?

    A. Tonic seizure
    B. Tonic–clonic seizure
    C. Atonic seizure
    D. Clonic seizure

184. Which of the following is NOT a pediatric sign of meningitis?

    A. Lethargy
    B. Irritability
    C. Poor feeding
    D. Headache

185. When teaching about stroke recognition, the acronym used as a mnemonic, FAST, stands for which of the following except:
    A. F = facial drooping
    B. A = arm weakness
    C. S = speech difficulties
    D. T = tinnitus or ringing ears

186. Which of the following areas of the brain is NOT easily identified as injured by using the National Institutes of Health Stroke Scale?
    A. Anterior cerebral artery
    B. Thalamic region
    C. Middle cerebral artery
    D. Posterior circulation

187. A brain tumor patient is experiencing nausea, vomiting, and headache from the cerebral edema. Which of the following would be the most appropriate initial treatment of the cerebral edema?
    A. Steroids
    B. Mannitol
    C. 3% saline
    D. Hyperventilation

188. Which of the following neurological injuries is known to result in the development of normal-pressure hydrocephalus?
    A. Subarachnoid hemorrhage
    B. Epidural hematoma
    C. Subdural hematoma
    D. Parenchymal contusion

189. Which of the following is NOT an educational stroke measure for stroke patients?
    A. Discharge medications for strokes
    B. Criteria for acute rehabilitation eligibility
    C. Signs and symptoms of stroke
    D. Personal risk factors for a stroke

190. Following a severe traumatic brain injury, the patient is intubated, agitated, and has elevated intracranial pressures. A sedative is ordered. Which of the following side effects of the sedative would be the most concerning for the nurse at this time?
    A. Hypotension
    B. Respiratory depression
    C. Urinary retention
    D. Constipation

191. Which of the following is a true statement regarding the use of steroids in traumatic brain-injured (TBI) patients?
    A. Steroids have been found to decrease cerebral edema following TBI.
    B. Steroids are recommended with severe TBI and require glucose monitoring.

C. Steroids are not recommended in TBI patients.
D. Steroids have been found to be more effective in minor brain injuries.

192. A child was just diagnosed with cerebral palsy (CP), and the parents are asking whether this is genetic and can affect any future children they were planning on having. Which is the best response of the nurse?
    A. You will need to discuss this with your physician.
    B. You will need to have genetic counseling before considering getting pregnant again.
    C. Yes, it is genetic and is most likely to affect your future children.
    D. It is not genetic, and you are not likely to have more children with CP.

193. A 13-month-old child had sudden extension of both arms and flexion of the trunk. These seizures repeat in clusters. Which of the following is the most accurate description of the seizure?
    A. Infantile spasms
    B. Lennox–Gastaut syndrome
    C. Febrile seizure
    D. Myoclonic seizure

194. Which of the following is the most common visual deficit with patients presenting with pituitary tumors?
    A. Homonymous hemianopsia
    B. Scotoma
    C. Complete blindness unilateral
    D. Bitemporal hemianopsia

195. Which of the following feeding methods would best decrease the incidence of ventilator-associated pneumonia following a traumatic brain injury?
    A. Percutaneous endoscopic gastrostomy tube
    B. Transpyloric jejunal tube
    C. Orogastric tube
    D. Bolus gastric feeding

196. After the physician left the patient's room, the family asked you to clarify what *pseudoprogression* means after receiving chemotherapy for a glioblastoma. What would be your best response?
    A. You will need to ask the physician the next time you meet with him.
    B. Chemotherapy is not an effective treatment for glioblastoma.
    C. The tumor appears to have worsened, but the tumor did not actually increase in size.
    D. This indicates that the tumor has become necrotic and progression will stop.

197. The addition of "BE" to FAST (BE FAST) is to improve the recognition of which of the following types of strokes?
    A. Anterior strokes
    B. Embolic strokes

C. Posterior strokes
D. Subarachnoid hemorrhage

198. A patient with a spinal cord lesion involving the spinal nerve root complains of severe pain. Which of the following medications is most appropriate for treating neuropathic pain?
    A. Hydromorphone (Dilaudid)
    B. Gabapentin (Neurontin)
    C. Ketamine
    D. Ketorolac (Toradol)

199. Which of the following is a true statement regarding amyotrophic lateral sclerosis (ALS)?
    A. ALS involves both motor and sensory abnormalities.
    B. ALS is sclerosis of the white matter in the frontal lobe.
    C. ALS involves both upper and lower motor neuron abnormalities.
    D. ALS affects the pons and results in locked-in syndrome.

200. Which of the following is the most significant complication of strict glycemic control (80–110 mg/dL) in patients following severe traumatic brain injuries?
    A. Worsening of the Glasgow Coma Scale score
    B. Increased cerebral edema
    C. Immunosuppression
    D. Hypoglycemia

201. Which of the following is NOT a true statement regarding cerebral palsy (CP)?
    A. CP is contagious.
    B. CP is not caused by a genetic abnormality or hereditary.
    C. CP is a chronic neurological disorder without a cure.
    D. CP is not always associated with mental impairment.

202. Which of the following is considered the single most important risk factor for a stroke?
    A. Hypertension
    B. Sedentary lifestyle
    C. Male gender
    D. Smoking

203. Which of the following is the surgical management used to manage the symptoms of normal-pressure hydrocephalus?
    A. Skull base surgery
    B. Long-term intracranial pressure monitor
    C. Ventriculoperitoneal shunt
    D. Vagal nerve resection

204. A traumatic brain-injured patient in the ICU has an intracranial pressure (ICP) monitor and is noted to have the following: blood pressure = 140/60 mmHg, MAP = 80 mmHg, and ICP = 15 mmHg. Which of the following is the correct calculated cerebral perfusion pressure?
    A. 95 mmHg
    B. 125 mmHg
    C. 65 mmHg
    D. 75 mmHg

205. Which of the following primary tumor locations most commonly metastasizes to the brain?
    A. Gastrointestinal tract
    B. Pancreas
    C. Lung
    D. Kidney

206. Which of the following presentations would most commonly be associated with autonomic seizures?
    A. Experiences of déjà vu
    B. Auditory hallucinations
    C. Feeling of being flushed and piloerection
    D. Repetitive movements

207. Which of the following goals for blood pressure management is recommended for both primary and secondary prevention in a nondiabetic person?
    A. Maintain systolic blood pressure (SBP) <160 mmHg and diastolic <100 mmHg
    B. Do not treat unless SBP >220 mmHg or diastolic >120 mmHg
    C. Manage BP within a normal pressure of 110/80 mmHg
    D. Maintain SBP <140 mmHg and diastolic <90 mmHg

208. What is a grade III astrocytoma called?
    A. Glioblastoma
    B. Neurofibromatosis
    C. Anaplastic
    D. Neuroblastoma

209. Which of the following reflexes require the cervical spine to be cleared of injury before being tested?
    A. Bulbocavernosus reflex
    B. Babinski reflex
    C. Oculocephalic reflexes
    D. Oculovestibular reflexes

210. Ergotamine is used to manage benign headaches. Which of the following is a complication of this drug therapy?
    A. Liver toxicity
    B. Acute myocardial infarction
    C. Increased intracranial pressure
    D. Acute kidney injury

211. An infant is born with a hypoplasia of the cerebellum. Which of the following is the correct classification of the Chiari malformation?

   A. Type I
   B. Type II
   C. Type III
   D. Type IV

212. Which of the following is NOT a route of exposure or cause of Creutzfeldt–Jakob disease?

   A. Sporadic
   B. Hereditary
   C. Exposure of infected person's tissue
   D. Casual contact

213. Which of the following would be considered a preventive intervention for cerebral palsy?

   A. Genetic counseling
   B. Administration of rubella vaccination prior to pregnancy
   C. Avoiding use of alcohol during pregnancy
   D. Participating in an exercise program during the pregnancy

214. Posttraumatic injury can involve cranial nerve (CN) injuries. Which of the following CNs is most commonly damaged with traumatic brain injury?

   A. CN I (olfactory nerve)
   B. CN V (trigeminal nerve)
   C. CN VII (facial nerve)
   D. CN VIII (acoustic nerve)

215. Which of the following should be stressed to the patient and family regarding best transportation to the hospital in case of a second stroke?

   A. EMS 9-1-1
   B. Personal vehicle
   C. Taxi
   D. Next-door neighbor

216. Which of the following does NOT increase the risk of seizures following severe traumatic brain injury?

   A. Penetrating head trauma
   B. Decreased level of consciousness
   C. Depressed skull fracture
   D. Linear skull fracture

217. What is a common complication of a pineal tumor?

   A. Hydrocephalus
   B. Visual field loss
   C. Hemiparesis
   D. Subarachnoid hemorrhage

218. Which of the following would be considered a "simple" definition or explanation of what a stroke is?

    A. A stroke is an ischemic event causing cerebral injury.
    B. Stroke happens when there is a lack of blood flow to the brain due to an obstruction.
    C. A stroke is a permanent injury to the brain tissue and areas of ischemia, which may be reversible injury.
    D. Stroke occurs when the penumbra converts to an infarcted area.

219. Cluster headaches may cause ipsilateral autonomic signs, which include all but which of the following?

    A. Nasal congestion
    B. Facial sweating
    C. Miosis
    D. Atrial fibrillation

220. Which of the following is not considered a route of entry for bacterial meningitis?

    A. Direct
    B. Sinusitis
    C. Airborne, droplet spread
    D. Eating undercooked pork

# 11

# Chapter Review Answers and Rationales

## CHAPTER 1: CHRONIC NEUROLOGICAL DISORDERS

1. **B**

    Rationale: Patients with subcortical dementia commonly due to Parkinson's disease present with alterations in complex attention and executive function. This includes tasks taking longer and the person makes errors performing routine tasks. Parkinson's disease is different than cortical injuries affecting the memory centers. Expressive aphasia and word finding affect the language center. Alteration in personality is a component of social cognition.

2. **D**

    Rationale: Normal-pressure hydrocephalus (NPH) is classified as a communicating hydrocephalus. The enlarged ventricles and large amount of cerebrospinal fluid (CSF) are caused by a decreased reabsorption in the arachnoid villi. NPH has normal to near-normal opening pressures. Noncommunicating hydrocephalus is due to obstruction of CSF flow in the ventricles. This is not NPH and typically has a high opening pressure. NPH is not congenital hydrocephalus.

3. **A**

    Rationale: Deep brain stimulation has been shown to improve motor movement in patients with Parkinson's disease. Normal-pressure hydrocephalus (NPH) is treated with ventriculoperitoneal (VP) shunt. Diastolic blood pressure treatment is not indicated for NPH, migraine headaches, and myasthenia gravis.

4. **A**

    Rationale: The subcortical region of the brain, especially the subthalamic nucleus, is the most common site to place the wire in deep brain stimulation. It is not commonly placed in the pituitary area, substantia nigra, or midbrain.

5. **C**

    Rationale: Levodopa used over several years can cause extreme, oftentimes incapacitating, dyskinetic movements. Parkinson's disease (PD) does not usually lead to muscle facility and is not considered a higher risk for an ischemic stroke. PD patients can develop dementia but it is typically Levy body dementia, not Alzheimer's disease.

## CHAPTER 2: CEREBROVASCULAR DISORDERS

1. C

   Rationale: A noncontrast CT scan of the brain is used initially in patients with stroke-like symptoms to identify hemorrhagic stroke. When the scan is negative in these situations, it just indicates there is no presence of hemorrhagic stroke. It does not rule out ischemic stroke nor is it used to diagnose a transient ischemic attack.

2. A

   Rationale: Angioedema is a known risk for administering intravenous (IV) alteplase and can cause partial airway obstruction. Bleeding is another potential complication, not thrombocytopenia. Leukocytosis and hypotension are not complications of IV alteplase administration.

3. C

   Rationale: Nimodipine is administered for 21 days after a subarachnoid hemorrhage caused by aneurysm rupture. It is used to reduce delayed ischemic injury and mortality with vasospasm and is administered throughout the period of time of vasospasm. Administering for only 48 hours would not be effective. There is no known benefit for longer administration of nimodipine.

4. D

   Rationale: Transcranial Doppler (TCD) is a noninvasive diagnostic test used to measure velocity of cerebral blood flow. Velocity correlates to vascular diameter. It is used to screen for vasospasms. Noncontrast CT scan does not identify vascular diameter or vasospasm. PET scan is not indicated in subarachnoid hemorrhage or vasospasms. Cerebral angiograms are diagnostic for vasospasms but are not routinely used to "screen" for vasospasm.

5. B

   Rationale: Ischemic injury to the right hemisphere or nondominant side results frequently in neglect or an unawareness of deficits on the affected side. Aphasia, both receptive and expressive, is more commonly associated with ischemic injury to the right or dominant hemisphere. Hemiplegia is contralateral, not ipsilateral.

6. A

   Rationale: The anterior cerebral artery (ACA) supplies blood to the medial portion of the frontal lobe. This is the location of the micturition center and can commonly result in incontinence following an ACA stroke. Middle cerebral artery, posterior cerebral artery, and vertebral artery strokes are not at as high of risk for incontinence.

## CHAPTER 3: TUMORS OF THE BRAIN AND SPINAL CORD

1. C

   Rationale: Neurofibromatosis type II is a genetic condition in which tumors develop bilaterally along cranial nerve VIII as acoustic neuroma (also called *schwannoma*).

A neuroendocrine tumor typically involves the pituitary gland. Embryonal tumors include medulloblastoma. Primary central nervous system lymphomas are tumors primarily composed of B lymphocytes.

2. D

Rationale: The frontal lobe is responsible for higher level functions, mood, personality, judgment, memory, and motor function. A tumor present in the frontal lobe can result in mood and personality changes and gait abnormality or loss of motor function. The presenting symptoms for a tumor in the hypothalamus involve the loss of certain regulatory functions such as temperature control and fluid balance. The pons is located in the brainstem and can present with motor changes but is not associated with mood or personality changes.

3. C

Rationale: The cerebellum is responsible for fine motor control and equilibrium. A tumor located in the cerebellum can result in ataxia. The symptoms will be ipsilateral because the cerebellum influences motor movement after the motor impulse has crossed into the pons. Cranial nerves originate primarily from the brainstem, not from the cerebellum. Cerebellum affects motor aspects and does not cause sensory deficits.

4. D

Rationale: There are no tumor markers available to identify primary brain tumors. A PET scan can be used to differentiate tumor regrowth from radiation necrosis. A functional MRI is used to identify areas of the brain responsible for language, higher level thinking, sensory and motor function. An MRI is the diagnostic test of choice to identify small lesions compared to CT scan.

5. C

Rationale: An MRI is considered the gold standard for diagnosing spinal tumors. Spinal x-rays can identify narrowing of the spinal canal but are not very accurate at identifying tumor. Myelogram can identify the level of spinal canal blockage but cannot identify etiology. CT scan can localize and identify an extradural lesion, but MRI is more diagnostic for spinal tumor.

6. B

Rationale: Brain biopsy is the most definitive diagnosis of a primary central nervous system (CNS) lymphoma. Initial treatment with glucocorticoids can produce rapid symptom resolution and dramatic radiographic changes, but this does not occur in all patients with CNS lymphoma. An MRI is better than CT scan in differentiating different brain tumors. Meningeal lymphoma cells can be isolated from the cerebrospinal fluid and can assist with the diagnosis but is not considered to be the most diagnostic tool.

## CHAPTER 5: IMMUNE INFECTIONS, PART 2

1. C

Rationale: Myasthenia crisis is an exacerbation of the symptoms of myasthenia gravis (MG) and commonly presents with ventilatory failure with the need to provide noninvasive or invasive ventilatory support. Serotonin syndrome is caused by certain serotonergic medications and includes symptoms such as agitation, high body temperatures, sweating, dilated pupils, and diarrhea. Refractory MG is seen when symptoms continue despite administration of corticosteroids and at least two immunosuppressive options for MG. Cholinesterase crisis: MG patients can present with cholinergic crisis with overdose of anticholinergic agents used to manage MG. Symptoms are lacrimation, salivation, urination, defecation, and emesis.

2. C

Rationale: The thymus gland controls the immune system, and an enlarged thymus or thymic tumor has been found to be associated with myasthenia gravis (MG). Even in patients without an abnormal thymus, thymectomy is a potential option in patients refractory to medical management. Adrenal, thyroid, and pituitary glands are not associated with MG.

3. B

Rationale: Bulbar symptoms include dysphagia (difficulty swallowing), dysarthria (difficulty speech), and dysphonia (abnormal speech sound). These can be the first presenting signs in amyotrophic lateral sclerosis (ALS). Heart rate changes, miosis/mydriasis, and sweating are autonomic nervous system symptoms, not bulbar symptoms. Memory loss and slowing cognition are not bulbar signs and are not associated with ALS.

4. B

Rationale: The trigger for posterior reversible encephalopathy syndrome (PRES) is acute hypertension and may be caused by loss of autoregulation (inability to constrict to protect the brain) when the systolic pressure is above a certain pressuret. Uncontrolled hypertension in the brain can lead to hyperperfusion and cerebral edema. It is reversible if the blood pressure is corrected early. Alcohol and hepatic failure can cause encephalopathy but do not present with bilateral occipital involvement. Ischemic stroke is not an etiology of PRES.

5. C

Rationale: Wernicke's encephalopathy is a result of vitamin B deficiency and commonly presents with a triad of symptoms. These include confusion, ataxia, and ophthalmoplegia. Dysphagia is a bulbar symptom and is not present with Wernicke's syndrome.

6. D

Rationale: Confusion, asterixis, and abnormal handwriting are signs of hepatic and uremic encephalopathy, but this patient has a history of hepatic failure, not renal. Posterior reversible encephalopathy syndrome (PRES) can be caused by hypertension and results in confusion but is not associated with asterixis. Encephalitis would present with fever, elevated white blood cell counts, and headache.

## CHAPTER 6: SEIZURES

1. B

Rationale: Severe behavioral and personality disorders are commonly associated with Lennox–Gastaut syndrome. These include hyperactivity, aggressiveness, and autism and can progress to psychosis. Sensory abnormalities (deafness and visual difficulties), ataxia, and gastrointestinal disorders are not commonly associated with Lennox–Gastaut syndrome.

## 11. CHAPTER REVIEW ANSWERS AND RATIONALES

**2. B**

Rationale: Nonconvulsive status epilepticus (NCSE) occurs when the patient is having epileptic changes on EEG but is not showing convulsive activity. NCSE may be suspected if the patient is exhibiting automatism activity, such as repetitive blinking. Headaches are not typically signs of NCSE. Repetitive jerking of an upper extremity is considered convulsive activity. No cerebral blood flow is a sign of brain death, not NCSE.

**3. C**

Rationale: Rhabdomyolysis is a result of muscle breakdown from repetitive muscle injury and myoglobinemia. Acute kidney injury as a result of rhabdomyolysis presents with "tea-colored" or "cola-colored" urine. Glomerulonephritis, nephritis, and chronic interstitial nephropathy do not present in such manner.

**4. C**

Rationale: Acute hippocampal swelling can be found on MRI followed by atrophy and mesial temporal sclerosis. Pyramidal cell loss occurs with general cognitive changes. Herniation of the cerebellum occurs in Chiari malformations. Patients with epilepsy do not commonly experience ischemic infarctions or atrophy of the frontal lobe (atrophy is primarily found in the hippocampal area).

**5. C**

Rationale: The Wada test has been used to evaluate the epilepsy patient's hemisphere of language and memory dominance prior to surgical excision of the epileptic focus. It has also been used to evaluate patients prior to brain tumor excision. Functional MRI can also be used to evaluate eloquent areas of the brain prior to surgery.

**6. D**

Answer: A vagal nerve stimulator (VNS) is indicated in patients with intractable or drug-resistant seizures. This is usually defined as having tried at least two appropriate antiepileptic medications. It is an add-on therapy, not used instead of pharmacological treatment. VNS does not affect the length of postictal time or number of falls that can be experienced by a person with seizures. VNS is not indicated in patients with nonepileptic activity.

**7. B**

Rationale: The "wand" is a magnet that is placed over the implanted generator to elicit additional burst stimulation to the vagal nerve stimulator (VNS.) The wand is used when the patient is having a seizure to help stop the seizure. It does not turn the VNS off and does not make it compatible with an MRI. The magnet does not affect the patient's heart rate. Some of the newer VNSs will sense an increase in heart rate and will deliver additional bursts of stimulation when this occurs.

**8. A**

Rationale: Neurogenic pulmonary edema is seldom a result of seizures or status epilepticus. Bilateral or unilateral fracture or dislocation of the humeral head of the shoulder is a common injury following a seizure. Rib fractures can occur and should be suspected if pain is present within the location. Aspiration pneumonia can occur and may be recognized with serial chest x-rays and hypoxic symptoms.

**9. D**

Rationale: Information regarding the type of seizure (partial vs. generalized) and severity of seizures is beneficial to be able to recognize the onset of the seizure and be prepared to prevent injury if a seizure should occur. Knowing whether the patient becomes postictal, whether he or she has psychiatric issues or a familial history of epilepsy is not going to improve the prevention of injury and safety of the patient.

## CHAPTER 7: PEDIATRIC AND DEVELOPMENTAL DISORDERS

**1. B**

Rationale: Myelomeningocele is associated with brain malformations, most commonly Chiari II malformations. There may be a genetic predisposition causing the association. Ischemic strokes and glioblastoma multiforme are not commonly associated with myelomeningocele. Chiari II malformations can cause hydrocephalus but that would be a high-pressure, not a normal-pressure, hydrocephalus.

**2. C**

Rationale: Hydrocephalus is common in Chiari malformations and is always due to obstruction of flow of cerebrospinal fluid (CSF). The cerebellum and fourth ventricle herniate through the foramen magnum, resulting in compression of lateral apertures of Luschka and obstruction of CSF flow into the subarachnoid space around the spinal cord. Hydrocephalus in Chiari malformations is not due to an increase in production of CSF. Herniation of the vermis alone is found in Chiari malformation type I and does not typically result in hydrocephalus. Hypoplasia of the cerebellum is a Chiari malformation type IV and does not result in hydrocephalus.

**3. B**

Rationale: The pathophysiological consequence of cerebellar herniation in Chiari malformations resulting in the patient's symptoms includes the compression of the cerebellar lobes, compression of the brainstem, particularly the medulla and upper spine. As the structures herniate, they obstruct cerebrospinal fluid flow out of the cranium, through the foramen magnum, into the spine subarachnoid space. Symptoms are not due to an increased intracranial pressure.

**4. D**

Rationale: Decompressive craniectomy is indicated in symptomatic Chiari malformations to manage the cerebellar herniation. Cerebellar masses and cerebrospinal fluid hypotensive syndrome can result in cerebellar tonsillar herniation but are not due to an abnormally large volume in the posterior fossa. Pons hemorrhagic stroke does not result in cerebellar tonsillar herniation, and decompressive craniectomy is not recommended.

**5. B**

Rationale: All neonates are at risk for hypothermia, but neonates with myelomeningoceles are at an even greater risk because of the incomplete skin coverage and exposure of internal structures. Close monitoring for hypothermia and prevention are key to managing these newborns. Dehydration, acidosis, and hypokalemia are not greater risks in neonates with myelomeningoceles than other neonates.

6. C

Rationale: All of the answers can be a complication of myelomeningocele, but developmental delay is more of a long-term than an immediate complication in a neonate with spina bifida.

## CHAPTER 8: NEUROLOGICAL TRAUMA: TRAUMATIC BRAIN INJURY

1. B

Rationale: Presence of symptoms associated with the subdural hematoma (SDH) frequently determines the need for surgical intervention. A shift noted on CT scan may be asymptomatic or minor neurological findings on clinical examination. Radiographic changes are not relevant as clinical signs. Bilateral SDH or acute or chronic SDH may require surgical intervention but this depends on clinical presentation.

2. A

Rationale: Elevate the head of the bed by 30 degrees or greater to lower intrathoracic pressure and facilitate venous drainage. Maintaining head alignment is recommended, but securing the cervical collar snugly can interfere with venous drainage. Elevating the foot of the bed may actually increase intrathoracic pressure and decrease cerebral venous return. Placement of a ventriculostomy is a physician's intervention and decreases cerebrospinal fluid, not venous drainage.

3. D

Rationale: Coughing, sneezing, pain, and agitation can cause transient and sustained elevations in intracranial pressure (ICP) following severe traumatic brain injuries. An upright position will decrease the ICP, not increase it.

4. C

Rationale: Preventing hypotension and hypoxia are the two main goals of prehospital management to prevent systemic insults, leading to secondary brain injuries. This is prevented with fluid resuscitation. Osmotic diuretics are not typically administered during the prehospital period. Hyperventilation is not currently recommended in managing traumatic brain-injured patients. Maintaining head of the bed by 30 degrees is recommended but reverse Trendelenburg is not.

5. C

Rationale: Glasgow Coma Scale is the most widely accepted scale used with traumatic brain injury (TBI). It is used for standardization of scoring severity of injury among different healthcare providers. National Institutes of Health Stroke Scale is the most widely accepted and used scale measuring the severity of a stroke, not TBI. Injury Severity Score and Apache scores are used to measure the acuity of trauma patients.

6. A

Rationale: Normal saline is an isotonic fluid, which is recommended for resuscitation following traumatic injuries. Lactated Ringers is also an isotonic solution that is used with trauma but is less commonly used in traumatic brain injury (TBI) patients. Dextrose should be avoided in TBI patients. Hyperglycemia has been found to worsen neurological outcomes.

7. C

Rationale: Gunshot wounds have metal bullet fragments that can heat with the MRI and cause significant damage. MRI is contraindicated in the presence of metal. Skull radiographs, CT scan, and Doppler ultrasound can be used to neurologically evaluate a patient with a gunshot to the head.

8. D

Rationale: The source of hemorrhage in epidural hematoma (EDH) is typically the middle meningeal artery. The middle cerebral artery, anterior cerebral artery, and posterior–inferior cerebral artery are commonly involved in ischemic strokes, not EDH.

9. A

Rationale: Rancho Los Amigos Scale includes an eight-level behavior/response scale. It determines the stage of recovery from the traumatic brain injury (TBI). It is commonly used to determine the level of rehabilitation required. Glasgow Coma Scale is used in TBI patients but in the acute period to determine their neurological function. Apache score is used in trauma patients for severity of injury but not to determine rehabilitation needs. Hunt and Hess score is used to evaluate the severity of a subarachnoid hemorrhage in patients with a ruptured aneurysm.

## CHAPTER 9: NEUROLOGICAL TRAUMA: SPINAL CORD INJURY

1. A

Rationale: Bladder training involves bladder scanning to determine the urine volume and performing intermittent straight cath procedures if a certain volume is met. If the patient voids, bladder scanning is recommended to determine the postvoid residual. An indwelling urinary catheter does not allow urine to stretch the bladder and trigger a reflex to void. It also has a high risk of infection. Suprapubic catheter placement has been used in patients with chronic retention but is not recommended for acute management of spinal cord–injured patients. Overfilling of the bladder will adversely affect bladder training and can cause complications. It is not recommended.

2. D

Rationale: Central cord injuries occur in the central portion of the spinal cord where the motor tracts for the upper extremity are located. Central cord-injured patients will have greater upper-extremity than lower-extremity weakness. Brown–Sequard syndrome is a hemisection of the cord and presents with ipsilateral loss of motor function and contralateral loss of sensory function. Anterior cord syndrome involves injury in the anterior portion of the cord, allowing for light touch, proprioception, and vibratory senses to be maintained.

3. C

Rationale: The American Spinal Injury Association impairment scale is used to assess spinal cord function following a traumatic spinal cord injury. It is a five-grade classification system (Grade A–E). Another grading system used to assess spinal cord function is the Frankel grade, also a five-grade classification system.

4. C

Rationale: Perfusion of the spinal cord is a high priority in the early management of both penetrating and blunt trauma if the injury is incomplete. Maintaining a higher mean arterial pressure can improve perfusion and prevent further neurological injury. Bowel and bladder training are important but are not the priority within the first 24 hours of injury. Administration of high-dose steroids is not recommended in spinal cord injury, especially with penetrating injuries. Venous thromboembolism prophylaxis is recommended immediately on admission, but in this patient, a mechanical compression device is the most appropriate intervention due to the increased risk of bleeding.

5. C

Rationale: The forced vital capacity (forced maximal breath in and maximal breath out) and negative inspiratory force are used to assess and measure the ability of the ventilatory muscles for breathing. Assessing tidal volume and respiratory rates can evaluate the patient's current ventilatory status. Forced expiratory volume in 1 second is used more frequently in assessing patients presenting with bronchospasm and airway narrowing.

6. D

Rationale: Abdominal binders are used to prevent orthostatic hypotension in spinal cord–injured patients. Abdominal binders may also improve respiratory function and voice. Vasopressors are used to increase blood pressure but not for preventing orthostatic hypotension in spinal cord–injured patients. Foot elevation may improve venous return but is not a technique used for orthostatic hypotension. A spine brace does not increase blood pressure.

7. D

Rationale: Following an injury to the spinal cord, patients develop an areflexic state with loss of motor and sensory function below the level of injury. This is temporary, and reflexes can return within 6 to 8 weeks. Neurogenic shock is vasodilation and bradycardia. Autonomic hyperreflexia is the presentation of hypertension due to pain stimulus below the level of injury.

8. A

Rationale: The loss of sympathetic innervation at the thoracic level (T1–T5) leads to inability to vasoconstrict and causes tachycardia. The results are vasodilation (hypotension) and bradycardia. Spinal cord concussion is a description of an injury to the spinal cord but is not the physiological cause of the neurogenic shock. Ischemic and reperfusion injuries can also happen to the cord but are not the cause of neurogenic fever. Compression of the spinal nerve roots causes injury to the peripheral nerves and does not result in neurogenic fever.

9. C

Rationale: The muscles and sphincters of the bladder are normally controlled by neurological input and spinal reflexes. Bladder dysfunction can be determined by the level of injury. Some patients have reflexive bladders, which contract the muscle when under pressure, and the patient will experience incontinence. Other spinal cord–injured (SCI) patients may have a loss of contractility that causes the bladder to stretch and retain urine. Some patients can have a combination of both. Obstruction to outflow is not a common issue with SCI patients.

10. **D**

    Rationale: Noxious stimuli below the level of injury can trigger autonomic hyperreflexia (AH), resulting in a medical emergency associated with severe hypertension that can be potentially fatal. When spinal shock is present, usually within the first 3 months, there is no AH. Spinal cord injury occurring at the level of T6 or above can result in the complication of AH within the first year of injury.

11. **A**

    Rationale: The most important nursing intervention in rehabilitation centers for prevention of autonomic hyperreflexia (AH) is to initiate bladder educational programs with patients and their families. Bladder distension is the primary cause of AH. Antihypertensives are not considered preventive therapy for the complication of AH. Bowel programs are important to initiate early to prevent AH, but bladder distension is a more common cause of AH. Alternatives to indwelling and straight catheterizations include condom catheters for male patients but these are not indicated in patients with urinary retention.

# 12

# Answers and Rationales for the Practice Exam

1. **B**

    Rationale: Both pilocytic astrocytoma and medulloblastoma brain tumors are more commonly found in the younger population. The incidence of these tumors will decrease with age. Glioblastomas are more frequently found in young adults. CNS lymphoma and metastasis will have an increased incidence with age.

2. **A**

    Rationale: Thrombotic strokes frequently present as a worsening neurological status over a short period of time. Patients may have experienced episodes of transient ischemic attacks (TIAs) before the onset of the ischemic strokes. Embolic strokes tend to have a more sudden onset without progression in symptoms. Subarachnoid hemorrhages (SAHs) are a sudden onset of headache without the history of transient neurological deficits. Vasospasms are associated with SAH, and symptoms occur most commonly between 7 and 10 days after thet SAH.

3. **A**

    Rationale: A coup injury occurs at the point of impact, and a contracoup injury occurs on the contralateral side. The mechanism of injury for acceleration injuries is commonly defined as a moving object hitting a stationary head, whereas a deceleration injury involves a moving head hitting a stationary object.

4. **C**

    Rationale: An epileptic seizure, which persists for greater than 90 minutes despite administration of anticonvulsants is called a *refractory seizure*. An epileptic seizure indicates the presence of EEG wave changes during the seizure activity. *Epilepsy* refers to repetitive seizures without a reversible cause such as hyponatremia. Nonepileptic seizure is the presence of seizure activity without the EEG changes.

5. **B**

    Rationale: Halo test (a positive result produces a yellow ring) is more accurate than a glucose test, especially with the presence of bloody drainage. A glucose test has been used to distinguish between sinus drainage and cerebrospinal fluid (CSF) because CSF has glucose but sinus drainage does not. But in this scenario, the drainage was "bloody," and blood has glucose. Bloody drainage may give a false positive with a glucose test. Testing for hemoglobin in the drainage does not determine the presence of CSF. Litmus test is used to test a pH of a fluid and is not used to distinguish CSF from nasal drainage.

6. **B**

    Rationale: Atrial fibrillation (AF) is the most common cause of an embolic stroke. Atrial septal defect (ASD) and calcified lesions can also result in embolic strokes but are significantly less common than AF. A complication of angioplasty can be distal embolization but again is not the most common cause of an embolic stroke.

7. **A**

    Rationale: Cranial nerve (CN) V (trigeminal nerve), VI (abducens nerve), VII (facial nerve), and VIII (acoustic nerve) originate from the pons. CNs IX (hypoglossal nerve), X (vagus), XI (spinal accessory nerve), and XII (hypoglossal nerve) originate from medulla. CNs III (oculomotor nerve) and IV (glossopharyngeal nerve) originate from the midbrain. No cranial nerves originate from the basal ganglia.

8. **B**

    Rationale: Hyponatremia is one of the most common electrolyte abnormalities that can cause a seizure. Hypocalcemia and hypomagnesemia can also cause seizures. Potassium is more likely to affect the myocardial electrical system, resulting in arrhythmias.

9. **C**

    Rationale: Traumatic brain injury (TBI) patients can experience "sympathetic storms" called *paroxysmal sympathetic hyperactivity*. The symptoms include fever, tachycardia, hypertension, profuse sweating, agitation, and increase respiratory rate. The "storm" is thought to be due to intermittent stimulation of the sympathoexcitatory centers located in upper brainstem and diencephalon. *Diencephalic seizure* is an incorrect term for the symptoms because the EEG is negative. Neurogenic fevers can occur following TBI but is not associated with the other symptoms of hypertension and tachycardia. Cerebral salt wasting syndrome (CSWS) is the loss of sodium through the kidneys and results in hypovolemic hyponatremia.

10. **C**

    Rationale: Failure to thrive is a complication of moderate to severe cerebral palsy (CP). It can result in malnutrition and death. CP is not associated with immunocompromise or coagulopathies. CP involves abnormal motor movements associated with spasticity or flaccidity, but does not develop locked-in syndrome.

11. **D**

    Rationale: The penumbra is the area surrounding an infarction that is ischemic or reversible ischemic tissue. Irreversibly damaged tissue is the area of tissue infarction and is the core of the infarction. Vasogenic cerebral edema is an increase in interstitial edema or fluid and is typically found surrounding the penumbra. Normal, healthy tissue is the area of brain tissue not affected by the ischemia or injury.

# 12. ANSWERS AND RATIONALES FOR THE PRACTICE EXAM

**12. B**

Rationale: Traumatic brain injury (TBI) patients can experience additional systemic injuries. Hypotension indicates hypovolemia from blood loss in trauma patients, but cerebral injury, even epidural hematoma, cannot account for the volume of blood loss. Scalp lacerations bleed profusely and may require sutures or staples to stop the bleeding. Neurogenic shock is associated with spinal cord injuries. Symptoms include hypotension and bradycardia (not tachycardia).

**13. C**

Rationale: Studies have shown warfarin is the best at preventing an embolic stroke but is associated with a greater risk of bleeding. Aspirin is also used in primary prevention of embolic strokes but has less efficacy in preventing embolic strokes. Aspirin has a lower risk of bleeding than anticoagulation therapy. Low-molecular-weight heparin (LMWH) and Plavix are not currently recommended in preventing embolic strokes.

**14. C**

Rationale: Karnofsky Performance Status Scale (KPS) is used to determine overall prognosis in patients with a brain tumor. It is used along with histopathology of the tumor, completeness of resection, presence of necrosis, and tumor size and location. CHADS2 score is used to determine the stroke risk of atrial fibrillation. Functional Independence Measure (FIM) is used to evaluate stroke patients in rehabilitation. PedsQL is a tool used to assess quality of life in pediatric patients with brain tumors but is not used for overall prognosis.

**15. C**

Rationale: Radiculopathy is compression of nerve roots due to the narrowing of foraminal processes. Osteoarthritis is the inflammation of bone and cartilage of the spinal joints. Myelopathy is compression of the spinal cord due to central stenosis. Spondylosis is the symptomatic degenerative change that occurs in osteoarthritis.

**16. B**

Rationale: The middle cerebral artery (MCA) supplies blood to the lateral portion of the cerebral cortex, which is where the motor strip for the upper extremities and face is located. The anterior cerebral artery (ACA) supplies blood to the medial portion of the cerebral cortex, which is where the motor strip for the lower extremities is located (results in lower-extremity weakness). The posterior cerebral artery (PCA) supplies blood to the occipital lobe, which results in visual deficits. The basilar artery is in the posterior circulation (brainstem) and may present with quadriplegia or "locked-in" syndrome.

**17. C**

Rationale: Never place a gastric tube nasally in a patient with a basilar skull fracture. The nasogastric (NG) tube may go through the cribriform fracture and enter the brain. A gastric tube can be placed orally, just not nasally. An enteral feeding tube may not be indicated at this time. Having the physician place the NG tube is not appropriate because the tube should not be placed nasally.

**18. C**

Rationale: The gaze abnormality in a middle cerebral artery (MCA) stroke is deviated toward the affected side. Seizures result in gaze away from the affected side. A dysconjugate or upward gaze is frequently associated with cranial nerve abnormalities but not commonly associated with strokes.

19. **A**

    Rationale: An aura is a simple partial seizure typically involving somatosensory symptoms such as hallucinations. People are aware of the aura prior to having a generalized seizure. Complex partial seizures result in a loss of awareness and are frequently manifested as motor or automatism behavior. Generalized seizures occur across both hemispheres at once and are most frequently tonic–clonic. Nonconvulsive seizure patients have epileptic EEGs, but no physical signs of a seizure.

20. **A**

    Rationale: Airway and breathing are the priorities of care. The ascending loss of muscle contraction can include the diaphragm and respiratory muscles. Vital capacity is commonly used to assess the effectiveness of ventilation in neuromuscular disorders. Electromyogram (EMG) testing may be ordered; the patient should be reassured, but the priority of care is airway and breathing. A CT of the spine may be ordered to rule out cord compression, but is not a priority over assessment of ventilatory capability.

21. **A**

    Rationale: Carotid artery dissections are associated with traumatic injuries at the cervical level. The flexion/extension mechanism of injury that causes vertebral fractures and spinal cord injuries can also cause carotid and vertebral dissections. Carotid dissections can cause cerebral infarctions with symptoms of contralateral motor loss of upper and lower extremities. Spinal cord injury and epidural hematoma would result in paralysis bilateral. There is no justification within the scenario to suspect cerebral edema as the cause of the symptoms.

22. **A**

    Rationale: Cerebrospinal fluid (CSF) leak is frequently managed by placing a lumbar drain to remove CSF. This lowers the CSF pressure and decreases the drainage. Mannitol is used to manage cerebral edema and increased intracranial pressure (ICP). Limiting fluid intake does not affect the CSF leak and is not recommended; head of the bed (HOB) is maintained flat, not elevated, to decrease the CSF leak.

23. **A**

    Rationale: The prognosis of pilocytic astrocytoma is good, with over a 90% survival rate in 10 years. It is commonly located in the cerebellum and can be surgically resected. It may not require follow-up radiotherapy if resection is complete. The tumor is not typically malignant.

24. **D**

    Rationale: The basilar artery provides blood to the ventral portion of the pons. The basilar artery is involved in the stroke, resulting in locked-in syndrome. The internal carotid artery typically presents with unilateral paresis or paralysis. The posterior communicating artery or anterior cerebral artery does not present with quadriplegia.

## 12. ANSWERS AND RATIONALES FOR THE PRACTICE EXAM

25. C

Rationale: Following a minor brain injury (concussion), patients may experience postconcussion syndrome. This is self-limiting, with neurological deficits that may last 6 months to a year after injury. Symptoms of postconcussion syndrome include (but not limited to) memory deficits, emotional outbursts, and difficulty concentrating. Periods of aphasia would be more likely transient ischemia attack. Swallowing deficit and ataxia are not associated with postconcussion syndrome and may indicate another neurological issue.

26. B

Rationale: A type II Chiari malformation is the downward displacement of cerebellar tonsils and inferior vermis, fourth ventricle, choroid plexus, and medulla.

27. D

Rationale: Priority of care is always airway and breathing. Patients presenting with a decreased level of consciousness (LOC) may be unable to maintain an airway, requiring the airway to be secured. The patient will need a CT scan and a National Institutes of Health Stroke Scale (NIHSS) assessment and may be a candidate for thrombolytic therapy, but airway and breathing are the priorities of care.

28. B

Rationale: The degeneration of the vertebral body includes increased bone formation of the subchondral bone adjacent to endplate and is called sclerosis. It is less able to absorb loads and causes formation of osteophytes, bony projections also known as spurs. These may compress on neurological structures and cause symptoms. Synovitis is inflammation of synovial joints. Foraminal stenosis causes the compression of exiting nerve roots. Lumbar disc compression can cause symptoms but is not an osteophyte.

29. B

Rationale: Anticholinesterase agents prevent the breakdown of acetylcholine by acetylcholinesterase. The effect of the anticholinesterase agents is to prolong the effect of the neurotransmitter acetylcholine. The agents do not increase secretion of the neurotransmitter acetylcholine or sensitize the receptors of acetylcholine. The postsynaptic muscle receptors are destroyed and cannot be regenerated.

30. C

Rationale: The benefits of MRI in evaluating acute spinal cord injury (SCI) are its ability to identify cord compression, soft-tissue injuries such as herniated disc and epidural hematoma, ligament instability, and intramedullary hematomas. Lateral C-spine radiographic studies can identify vertebral fractures and can assess for misalignment of the cervical spine but cannot identify cord or soft-tissue injuries. CT scans are not considered as beneficial as MRI in identifying injury to the spinal cord, soft tissue, or ligaments. Flexion/extension radiographs are used in certain patients to identify misalignment of the spine (ligament injury) but are not able to identify actual injury to the cord, soft tissues, or ligaments.

31. A

Rationale: The preictal state is the "warning" sign of an impending seizure that may occur days prior to the seizure. This may include feelings of general irritability or depression, mood changes, anxiety, headaches, lethargy, change in appetite, and lightheadedness. An aura is the actual start of the seizure. Intraictal is the period of time during the seizure. Postictal is after the seizure.

## 32. B

Rationale: Current research has found the two most important determinants of outcome following a traumatic brain injury are hypoxia and hypotension. They both are considered secondary injuries and determine cerebral perfusion. Hyperglycemia, hyperthermia, hyponatremia, and metabolic acidosis are secondary injuries and can affect outcomes but are not as severe as secondary injuries affecting cerebral perfusion.

## 33. A

Rationale: Eliquis is classified as a novel anticoagulant. A National Institutes of Health Stroke Scale (NIHSS) score of 10 is not a contraindication for alteplase. Depending upon other criteria, it would be an indication. Antiplatelet agents, such as aspirin, are not a contraindication to alteplase in acute stroke. An acute ischemic stroke will have a negative CT scan initially.

## 34. C

Rationale: Aneurysm rupture results in subarachnoid hemorrhages (SAH) and intraventricular hemorrhage (IVH), not primarily intracerebral bleeds. Anticoagulated patients, hypertensive crisis, and vascular tumors will typically cause bleeding into the parenchyma and are called intracerebral hemorrhage (ICH).

## 35. D

Rationale: There is no cure for cerebral palsy (CP). It is preventable in some cases such as those due to maternal infections (vaccinations) or Rh incompatibility (use of Rhogam). CP can be at birth or acquired at a very young age. CP may shorten life expectancy, but many children with CP live into adult ages.

## 36. B

Rationale: Guillain–Barré is an autoimmune disorder. Plasmapheresis involves the exchange of serum plasma to remove the antibodies. Plasmapheresis does not exchange red blood cells, wash white blood cells, or filter immunoglobulins.

## 37. D

Rationale: Moyamoya disease is the progressive narrowing or occlusion of the internal carotid artery with the development of collateral circulation called *Moyamoya vessels*. Presence of multiple, small aneurysms in the microcirculation is called Charcot-Bouchard. Hyperlipidemia results in the formation of plaque and the narrowing of the vessel but is not called Moyamoya vessels. Arteriovenous malformations (AVMs) are congenital vascular anomalies in which the arteries feed directly into draining veins.

## 38. D

Rationale: MRI of cervical spine can be used to clear a cervical spine injury (C-spine) in certain circumstances but is not required. Maintaining cervical immobilization until ligament injuries can be cleared is required to prevent subluxation and cord compression if an injury is present. Awake, asymptomatic patients require evaluation (radiographs or physical assessment) of flexion and extension capability to determine if potential ligament injury since plain radiographs cannot identify ligament unless some degree of subluxation is noted. Lateral C-spines require visualization of C1–C7 and the tip of T1 to clear the C-spine of bony fractures.

### 39. B

Rationale: Overall, causes of brain tumors are unknown. Exposure to ionized radiation is a known risk factor, which can be modified. Cell phones produce a very low magnetic radiation and have not been found to increase the risk of brain tumor. Environmental risks such as ingestion of high mercury and food cooked in microwave have not been found to increase risk of brain tumors.

### 40. B

Rationale: A decrease in level of consciousness is frequently associated with lobar intracerebral hemorrhage. A bleed within the brainstem frequently presents with cranial nerve deficits, pinpoint pupils, and Horner's syndrome.

### 41. C

Rationale: A common complaint by patients is a "roaring" sound in their ears as well as aural fullness. Urinary incontinence is associated with normal-pressure hydrocephalus (NPH). Subarachnoid hemorrhage (SAH) presents with the "worst headache of their life." Mèniére's disease is not associated with frequent ear infections but can have hearing losses.

### 42. A

Rationale: The goal to prevent injury of the patient is to move objects that can potentially injure the patient away from the patient. Restraining or attempting to move the patient can cause injury to the patient. Just monitoring without attempting to protect the patient is incorrect and can cause great injury to the patient.

### 43. D

Rationale: Cholinergic side effects of anticholinesterase medications include diarrhea, increased salivation, and nausea and vomiting. Urinary retention is not considered a side effect of anticholinesterase agents.

### 44. D

Rationale: Cerebral edema is classified as vasogenic and cytotoxic. Cytotoxic cerebral edema involves intracellular swelling and is caused by hypoxic and/or anoxic brain injuries. Vasogenic cerebral edema is interstitial swelling and is usually caused direct trauma or injury to the brain tissue. The "steal" phenomenon involves inappropriate distribution of blood flow to areas of injury following traumatic brain injury. Neurogenic cerebral edema is not a classification of brain swelling.

### 45. A

Rationale: Cerebellar hemorrhage frequently presents with nausea, vomiting, and ataxia. Thalamic hemorrhage presents with loss motor and/or sensory. Headache and sudden loss of consciousness is sign of lobar (frontal lobe) hemorrhage. Pituitary hemorrhage causes sudden onset of headache and visual field deficits.

**46. D**

Rationale: Cervical flexion extension radiographs are used to evaluate vertebral segmental stability. Diffusion weighted imagery is used to identify brain hypoperfusion in stroke patients. Myelogram is utilized to view central and lateral recesses and can visualize compression of individual nerve roots.

**47. C**

Rationale: Rehabilitation begins on admission into an acute care facility. A major component of rehabilitation is the prevention of secondary injuries that can adversely affect outcome. A goal of rehabilitation is to improve the patient's independence in activities of daily living, but it is not realistic to have the goal of returning to their prior level of function in spinal cord–injured (SCI) patients. Rehabilitation is to assist with reintegration of the patient into society with good resources, but it is not to provide long-term care and assistance to the patient.

**48. C**

Rationale: The primary characteristic of paralysis in Guillain–Barré (GB) is bilateral, ascending paralysis. It may or may not involve ventilatory muscles and requirement for mechanical ventilation. It is bilateral, not unilateral, paralysis. GB presents in an ascending manner, not in a descending manner.

**49. D**

Rationale: Genetic syndromes, such as neurofibromatosis types I and II, have been associated with brain tumor risk in families. Glioblastoma has a less than 1% with a genetic predisposition. Allergies and immune disorders may protect against brain tumors. Down syndrome has a very low association with brain tumors.

**50. C**

Rationale: Airway and breathing are always the priorities. Following a seizure, patients may have altered mentation and are unable to maintain airway. All of the other answers are interventions following a seizure, but the priority is airway.

**51. A**

Rationale: Brudzinski's and Kernig's signs are both signs of meningeal irritation and can be present in patients with meningitis. The Brudzinski's sign is seen when the flexion of the neck causes knees to passively flex. The Kernig's sign is pain or hamstring spasm upon straightening the bent leg. Romberg's sign is found in patients with vertigo. Kehr's sign is found in splenic injuries.

**52. C**

Rationale: The goal in a hemorrhagic stroke is to keep the systolic blood pressure (SBP) low to prevent a rebleed but high enough for perfusion of the brain tissue. Frequently, the BP will be ordered as a range such as between 130 and 150 mmHg. An SBP > 220 mmHg will increase incidence of rebleeding. Less than 100 mmHg will increase

## 12. ANSWERS AND RATIONALES FOR THE PRACTICE EXAM   231

ischemic injury. The BP should be managed to prevent complications such as rebleeds, not to treat them only when they occur.

### 53. D

Rationale: The procedure of carotid endarterectomy (CE) involves clamping of the carotid artery, which can lead to cerebral ischemia. Placing a catheter into the carotid artery to perform the CE can cause embolic showers. When the carotid artery is opened and perfusing, reperfusion hyperemia can predispose the patient to brain edema. Subdural hematoma is not a common complication of CE.

### 54. C

Rationale: The elderly, alcoholics, and dementia patients are prone to experiencing chronic subdural hematomas. These patient populations have atrophy of brain, resulting in a greater capacity to hold the volume of venous blood, delaying the onset of symptoms. Patients on anticoagulation are more likely to experience an intracerebral hemorrhage or an acute to subacute bleed.

### 55. B

Rationale: An aura has been found to frequent migraine headaches. It is not associated with cluster, stress, or daily headaches.

### 56. A

Rationale: A benign tumor in the brain may be more life-threatening than a malignancy due to several factors. The location is very important because the tumor may be benign but is present in an eloquent area of the brain or a difficult location to reach with surgery or radiation. Tumor behavior or growth is important to the development of symptoms. Patient's comorbidities, including health and age, play a significant role in outcomes with brain tumors.

### 57. A

Rationale: An aneurysm with a neck is called a *saccular* or *berry aneurysm*. A fusiform is more of an outpouching of the vessel wall. A giant aneurysm is based upon the size of the aneurysm, measuring greater than 2.5 cm in diameter. A mycotic aneurysm is classified based upon origin being an infectious source such as endocarditis.

### 58. B

Rationale: Disc protrusion or propulsion involves the rupture of the outermost fibers of the annulus. This results in bulging outward of the disc. Disc nuclear herniation without protrusion involves injury to the inner annulus without disruption of the outer. Nuclear extension is the complete split of the annulus allowing nuclear material to leak into surrounding spaces, but protruded material remains attached. Extruded nuclear substances, which are not attached and float around the spinal cord, are called sequestered nuclei.

### 59. B

Rationale: Paraplegic patients are taught to perform frequent chair shifting to prevent prolonged pressure and pressure ulcers (redistribution techniques). Cushions can be used in chair to lower the risk, but shifting frequently is more important. Hoyer lifts can be used, but paraplegic patients can usually shift themselves with their upper extremities. Massaging can improve circulation to skin but is not a technique to prevent pressure ulcers while sitting in the wheelchair.

60. **B**

Rationale: When there is an obstruction to cerebrospinal fluid (CSF) flow resulting in hydrocephalus, it is called *noncommunicating hydrocephalus*. Communicating hydrocephalus is a result of overproduction or decreased reabsorption of the CSF. Degenerative and productive hydrocephalus is not a classification of hydrocephalus.

61. **B**

Rationale: When trigeminal neuralgia (TN) is found in the younger population without other risk factors, they will frequently test for multiple sclerosis (MS). TN and MS are associated disorders, which frequently occur together. Lupus, crest syndrome, and myasthenia gravis are autoimmune disorders but are not frequently associated with TN.

62. **D**

Rationale: Mycotic aneurysms are a result of a septic source such as endocarditis showering septic emboli. Charcot–Bouchard is the presence of multiple tiny aneurysms within the deep structures of the brain. A giant aneurysm measures greater than 2.5 cm in diameter. Ehlers–Danlos syndrome is a connective tissue disease resulting in formation of aneurysms throughout the vasculature.

63. **B**

Rationale: Carbon dioxide ($CO_2$) is a potent vasodilator in the cerebral circulation. A decrease in $PaCO_2$ causes cerebral vasoconstriction, thus lowering ICP. An increase in $PaCO_2$ causes cerebral vasodilation resulting in an increase in the intracranial pressure (ICP). The lowering of the $PaCO_2$ does not increase cerebral edema.

64. **D**

Rationale: The pain of trigeminal neuralgia (TN) is neuropathic pain. It is frequently described as shock-like or electrical pain, which comes in volleys, or episodes of pain. It usually occurs unilateral. It is not described as dull, constant, or a cramping-like pain.

65. **A**

Rationale: Intracranial aneurysm rupture causes bleeding into the subarachnoid and intraventricular spaces. Epidural and subdural hematomas can be caused by trauma to the vascular but are not related to aneurysm rupture. Intracerebral hemorrhage (ICH) is bleeding into the brain parenchyma and is more likely caused by hypertension or anticoagulation.

66. **B**

Rationale: Meningococcal meningitis is spread through an airborne route and can become an epidemic in close quarters. A vaccination has been developed against one strain of meningococcal meningitis and is recommended in people living in close quarters such as military barracks or college dorms.

# 12. ANSWERS AND RATIONALES FOR THE PRACTICE EXAM

**67. D**

Rationale: Gamma-aminobutyric acid is an inhibitory neurotransmitter in the brain and has been found to inhibit seizures. Glutamine is an excitatory neurotransmitter and has been found to stimulate seizures. Dopamine inhibits motor tone and is found to be diminished in Parkinson's disease. Acetylcholine is a neurotransmitter at the level of the neuromuscular junction and is required for muscular contraction.

**68. B**

Rationale: A postural tremor occurs due to a fixed posture against gravity. Kinetic intentional tremor occurs during goal directed movement. Magnetic gait occurs with normal-pressure hydrocephalus (NPH). Ataxia is an abnormal balance or coordination and is not considered a tremor.

**69. D**

Rationale: Osmotic diuretics increase serum osmolality, resulting in hemoconcentration. As the serum osmolality increases greater than 320 mmol, neurological injury can occur. As the serum becomes hemoconcentrated, serum $Na^+$ levels increase. Thus, monitoring of both serum osmolality and $Na^+$ levels is recommended. Hgb, hct, $Ca^+$, $PO4^+$, creatinine, and blood urea nitrogen (BUN) may also be ordered but are not as greatly affected.

**70. B**

Rationale: Spina bifida occulta is just the identifiable gap between vertebral bodies found on radiographic studies. It does not involve injury to the spinal cord or spinal nerve roots. Meningocele and myelomeningocele are also forms of spina bifida and are more severe due to the involvement of the spinal cord and spinal nerve roots. Syrinx is the fluid accumulation within the central portion of the spinal cord and is not considered a form of spina bifida.

**71. A**

Rationale: About 80% of cerebral aneurysms occur within the anterior circulation, including the intracranial portion of the internal carotid artery (ICA), middle cerebral artery (MCA), and anterior cerebral artery (ACA). Of the vessels in the anterior circulation, the intracranial internal carotid artery (ICA) has the highest frequency. Injury to extracranial portion of the ICA is more commonly caused by a traumatic dissection versus an aneurysm formation. The basilar artery and vertebral arteries make up the posterior circulation and account for about 20% of the cerebral aneurysms.

**72. C**

Rationale: An oligodendrioglioma, astrocytoma, and ependymoma all gliomas arise from glial cells. They are classified as intraaxial tumors because they are actually located in brain tissue. A pituitary adenoma is a tumor involving the pituitary gland in the brain but is not composed of brain tissue cells. This is classified as an extraaxial tumor.

**73. A**

Rationale: Neuropathic pain is treated most effectively with antiepileptics (such as gabapentin) or tricyclic antidepressants. Nonsteroid anti-inflammatory drug (NSAID) can be a first-line treatment of neuropathic pain but is not as effective as antiepileptics. Neuropathic pain is not as responsive to opioids or anxiolytics in managing pain.

74. **C**

Rationale: The most common sign of a subarachnoid hemorrhage (SAH) is "the worst headache" of their life. They may also experience some focal neurological deficits and nausea and vomiting. Paralysis is not a common presenting sign of an SAH. Aphasia is more commonly associated with an ischemic stroke.

75. **D**

Rationale: CN VIII (acoustic) is the most commonly damaged cranial nerve (CN) as a result of bacterial meningitis. Hearing loss is a long-term complication of bacterial meningitis. Other CNs frequently injured in meningitis include CN III (oculomotor), IV (trochlear), and VI (abducens), which are involved in extraocular eye movement and CN II (optic).

76. **A**

Rationale: Elevating the head of the bed facilitates venous drainage, thus lowering volume and pressure in the intracranium. Elevating the foot of the bed may actually increase the intracranial pressure (ICP). Carotid massage can cause bradycardia but is not used to lower the ICP. Maintaining head alignment is appropriate to facilitate venous drainage, but a rolled towel is not as effective as a soft cervical collar.

77. **A**

Rationale: Simple partial seizures are localized seizures to one area of the brain in which the patient maintains consciousness. Complex partial seizures are also localized seizures but with the loss of consciousness. Generalized seizures occur across both hemispheres at once and are associated with a loss of consciousness. Nonepileptic seizures may be caused by subclinical or psychological seizures.

78. **A**

Rationale: Treatment of sleep apnea improves the outcomes of stroke patients with sleep apnea. Treatment of sleep apnea includes the use of continuous positive airway pressure. Intubation and mechanical ventilation is invasive management of an airway but is not indicated to treat sleep apnea. Monitoring $EtCO_2$ can be used to assess for $CO_2$ retention but is not an intervention to improve outcomes. A ketogenic diet is not a known therapy for sleep apnea.

79. **A**

Rationale: The most common neurological side effects of neuroleptic agents are dystonic movements (twisting or posturing), tremors, and involuntary movements. Weight loss is also a side effect of neuroleptic agents but it is not a neurological side effect. Acute renal failure and angioedema are not common side effects of neuroleptic agents.

80. **D**

Rationale: Prolactinoma is a pituitary adenoma, which secretes prolactin. Medical management is recommended to shrink the tumor. All of the other pituitary adenomas typically require surgical resection.

81. **D**

Rationale: A hyperflexion injury in the cervical region causes stretching of the posterior ligament with ligament disruption. The compressed area is anterior, causing anterior

## 12. ANSWERS AND RATIONALES FOR THE PRACTICE EXAM 235

vertebral body fractures. Anterior ligament disruption with posterior vertebral body fracture is caused by cervical hyperextension injuries. Central cord injuries are usually a result of hyperextension and may not be associated with vertebral fractures. Brown-Sequard cord syndrome is caused by an injury resulting in hemisection of the spinal cord.

**82. D**

Rationale: In myelomeningocele cases, the fetus's spinal canal remains open along several vertebrae in the low to middle back with protrusion of meninges and spinal cord. The cord compression and spinal nerve root injuries result in greater number and severity of complications over the other forms of spina bifida. Chiari malformation type I is not a form of spina bifida.

**83. D**

Rationale: A grade III subarachnoid hemorrhage (SAH) based upon the Hunt and Hess scale includes a patient presenting with an altered mental status, including being drowsy or confused. Asymptomatic presentation would be a grade 0, and the unruptured aneurysm may be found incidentally. Posturing is a grade IV, and unresponsive is a grade V.

**84. C**

Rationale: In benign essential tremor (BET), the tremors occur with intentional activity, not at rest. This is different than Parkinson's disease, in which tremors occur at rest and improve during intentional activity. Stress will worsen tremors, but it is not the only time when the tremors occur in BET.

**85. D**

Rationale: Axial loading or vertical compression of the spine causes the vertebral body to burst. Hyperflexion injuries cause posterior ligament disruptions and anterior vertebral compression fractures. Hyperextension injuries cause fracture of posterior vertebral body components and disruption of anterior longitudinal ligament. Torsion injury is associated with sprain or muscle injury of the neck.

**86. C**

Rationale: MRI with and without contrast is considered the gold standard in diagnosing central nervous system tumors, including determining the location and characteristic of the tumor. CT with and without contrast is typically a screening and can identify mass lesions and shifts. Magnetic resonance angiography (MRA) is used more to identify vascular anomalies such as a cerebral aneurysm or arteriovenous malformation (AVM).

**87. A**

Rationale: Anterior cord syndrome results in the loss of motor, pain, and temperature but spares some of the sensory tracts such as proprioception and light touch. Central cord syndrome results in greater upper-extremity than lower-extremity weakness. Brown–Sequard cord syndrome is a hemisection of the cord and results in ipsilateral loss of motor and contralateral loss of pain and temperature. A complete cord injury is a loss of all motor and sensory below the level of injury.

88. **A**

Rationale: A prion disease is an abnormal infectious protein. It results in a fatal encephalopathy. Prion diseases are not related to protozoa infections and tapeworm and are not transmitted by ticks.

89. **D**

Rationale: Atonic seizures are classified as generalized seizures. The epileptic focus initiates throughout both hemispheres. Somatosensory, psychic, and autonomic seizures are classified as simple partial seizures due to epileptic focus occurring within a focal area of the brain.

90. **A**

Rationale: Following a lumbar puncture, herniation can occur if the patient has an increased intracranial pressure (ICP). The positive pressure in the brain can herniate brain structures following a negative pressure in the lumbar region caused by the lumbar puncture. Kernig's and Brudizinski's signs are associated with meningitis or meningeal irritation. Aphasia is associated more commonly with ischemic strokes.

91. **A**

Rationale: Prone positioning for spine surgery puts one at a high risk for visual losses. The addition of the patient experiencing a significant blood loss and who is hypotensive increases the risk of visual losses. Blood loss and hypotension can cause mesenteric ischemia and acute kidney injury, but in this scenario with the patient being in the prone position for a prolonged period of time, it is more likely to cause visual losses. A complication would more likely be an ischemic versus a hemorrhagic stroke.

92. **C**

Rationale: Subarachnoid hemorrhage (SAH) complication of vasospasms has its highest incidence 7 to 10 days post SAH. Vasospasms are not typically seen before day 4 or after day 21 post SAH.

93. **A**

Rationale: Corticosteroids are commonly used to manage the vasogenic edema surrounding cerebral tumors. Dexamethasone (Decadron) is the drug of choice. In severe edema and increased intracranial pressure (ICP), osmotic diuretics (such as mannitol and hypertonic saline) may be used to lower the ICP. Therapeutic hypothermia is used in patients with cytotoxic cerebral edema caused by an anoxic brain injury (postresuscitation).

94. **B**

Rationale: Hypertension is used to provide perfusion to the brain tissue distal to the narrowed vessel experiencing vasospasm. Hypervolemia is no longer recommended due to situations of volume overload. It is recommended to optimize hemodynamic parameters and assure euvolemic status. Hypothermia is not recommended for subarachnoid hemorrhage (SAH) patients. Hemodilution is not recommended because of the effect on ability to carry oxygen to the tissues.

95. **C**

Rationale: The treatment of benign essential tremor (BET) does not cure or stop the tremors. The goal of treatment is to decrease the amplitude of the tremors.

Improvement of the emotional side may occur following the reduction in amplitude but is not the primary goal of treatment.

96. **B**

    Rationale: In bacterial meningitis, cerebrospinal fluid (CSF) analysis results in elevated protein, elevated white blood cell (WBC) neutrophils, increased lactate, and low glucose. Bacterial meningitis causes low glucose, not high. Viral meningitis typically has a normal CSF glucose level.

97. **D**

    Rationale: Evidence suggests that increased body temperature in the early months of pregnancy may increase the risk of spina bifida (SB). Elevated core body temperature by about 2°C (about 3–4°F) above normal caused by fever or the use of saunas and hot tubs can result in development of SB. Vitamin B9 deficiency, not vitamin C, may increase the risk of SB. Maternal trauma is not as known of a risk for SB as for cerebral palsy. Exercise is not a risk for SB.

98. **B**

    Rationale: Hyponatremia is the most common electrolyte abnormality following subarachnoid hemorrhage. It can be due to cerebral salt wasting syndrome or syndrome of inappropriate antidiuretic hormone.

99. **C**

    Rationale: It is currently not recommended for a patient with transient ischemic attack (TIA) to be immediately taken for angioplasty and stent placement. Medical management with dual antiplatelets, BP control, and high intensity statins is recommended as a first-line intervention. If TIA reoccurs or stroke occurs, then invasive management with stents or endarterectomy may be considered.

100. **B**

    Rationale: Flu vaccines can cause the onset of Guillain–Barré (GB). Other known causes include viral infections and trauma. Urinary tract infections (UTIs) are typically bacterial infections and are not associated with GB. Hyperthyroidism and bacteremia are not associated with triggering GB.

101. **A**

    Rationale: Brown–Sequard cord syndrome involves the hemisection of the spinal cord. The resulting symptoms include ipsilateral loss of motor function and contralateral loss of pain and temperature control. In a complete cord injury, there is a complete loss of motor and sensory function below the level of injury. Central cord syndrome presents with greater loss of upper-extremity motor function than lower extremity motor function. A loss of sensory function without motor function is not indicative of Brown–Sequard syndrome.

102. **C**

    Rationale: Neurocysticercosis involves pig tapeworm larvae entering the brain. Pig tapeworm larvae are acquired by eating undercooked pork or improper hand washing while preparing food of an infected person of tapeworm. Tick bites can cause Lyme disease. Swimming in stagnant water may expose children or immunosuppressed patients to protozoa, which results in severe cerebral edema and death. A mosquito bite can spread encephalitis.

103. A

Rationale: Deep, intraaxial tumors in the brainstem, vascular tumors, and tumors located in eloquent areas (i.e., Broca's area) are not amendable to surgical resection and biopsy due to the location or risk of hemorrhage. A glioblastoma located in the frontal lobe is a candidate for resection.

104. C

Rationale: Cerebral palsy (CP) is considered to be nonprogressive. The abnormal movement may change as the child matures but is not progressive. There are multiple causes and underlying etiologies besides just hypoxic injuries that can result in CP. CP is a permanent neurological disorder that is not reversible.

105. B

Rationale: The complementary medicine most commonly used to manage pain in trigeminal neuralgia (TN) is acupuncture. Spinal manipulation is not a pain management technique used in treating TN. Meditation can be an effective treatment for pain, but acupuncture is more effective in TN. Herbal supplements are not common for managing TN.

106. B

Rationale: C4 is the level at which the diaphragm is innervated. Injury occurring at the level of C4 or above will affect the patient's ability to have spontaneous ventilation. C2 level injury, above the level of the diaphragm, results in a complete loss of ventilation, and the patient will become ventilator dependent. C6 and T1 injury level injuries occur below the level of diaphragm innervation and should be able to ventilate spontaneously once edema has resolved.

107. C

Rationale: All of the answers are complications of subarachnoid hemorrhage, but hydrocephalus is the only long-term complication and may even require the placement of a ventriculoperitoneal (VP) shunt. Vasospasms occur most frequently between day 7 and 10 post subarachnoid hemorrhage (SAH). Cerebral edema and nausea and vomiting commonly occur within the first 48 hours.

108. D

Rationale: Disequilibrium syndrome with hemodialysis is a sudden onset of cerebral edema caused by a rapid removal of blood urea nitrogen (BUN), resulting in a rapid decrease of serum osmolality. Septic encephalopathy is a result of sepsis and leukocytosis. Septic patients can develop altered mentation, but it is due more to the disruption of the blood–brain barrier. Drug-induced delirium is temporary due to the drug and resolves when the drug leaves the system. Hepatic encephalopathy is due to elevated ammonia levels and alterations of the blood–brain barrier.

109. C

Rationale: Todd's paralysis is a temporary neurological deficit following a seizure. It may include temporary loss of motor or sight. A postictal period is the time after a

## 12. ANSWERS AND RATIONALES FOR THE PRACTICE EXAM 239

seizure in which the patient may be drowsy or lethargic. It does not involve a paralysis. An aura comes before the generalized seizure and is considered to be a simple partial seizure. Electromechanical dissociation is the physical presence of seizure activity without the electrical activity on EEG.

110. A

Rationale: Normal-pressure hydrocephalus (NPH) presents as "wet," "wacky," and "wobbly." Wet is incontinence (urinary symptoms), wacky is dementia, and wobbly are the abnormal gait disturbances. Nausea and vomiting is a sign of increased pressure hydrocephalus, **not** in NPH.

111. A

Rationale: Maternal serum alpha-fetoprotein (MSAFP) is the most commonly used screening test for spina bifida (SB). Estriol, human chorionic gonadotropin (HCG) and amniocentesis may be used if the MSAFP is positive for a high risk of the fetus having SB and confirmation is needed.

112. C

Rationale: There are seven vertebral bodies in the cervical region, but there are eight paired cervical nerve roots exiting the spinal cord. The spinal nerve roots exit above the corresponding vertebral body until the level of C7 in which the spinal nerve root changes to exit below the vertebral body. There are two sets of paired cervical spinal nerve roots at the level of C7.

113. D

Rationale: A fusiform aneurysm is an outpouching of the vessel wall. A saccular or berry aneurysm has a neck. A giant aneurysm measures greater than 2.5 cm in diameter. Tiny, multiple aneurysms in microcirculation are called Charcot–Bouchard aneurysms.

114. A

Rationale: Multiple sclerosis (MS) is a demyelinating disorder of the central nervous system (CNS). The most common form of MS involves relapses and remissions. Myasthenia gravis (MG) affects the neuromuscular junction. Amyotrophic lateral sclerosis (ALS) is a pure motor neuron disorder. Guillain–Barré presents with the ascending paralysis bilateral.

115. C

Rationale: Pseudotumor cerebri is considered a benign intracranial hypertension. It commonly presents with visual changes, headaches, nausea and vomiting, tinnitus, forgetfulness, and depression. Viral encephalitis commonly presents with altered mentation. Meningioma presentation may include headaches and visual changes (depending upon the location of the tumor) but is not typically associated with depression. Normal-pressure hydrocephalus (NPH) presents with gait abnormalities, incontinence, and dementia.

116. C

Rationale: The goal of brain tumor resection is to remove as much tumor as possible without increasing morbidity or adversely affecting quality of life. Eloquent areas of the brain, such as the language and speech center, affect quality of life. If the goal was to always resect the complete tumor, areas of eloquence would be damaged and quality of life would be affected. It is recommended to resect as much of the tumor as feasible. Surgical resection is typically the first-line treatment followed by chemotherapy and/or radiation in primary brain tumors.

117. C

Rationale: Nausea and vomiting are not common side effects of most antiepileptics. Drowsiness, dizziness, and diplopia are common side effects of antiepileptics.

118. A

Rationale: Central venous thrombosis (CVT), like any other venous thrombotic events, is the result of a hypercoagulable state. The venous clot is occurring in the venous sinuses of the central nervous system (CNS). It is venous in nature, not arterial, so it does not involve the dural arterial system. CVT can present as an ischemic or hemorrhagic stroke and sometimes can be a combination of both. The venous sinuses (cavernous sinus, sagittal sinus, and lateral sinus) are the most common locations of the central venous thrombosis, not the external jugular vein.

119. D

Rationale: Not all patients with normal-pressure hydrocephalus (NPH) will show significant improvement with the placement of a ventriculoperitoneal (VP) shunt. Typically, a test will be performed in which cerebrospinal fluid (CSF) is removed, and the patient is reevaluated to determine whether the procedure will be effective before the VP shunt is placed. This can include lumbar drain trials in a hospital setting or high-drainage test with a lumbar puncture. VP shunts can improve the symptoms in some patients. It is not recommended to place a ventriculostomy or intracranial pressure (ICP) monitor to determine the ICP while making the diagnosis of NPH.

120. C

Rationale: The Lhermitte's sign is a sign of neuropathy pain. It is described as an electric- shock sensation. It is not paresthesia, head tremors, or difficulty with word finding.

121. C

Rationale: Spinal shock results in a loss of motor, sensory, and deep tendon reflexes. A loss of anal tone is a sign of loss of reflexes. Hyperspasticity, hyperreflexia, and hypertension occur after spinal shock has resolved, and the patient is at risk for autonomic hyperreflexia.

122. C

Rationale: Seizure risk is based upon location and the type of tumor. The temporal lobe is most susceptible to seizures and epilepsy. Tumors located in the temporal lobe commonly present with seizures.

123. C

Rationale: A factor VIII deficiency would cause the patient to have a coagulopathy with a decreased ability to clot. The patient would not be at risk for central

## 12. ANSWERS AND RATIONALES FOR THE PRACTICE EXAM  241

venous thrombosis (CVT). Malignancy, infections (especially, eyes, ears, and scalp), and pregnancy can all cause hypercoagulable states and are known risk factors for CVT.

124. **B**

    Rationale: Venous thrombosis strokes are venous, not arterial. Arterial strokes most commonly present acutely, within hours of onset of the stroke symptoms. Venous strokes can present as acute, subacute, or chronic, but are most commonly subacute.

125. **C**

    Rationale: High levels of maternal serum alpha-fetoprotein (MSAFP) and amniocentesis measuring fetal alpha-protein are able to identify a fetus with spina bifida (SB), but advanced ultrasonography is the diagnostic examination used to visualize the spine and assist with determining the severity of the SB.

126. **A**

    Rationale: The Valsalva maneuver, nose blowing, sneezing, and coughing can cause a subsequent cerebrospinal fluid (CSF) leak. If the patient needs to cough, an open mouth cough or sneeze is recommended. Packing the nose with a CSF leak increases the risk of CNS infection.

127. **A**

    Rationale: Anticoagulation therapy is the recommended management of central venous thrombosis (CVT), even if there is a hemorrhagic component to the stroke. CVT is treated like other venous thromboembolisms (VTEs). Steroid therapy is not recommended in CVT. Decompressive craniotomy is reserved for severe cerebral edema and poor neurological function. This patient is awake and communicating. Statin therapy is not recommended due to the hemorrhagic stroke.

128. **B**

    Rationale: Multiple sclerosis (MS) is an autoimmune disorder and is frequently treated with immunosuppressant medications. Commonly ordered medications include steroids, immunosuppressive agents, and interferon. Acetylcholinesterase inhibitors are primarily used in myasthenia gravis (MG).

129. **B**

    Rationale: Obesity is the most common link associated with pseudotumor cerebri. A weight-loss program is often used in managing symptoms. Other associated risks include women greater than men, pregnant women, thyroid condition, and chronic kidney disease. Hyperlipidemia, Hispanic race, and exposure to pet dandruff are not considered higher risks for pseudotumor cerebri.

130. **B**

    Rationale: Sudden twisting or head movements can cause vertebral or carotid dissections, but the most common location is extracranial. Extracranial vertebral would be more common with trauma and neck manipulations than an intracranial carotid dissection. The scenario is not likely to have resulted in a basilar artery occlusion or a central venous thrombosis (CVT).

131. **B**

Rationale: The benzodiazepines work to stop a seizure by enhancing the inhibitory effects of the neurotransmitter gamma-aminobutyric acid (GABA). Phenytoin works by blocking by sodium (Na$^+$) channels and can be used to increase the seizure threshold. Vagal nerve stimulators are used like pacemakers in the heart. They can overdrive the neuronal impulses to control and inhibit the firing of the neurons. Barbiturates are used to induce a medical coma in a refractory seizure.

132. **B**

Rationale: Trigeminal neuralgia (TN) most commonly affects the mandibular and maxillary division of the trigeminal nerve and rarely affects the ophthalmic division only. TN is typically unilateral and difficult to diagnose. MRI does not typically identify the cause of TN. Pain is intermittent with paroxysmal attacks. It occurs in cycles with remissions.

133. **B**

Rationale: Signs of autonomic hyperreflexia include hypertension, headache, and sensation of stuffy nose. Autonomic hyperreflexia results from an obnoxious stimulus below the level of injury. Putting the head of the bed (HOB) up will lower blood pressure (BP) due to orthostatic hypotension experienced by patients with spinal cord injuries. This allows time to find the painful source and remove it. Administering an antihypertensive initially will cause hypotension once the painful source is found and removed. Without treatment, the hypertension can be life-threatening.

134. **A**

Rationale: Radiation affects both normal and brain tumor cells. The mechanism of radiation to treat tumor cells is irreversible necrosis. Certain brain structures are more radiosensitive such as optic nerve and brainstem.

135. **D**

Rationale: Horner's syndrome includes ptosis (eyelid drooping), miosis (small pupils), and unilateral facial anhydrosis (inability to sweat). This is a result of injury to the sympathetic innervation of the face. Locked-in syndrome is a result of basilar artery occlusion. Duvet's syndrome does not result in the symptoms mentioned here. There is not a neurological disorder called Chagall's syndrome.

136. **C**

Rationale: Injury to the motor cortex during the maturation of the brain can result in cerebral palsy (CP). This injury can occur before birth, during the birthing process, or after birth during maturation of the motor cortex. CP is not always associated with mental delays or retardation.

137. **C**

Rationale: Spinal cord–injured patients are at risk for the development of autonomic hyperreflexia. Symptoms of autonomic hyperreflexia include hypertension, headache, and diaphoresis above the level of injury. Spinal shock is a loss of motor and sensory below the level of injury in acute spinal cord–injured patients. Neurogenic shock occurs in acute spinal cord–injured patients and results in hypotension and

## 12. ANSWERS AND RATIONALES FOR THE PRACTICE EXAM  243

bradycardia. Lacunar stroke is a type of ischemic stroke caused by chronic hypertension and is not related to spinal shock.

138. **B**

    Rationale: Abnormal infectious prions are not susceptible to normal disinfection agents or autoclaving. When instruments have been used on contaminated brain tissue, they need to be destroyed.

139. **B**

    Rationale: Temozolomide (Temodar) is a first-line chemotherapy treatment in a glioblastoma. It is used in brain tumors because it does cross the blood–brain barrier. Bevacizumab (Avastin) is used in treating several different types of cancer, including glioblastoma. It is used more often in recurring glioblastomas than as a first-line treatment. Doxorubicin (Adriamycin) is a chemotherapy drug commonly used to treat breast cancer. Paclitaxel (Taxol) is a chemotherapy drug used to treat lung cancer.

140. **D**

    Rationale: Spina bifida occulta is a deformity in the closure of the vertebral bodies, but the spinal canal is intact. There is no spinal cord involvement and does not require surgery. Myelomeningocele and meningocele have opening in the spinal canal with protrusion of meninges and, in the severe cases, protrusion of the spinal cord. This does require surgery to replace the meninges and close the spine. Chiari malformations type II frequently require surgical management due to the severity of the herniation.

141. **C**

    Rationale: Myasthenia gravis (MG) has been found to be associated with thyroid disorders. Thymectomy procedures have been shown to improve clinical function. Vaccinations have been associated with Guillain–Barré (GB). Lyme disease and renal disease are not associated with MG.

142. **C**

    Rationale: Ehlers–Danlos is a connective tissue disease that causes a weakening of the medial layer within the vasculature. This places the person at a greater risk for arterial dissections (vertebral and carotid) and aneurysm formation (intracerebral). Arteriovenous malformation (AVM) is congenital and is present at birth. These are not commonly associated with Ehlers–Danlos.

143. **D**

    Rationale: The cerebrospinal fluid (CSF) analysis is considered the gold standard for diagnosing leptomeningeal tumor. The presence of malignant tumor cells in the CSF is diagnostic. Neuroimaging can be used to assist with the diagnosis based upon the pattern of findings. The MRI would be a better imaging technique than the CT scan. PET scans are not used as often with identifying location of brain tumors. Rarely would a biopsy be indicated to diagnose a leptomeningeal tumor.

144. **A**

    Rationale: Orthostatic hypotension occurs in spinal cord–injured patients. Abdominal binders have been found to reduce incidence of orthostatic hypotension. A halo test is used to stabilize an unstable fracture but does not have an effect on orthostatic hypotension. A "quad" cough is performed to improve the effectiveness of the cough in spinal cord–injured patients with limited ventilatory effort. Bowel stimulation is a part of the bowel program in spinal cord–injured patients.

145. **D**

    Rationale: Cavernous malformations frequently result in small hemorrhages separated by months to years. Gradient echo MRI is the best tool for identifying small hemorrhage and identifying various ages of the bleeds. Transcranial Doppler is used to identify focal narrowing of the cerebral arteries and does not contribute to the diagnosis of cavernous malformations. The vascular anomalies are low flow states and are not easily identified with cerebral angiogram. Noncontrast CT is not as specific as gradient echo MRI in identifying small areas of blood.

146. **B**

    Rationale: Ménière's disease is characterized by episodes of vertigo. Symptoms include vertigo, nausea, and feeling of "fullness" in the ear. Ménière's disease is not associated with dementia and is not considered a sensory abnormality such as facial numbness or neuropathic pain syndrome of the face.

147. **B**

    Rationale: Phenytoin (Dilantin) should not be administered too rapidly intravenously (IV). Dilantin administered via IV too rapidly can cause cardiac arrest. The recommended rate of administration is no faster than 50 mg/minute. It should never be given rapid IV push. The bolus does not require 4 hours to administer. Dilantin is available and is frequently administered in the IV route.

148. **C**

    Rationale: Primary central nervous system (CNS) vasculitis is commonly diagnosed with bilateral temporal artery biopsy. Brain biopsy may be the gold standard but can have a higher risk. Transcranial Doppler is used to identify vasospasms following a subarachnoid hemorrhage. Cerebrospinal fluid drainage is a technique used to evaluate improvement in patients with normal-pressure hydrocephalus (NPH). MRI is not effective in identifying primary CNS vasculitis.

149. **C**

    Rationale: Myasthenia gravis (MG) is the result of muscle receptor sites being destroyed by antibodies, thus significantly limiting the number of receptor sites for acetylcholine. Repetitive movements begin to weaken the muscular contraction, resulting in weaker movement with repetitive activity. Testing large muscle repetitive muscles assist with determining the effectiveness of treatment.

150. **D**

    Rationale: The leptomeningeal tumors are located in the meninges and subarachnoid space. Administration of a chemotherapy medication directly into the cerebrospinal fluid (CSF) (intrathecal) would assure that the medication more likely reaches the tumor bed. Central nervous system (CNS) lymphomas, gliomas, and pituitary tumors are not within the meninges or CSF and would not benefit from the intrathecal route.

# 12. ANSWERS AND RATIONALES FOR THE PRACTICE EXAM    245

**151. D**

Rationale: Moyamoya disease is the formation of abnormal collateral circulation due to the bilateral narrowing of the internal carotid and anterior cerebral arteries bilaterally. The gold standard for diagnosis is cerebral angiogram. When the contrast is injected, hazy, smoke-like puffs are seen in the carotid and anterior cerebral arteries bilateral. Leptomeningeal fibrosis is not a disease process. Neurofibromatosis can be a risk for Moyamoya but is not identified by the cerebral angiogram. Ehlers–Danlos disease is a connective tissue disease more commonly associated with vascular anomalies such as aneurysms and dissections.

**152. B**

Rationale: Bell's palsy involves the terminal branches of the facial nerve (cranial nerve [CN] VII). It results in a loss of motor especially involving the muscles required for facial expressions. It is usually unilateral and will not spare the forehead muscles. Lyme disease is an encephalopathy. Trigeminal neuralgia is a pain syndrome, which involves the trigeminal nerve (CN V). Ischemic stroke causing facial droop and unilateral facial paralysis will not involve the forehead.

**153. B**

Rationale: Following administration of alteplase in acute stroke patient, the American Heart Association/American Stroke Association (AHA/ASA) recommend maintaining the systolic blood pressure (BP) less than 180 mmHg and the diastolic BP less than 100 mmHg. If the patient did not receive alteplase and it is an ischemic stroke, the systolic BP is allowed to increase to 220 mmHg before treatment. Hemorrhagic strokes, not ischemic with alteplase administration, will have the systolic BP maintained below 160 mmHg.

**154. B**

Rationale: The most common cause of spina bifida (SB) is dietary deficiencies, especially of folic acid (vitamin B9). Fortifying or supplementing the diet with vitamin B and other required vitamins significantly lower the incidence SB. Genetic testing for abnormal variances is not consistent or reliable. Maternal vaccinations can help prevent cerebral palsy caused by maternal infections. Use of seatbelts is protective but does not prevent SB.

**155. C**

Rationale: The standard of care for a single unprovoked seizure is avoidance of typical precipitants such as alcohol and sleep deprivation. An anticonvulsant is not recommended unless the patient has risk factors for recurrence. Admission for video EEG monitoring is typically for patients with intractable episodes or to evaluate the etiology of the seizure. A patient with a seizure, even the first episode, should have follow-up with a neurologist.

**156. C**

Rationale: Decompressive hemicraniectomy is the surgical removal of a large portion of the skull to allow room for swelling. It is used to prevent herniation within the closed space or medically retractable increased intracranial pressure. Contusions are not an indication for decompressive craniectomy unless accompanied by increased intracranial pressure. Following brain death and while maintaining the patient for organ donor, a hemicraniectomy is not recommended. Adults and pediatric patients have been found to improve outcomes in certain circumstances.

157. B

Rationale: Hyperthermia can worsen outcomes in a patient following an ischemic stroke. Strict normothermia should be maintained, treating body temperature greater than 38°C. Hyperglycemia can also worsen neurological outcomes but is not usually treated until greater than 140 mg/dl. A $Na^+$ of 142 is normal, so obtaining urine osmolality and specific gravity to diagnose water imbalances is not required at this time.

158. C

Rationale: Anticholinergics, which are used frequently to manage Mèniére's disease, may produce blurred vision. It decreases oral secretions and nausea and can cause bradycardia, not tachycardia.

159. B

Rationale: Astrocytoma, even a low-grade "benign" tumor, can be very invasive, difficult to treat, and can progress to a higher grade "malignant" tumor. Brain tumor prognosis is based more upon the cell origin and location of the tumor than labeling the tumor benign or malignant. Astrocytoma typically requires follow-up treatment with either or both radiation and chemotherapy. Astrocytoma does not commonly metastasize to the lungs.

160. D

Rationale: A bedside swallow test should be performed on all stroke patients prior to any oral intake, including oral medications. If they fail a bedside swallow, they should remain NPO until speech therapy can evaluate them. Supplemental oxygen should be administered if the oxygen saturation is less than 94%. It is not recommended to administer to all stroke patients. Prophylactic anticonvulsants are not recommended in stroke patients. Following an ischemic stroke, permissive hypertension is recommended for perfusion unless the patient had received fibrinolytic agent. Systolic blood pressure (BP) may not be treated unless greater than 220 mmHg.

161. D

Rationale: Allodynia is a sensory abnormality in which light touch can become painful. People with cerebral palsy (CP) may experience allodynia. The inability to control body temperature is not typically an issue with CP and is called poikilothermia.

162. D

Rationale: Partial-onset seizure carries a higher risk of recurrence than generalized seizures. Epileptiform or slowing on the EEG findings is associated with the highest risk of recurrence. Abnormal findings on MRI, including hydrocephalus, can increase the risk of reoccurrence of seizures.

163. B

Rationale: Even though the patient may have passed the bedside swallow examination prior to admission, if a stroke patient begins to cough with oral intake, they should be place NPO and speech therapy are consulted for further swallow evaluations. Stroke patients with abnormal swallowing are at high risk for aspiration pneumonia. The speech therapist will evaluate the stroke patient and make a decision on the most appropriate follow-up diagnostic study. The patient does not require supplemental oxygen unless the oxygen saturations are less than 94%.

164. **B**

    Rationale: The diagnosis of diabetes insipidus (DI) is made when the urine is dilute (urine specific gravity <1.005 and urine osmolality <200 mOsm/L) and the serum is concentrated (serum $Na^+$ >145 dg/L). Serum osmolality of <200 mOsm/L indicates a hypotonic serum.

165. **C**

    Rationale: There is very little research data supporting the use of therapeutic hypothermia in severe traumatic brain injury (TBI) and it is currently not a recommended treatment. Mannitol and hypertonic saline are both hyperosmolar agents that can lower the intracranial pressure (ICP) and are recommended to treat increased ICP in severe TBI patients. Cerebrospinal fluid (CSF) drainage is used to lower the CSF volume and decrease ICP.

166. **C**

    Rationale: Heparin is the most common cause for a drug-induced thrombocytopenia. The decrease in platelet count typically occurs between 5 and 10 days of being on heparin and is greater than a 50% decrease. The scenario had the patient on heparin, so heparin-induced thrombocytopenia (HIT) was more likely the cause over idiopathic thrombocytopenic purpura (ITP). An elevated INR does not cause platelet counts to decrease. Suppression of bone marrow production can decrease platelets, but there is no risk identified in the patient's scenario.

167. **D**

    Rationale: Traumatic brain injury (TBI) is not considered a common cause of trigeminal neuralgia (TN). Compression of the trigeminal nerve by tumor or aneurysm is a known cause of TN. One of the first signs of multiple sclerosis (MS) is TN due to the demyelination of the cranial nerve.

168. **C**

    Rationale: Of the 12 cranial nerves (CNs), 10 CNs originate from the brainstem. CN assessment is important with brainstem involvement. The pons originates in CN s V through VIII, so a tumor involved in the pons commonly presents with deficits in those CNs and those CNs should be assessed. CNs I and II originate from the cerebral cortex. CNs III and IV originate from the midbrain. And CNs IX, X, and XII originate from the medulla.

169. **D**

    Rationale: If a patient is allergic to acetylsalicylic acid, the recommendation is to use clopidogrel (Plavix). The patient should receive an antithrombotic medication following an acute ischemic stroke. It would not be appropriate to encourage a patient to take a medicine that the patient states is an allergy. Documentation of the allergy (not that the patient is refusing the acetylsalicylic acid) is appropriate, but the best response to contact the physician for discussion about another antithrombotic agent.

Calling the pharmacy about acetylsalicylic acid allergies may be for informational purposes but is not as appropriate as giving the best care to the patient.

170. C

Rationale: The entral nervous system, including the brain and spinal cord, is an upper motor neuron (UMN). UMN injury results in symptoms of spasticity, increased muscle tone, increased deep tendon reflexes (DTRs), and less muscle atrophy. Lower motor neuron (LMN) injury results in flaccid paralysis with a decrease in muscle tone, decreased DTRs, and significant muscle loss.

171. B

Rationale: Tonic activity in motor seizures involves sustained focal stiffening. Atonicity is the focal loss of muscle tone. Myoclonic activity is irregular brief focal jerking movements. *Clonic activity* refers to the focal rhythmic jerking movement. It is more rhythmic than the myoclonic activity.

172. A

Rationale: Simple and complex involuntary motor movements and vocalizations are signs of Tourette's syndrome. Tourette's can be associated with attention deficit hyperactivity disorder (ADHD) and obsessive-compulsive behaviors. Miller Fisher syndrome is a variant presentation of Guillain–Barré. Absence seizures are found in children but are demonstrated by periods of blank stares, not involuntary movements. Dravet's syndrome is frequent and prolonged seizures in children within the first year of life.

173. B

Rationale: The INR goal for ischemic stroke patients with atrial fibrillation is between 2 and 3. An international normalized ratio (INR) below 2 is too low and will increase their chance of another embolic event. An INR greater than 3 is too high and will increase the risk of bleeding.

174. B

Rationale: The patient is hyponatremic ($Na^+$ 130), and administration of hypertonic saline (3% or 7.5%) to treat an increased intracranial pressure (ICP) can be detrimental to hyponatremic patients. Sodium levels should be corrected slowly over 24 hours to prevent complications. Administration of hypertonic saline to treat increased ICP can change too rapidly the serum sodium. Mannitol is recommended over hypertonic saline in hyponatremic patients when treating an increased ICP. Glycerol is not commonly used to lower an ICP.

175. B

Rationale: An acoustic neuroma involves a tumor invading the neural sheath surrounding cranial nerve (CN) VIII (acoustic). CNs VIII, VII (facial), and V (trigeminal) lie adjacent to each other, so damage to CN VII is commonly associated with acoustic neuroma.

176. D

Rationale: Automatism can be found in focal and absence seizures. It involves less coordinated, purposeless repetitive movements. Motor arrest is the cessation of motor movement and unresponsiveness. Hyperkinetic activity is an increase in activity such as pedaling or thrashing. Irregular, brief focal jerking movement is myoclonic activity.

177. **A**

Rationale: A potential complication of statin administration includes rhabdomyolysis. Patient education regarding rhabdomyolysis, including the color change of urine, is recommended. It is actually recommended to avoid grapefruits and grapefruit juice due to the effect on drug levels. A statin may be ordered even if the patient has a normal cholesterol level. Liver function tests, not kidney function, are monitored when placed on a statin.

178. **D**

Rationale: Mannitol is effective in lowering intracranial pressure (ICP) and may be administered in severe traumatic brain injury (TBI), but the diuresis can result in hypovolemia and hypotension. This can be detrimental in multisystem trauma patients due to loss of blood. Hypertonic saline may be preferred in multisystem trauma patients over mannitol. Hypokalemia is a potential side effect of mannitol and does require treatment, but this is not specific to multisystem trauma patients. Increased serum osmolality and potentially some increase in sodium can occur but is not the concern with multisystem trauma patients as the diuresis, hypovolemia, and hypotension.

179. **A**

Rationale: The approach for the decompression of the vestibular nerve is base skull surgery. This surgical approach is an increased risk for cerebrospinal fluid (CSF) leaks and central nervous system (CNS) infections. Epidural hematoma is not considered a potential complication of base skull surgeries. Cushing's triad is the symptoms of increased intracranial pressure and herniation. This is not a complication of vestibular nerve resection. Cerebellar herniation is the physiological effect of Chiari malformations.

180. **C**

Rationale: Pituitary tumors and resections of the tumor by the transphenoidal route can affect the pituitary–hypothalamus axis, resulting in water imbalances postoperative. A sudden increase in urine output would more likely be due to a lack of production of antidiuretic hormone (ADH). Syndrome of inappropriate antidiuretic hormone (SIADH) is also a water imbalance associated with the pituitary gland but would result in a decrease in urine output and hyponatremia. Cerebral salt wasting syndrome (CSWS) is not associated with ADH and causes a hyponatremia. Fluids can shift from interstitial space back into the vascular space 24 to 48 hours postoperatively. This will increase the urine output due to an increase in circulating volume but would not typically cause the sudden increase in urine output within 1 hour.

181. **B**

Using the technique of "Teach Back" in which information is provided to the patient followed by the patient repeating the information back in his or her own words. This can be utilized to assess the patient's understanding of what is being taught. Documentation is important but is not used to determine the patient's understanding.

It is recommended that a variety of methods are used to teach the patient, but it does not necessarily evaluate the understanding of the material being taught. Providing large amounts of information in a short period of time is not recommended due to the inability to take it all in and understand the information.

182. **B**

    PaCO$_2$ is considered the most powerful determinant of cerebral blood flow (CBF) by controlling the cerebral vascular diameter. CBF responds in a linear fashion to the PaCO$_2$ levels. As the PaCO$_2$ decreases, so does CBF. PaO$_2$ and pH also play a role in cerebral vascular diameter but is not as potent. Bicarbonate levels do not affect CBF.

183. **B**

    Rationale: In tonic–clonic seizures, the initial onset of the seizure involves muscle-stiffening (tonic) phase, which is followed by rhythmical motor activity, called clonic. A tonic seizure would begin and end with muscle stiffening and no other motor activity. Atonic seizure is a loss motor tone and is commonly associated with dropping or falling. Clonic seizure begins and ends with rhythmical motor activity.

184. **D**

    Rationale: Lethargy, irritability, and poor feeding are signs of meningitis in pediatric patients. Pediatric patients cannot complain of headaches, and it is not considered a sign of pediatric meningitis.

185. **D**

    The "T" in the acronym of FAST stands for *time to call 911*, not *tinnitus*. The acronym of FAST is used to teach the public to recognize common symptoms of strokes.

186. **D**

    Rationale: Posterior strokes, such as in the vertebral–basilar region, are not easily identified by using the National Institutes of Health Stroke Scale (NIHSS). The NIHSS is designed to identify anterior stroke syndromes such as middle cerebral and anterior cerebral artery territory. The thalamic infarction is more readily identified with the NIHSS than the posterior strokes.

187. **A**

    Rationale: The cerebral edema most commonly experienced by patients with brain tumors is focal, surrounding the tumor bed. The initial medical management includes steroids, such as dexamethasone. Mannitol and 3% saline can be used in patients with cerebral edema and increased intracranial pressure (ICP) but would not be the initial first-line therapy in brain tumor patients. Hyperventilation is not a recommended therapy for routine management focal edema.

188. **A**

    Rationale: A subarachnoid hemorrhage (SAH) results in blood being introduced into the cerebral spinal fluid (CSF) causing obstruction to the reabsorption of CSF through the arachnoid villi. Damage to the arachnoid villi causes chronic hydrocephalus, resulting frequently in normal-pressure hydrocephalus (NPH). Epidural hematoma, subdural hematoma, and parenchymal contusions are not typically associated with NPH.

# 12. ANSWERS AND RATIONALES FOR THE PRACTICE EXAM

189. **B**

Rationale: It is important for patients and families of stroke patients to understand the eligibility and criteria for acute stroke rehabilitation but is not considered a measurement for strokes. Stroke measures for education include discharge medications, symptoms of stroke, and risk factors personalized to the patient.

190. **A**

Rationale: A sedative or analgesic can cause hypotension, which would adversely affect cerebral blood flow (CBF) and perfusion. Blood pressure must be monitored closely following administration. Respiratory depression can be a life-threatening side effect, but this patient is already intubated and being ventilated. Urinary retention or constipation is not an immediate concern at this time.

191. **C**

Rationale: Steroids have not been found to decrease cerebral edema or improve outcomes in patients with traumatic brain injury (TBI). The use of steroids for TBI patients (minor or severe) is not recommended. High-dose steroids have been found to increase morbidity and mortality in severe TBI patients.

192. **D**

Rationale: Cerebral palsy (CP) is not genetic. The chances a second child of the parents will have CP are unlikely unless exposed to the same situation during the pregnancy or delivery. Genetic counseling is not recommended following the diagnosis of CP.

193. **A**

Rationale: The term *infantile* is used because the spasms occur during infancy. The description provided of the seizure is typical of a spasm and can affect just legs or legs and body. Lennox–Gastaut syndrome usually begins between 3 and 5 years of age and commonly presents with myoclonic or abnormal absence seizures. Febrile seizures occur in infants and pediatric patients, but no temperatures or fever was provided in this scenario. Myoclonic seizure is more a rhythmical jerkin than spastic extension of arms or trunk.

194. **D**

Rationale: The pituitary gland is centrally located and adjacent to the optic chiasm. The lateral (temporal) vision crosses in the optic chiasm and travels through the contralateral optic nerve to the occipital lobe. A pituitary tumor can cause compression of the optic chiasm, resulting in bitemporal hemianopsia (loss of half vision in the peripheral in both eyes). This causes a "funnel" vision. A scotoma is a blind spot located anywhere within the visual field. Homonymous hemianopsia is the loss of half vision, medial (nasal) vision in one eye, and lateral (temporal) vision in the other. This commonly involves the occipital lobe. A complete loss of vision in one eye (unilateral) is typically caused by an injury that occurs before the optic chiasm.

195. **B**

Rationale: Early gastric feeding (percutaneous gastrostomy tube [PEG] or orogastric tube [OGT]) can pose the risk of delayed gastric emptying and an increase in gastric residuals and aspiration of gastric contents. This increases the risk of ventilator-associated pneumonia (VAP) or hospital-acquired pneumonia (HAP). Placing the feeding tube postpyloric or in the jejunum decreases gastric residuals and lowers the risk of VAP.

**196. C**

Rationale: Following chemotherapy with temozolomide (TMZ), the glioblastoma tumor may appear to have worsened on radiographic studies, but the tumor progression has actually decreased. There is currently no noninvasive technique to determine pseudoprogression versus actual progression. Nurses should be familiar with management issues of brain tumors to clarify questions of the patients and family members. TMZ has been found effective in some glioblastoma tumors to increase life expectancy. The appearance of pseudoprogression may actually be a good prognosis, but because it cannot be differentiated from actual tumor growth, false reassurance is not recommended.

**197. C**

Rationale: The use of FAST as an acronym used to remember signs of a stroke had been focused on anterior strokes. The addition of *BE* to the acronym is meant to improve the recognition of posterior stroke and stands for *balance* and *eyes*. Frequently, posterior strokes present with dizziness and visual deficits. An embolic stroke most often involves the middle cerebral artery and is considered an anterior stroke. This acronym is not as beneficial for recognizing a subarachnoid hemorrhage.

**198. B**

Rationale: Neuropathic pain is most amendable to anticonvulsant medications, such as gabapentin. Other classes of medications used to manage neuropathic pain commonly include tricyclic antidepressant. Nonsteroidal medications, such as Toradol, can be used in the initial pain management but are not the most appropriate pain management for neuropathic pain. Opioids, such as Dilaudid, are not as effective in neuropathic pain and can lead to opioid addictions. Ketamine is an anesthetic with pain properties but is not recommended for the management of neuropathic pain.

**199. C**

Rationale: Amyotrophic lateral sclerosis (ALS) involves both upper motor neurons and lower motor neurons. There is no sensory involvement in ALS. It is considered a pure motor neuron disease. It is not a sclerosing disorder of white matter. ALS does not affect the pons but can progress to similar paralysis like locked-in syndrome.

**200. D**

Rationale: Hyperglycemia is common following the severe stress, including in traumatic brain injury (TBI) patients. Hyperglycemia is thought to worsen outcomes, but strict glycemic control (range 80–110 mg/dL) results in frequent hypoglycemic episodes. Hypoglycemia can also negatively affect outcomes following neurological injury. Strict glycemic control itself does not cause a worsening of Glasgow Coma Scale (GCS) score unless periods of hypoglycemia (brain requires glucose and cannot store it). Immunosuppression and increased cerebral edema are not complications of insulin administration or strict glycemic control.

**201. A**

CP is not contagious. It is chronic without a known cure. It is not related to a genetic abnormality and cannot be passed along generation to generation. It can be associated with mental impairment but not always.

## 12. ANSWERS AND RATIONALES FOR THE PRACTICE EXAM

202. **A**

Rationale: Hypertension is considered the single most important risk factor of both ischemic and hemorrhagic strokes. Sedentary lifestyle contributes to obesity and other known risk factors of stroke but is not the single most important risk factor. Male gender is a higher risk of most strokes than female, but both are at risk for strokes. Smoking is the most preventable risk for a stroke.

203. **C**

Rationale: A ventriculoperitoneal (VP) shunt may be placed to manage the symptoms of normal-pressure hydrocephalus (NPH) including patient's gait and urinary continence. Base skull surgeries and vagal nerve resections are not surgical procedures used to manage NPH. Intracranial pressure (ICP) monitors are not placed for long term or chronic use.

204. **C**

Rationale: Cerebral perfusion pressures (CPPs) are calculated by subtracting the intracranial pressure (ICP) from the mean arterial pressure (MAP). So, MAP – ICP = CPP. This patient's MAP = 80 and ICP = 15. The CPP is 65 mmHg.

205. **C**

Rationale: Tumors arising from the lungs commonly metastasize to the brain. Kidney and gastrointestinal tract tumors can also metastasize to the brain but not as commonly as lung. Pancreas is not as well known to metastasize to brain tissue.

206. **C**

Rationale: Autonomic seizures are commonly classified as simple partial or focal seizures with maintenance of awareness. Symptoms include feelings of being flush, piloerection (hair on the arms standing on end), pallor, and sweating. Auditory hallucinations and experiences of déjà vu occur in simple partial (focal) seizures but are commonly called *somatosensory* or *psychic*, respectively. Repetitive movements are called *automatisms* and are commonly found in complex partial seizures.

207. **D**

Rationale: The recommendation by the American Heart Association/American Stroke Association (AHA/ASA) is to initiate blood pressure (BP) therapy with antihypertensive agents for a systolic BP > 140 mmHg and diastolic > 90 mmHg. There are no studies to support maintaining the BP less than 140/90 in nondiabetic patients. Not treating systolic BP unless greater than 220 mmHg and diastolic greater than 120 mmHg is only recommended in an acute stroke patient not eligible for thrombolytic therapy. It is not recommended for primary or secondary stroke prevention.

208. **C**

Rationale: An anaplastic astrocytoma is a grade III astrocytoma. A glioblastoma is a grade IV astrocytoma. Neurofibromatosis is a familial tumor syndrome. Neuroblastoma is a solid tumor occurring on a peripheral nerve, commonly involving the sympathetic nervous system.

209. **C**

Rationale: Moving the head side to side to assess for eye movement is performed to identify the presence of the oculocephalic reflex. Cervical spine should be cleared of injury prior to performing this reflex evaluation. Bulbocavernous reflex is used to evaluate spinal cord–injured patient and does not involve manipulating the neck. Running an object up the bottom of the foot tests Babinski reflex, assessing the movement of the toes. Oculovestibular reflex involves irrigation of iced cold water into the ear. This does not involve movement of the neck, and cervical injury does not need to be cleared before assessment. Both oculocephalic and oculovestibular reflexes are used to evaluate comatose patients for brain death. Assessment of oculovestibular reflex is safer in comatose patient.

210. **B**

Rationale: Ergotamine causes vasoconstriction in the cerebral circulation but also causes vasoconstriction in the coronary arteries. This coronary vasoconstriction may increase the risk of acute myocardial infarction. Liver toxicity, increased intracranial pressure, and acute kidney injury are not common complications found with the administration of ergotamine.

211. **D**

Rationale: The type IV Chiari malformation refers to a hypoplasia, which is an incomplete development of the cerebellum, or an aplasia, which is a lack of development of a portion of the cerebellum. These do not involve an actual herniation like the Chiari malformations type I and type II.

212. **D**

Rationale: Creutzfeldt–Jakob disease (CJD) can be acquired through sporadic alteration of protein, hereditary, or exposure of the infected person's tissue. Casual contact is not a route of exposure to CJD.

213. **B**

Rationale: One of the known causes for cerebral palsy (CP) is maternal infection, such as Rubella (German measles), during pregnancy. Prevention of CP includes vaccinations to prevent maternal infections. Genetic counseling is not considered preventive in CP. Avoiding alcohol and participating in exercise programs during pregnancy are always recommended for the health of the newborn but do not necessarily prevent CP to the degree of preventing maternal infections.

214. **A**

Rationale: CN I, the olfactory cranial nerve, is commonly damaged due to shearing of the olfactory fibers at the cribriform plate during the trauma. This can result in loss of smell (amnosia) permanent, with some return and regeneration. CN V (trigeminal), CN VII (facial), and CN VIII (acoustic) are not commonly injured in traumatic brain injury (TBI).

215. **A**

Rationale: Activating the EMS 9-1-1 system allows a more rapid transport to the hospital and allows for the prehospital identification of stroke symptoms, transport to designated stroke centers, and an early alert for the hospital to have the stroke team ready.

## 12. ANSWERS AND RATIONALES FOR THE PRACTICE EXAM   255

216. **D**

Rationale: Linear skull fracture is associated with traumatic brain injury (TBI) but does not carry the high risk of seizures as in patients with penetrating head trauma, decreased level of consciousness, and depressed skull fractures. Other high risks for seizures include large parenchymal contusions and hematomas (epidural and subdural).

217. **A**

Rationale: Pineal tumors commonly cause the obstruction of cerebrospinal fluid, resulting in noncommunicating hydrocephalus. Visual field losses, hemiparesis, and subarachnoid hemorrhage are not commonly found in patients with pineal tumors.

218. **B**

Rationale: Keep the definitions and explanations simple, at a fourth-grade level. Use common words and limit words with multiple syllables. Avoid medical jargon in definitions. However, you may develop a list of medical terms and definitions to assist the patient with medical jargon in the hospital.

219. **D**

Rationale: Autonomic signs may be present with cluster headaches. These signs include nasal congestion, facial sweating, and miosis. Atrial fibrillation is not an autonomic sign.

220. **D**

Rationale: Introduction of bacteria into the meninges can occur through the direct route such as a surgical site, sinusitis, and, in some type of meningitis, via an airborne or droplet route. Eating undercooked pork does not cause meningitis but can increase the risk of neurocysticercosis.

# 13

# Bonus Exam Questions

Disclaimer: These questions are intended for extra practice. The questions may include topics that are not covered in the review.

## CHAPTER 1: CHRONIC NEUROLOGICAL DISORDERS

1. Which of the following LEAST describes Huntington's disease?

    A. Incurable and progressive
    B. Eventually fatal genetic disorder
    C. Affects memory and motor control
    D. Classified as cortical dementia

2. In Huntington's disease, the person may present with abnormal motor movements. Commonly, these are involuntary, jerking movements of the extremities and face. What is the name for these abnormal movements?

    A. Blepharospasm
    B. Athetosis
    C. Fasciculations
    D. Chorea

3. Which of the following is the most definitive diagnosis of Huntington's disease?

    A. MRI
    B. Genetic testing
    C. Lumbar puncture with cerebrospinal fluid analysis
    D. Electromyography testing

4. In the late stages of Huntington's disease, which of the following is a common problem associated with the disease progression?

    A. Urinary retention
    B. Inability to comprehend language
    C. Dysphagia and aspiration
    D. Inability to recognize family

5. Suicide has been found to be a higher risk than normal in patients with Huntington's disease. Which of the following stages would carry the highest risk of suicide?
   A. Early stages
   B. Middle stages
   C. Late stages
   D. End of life

6. Which of the following statements best describes restless leg syndrome (RLS)?
   A. RLS is a pure motor disorder of involuntary movement.
   B. Uncomfortable sensations in lower extremities accompanies RLS.
   C. RLS occurs only at night during sleep.
   D. RLS is constant and progressive.

7. Which of the following neurological disorders frequently experience restless leg syndrome?
   A. Alzheimer's dementia
   B. Huntington's disease
   C. Parkinson's disease
   D. Myasthenia gravis

8. A patient presents with restless leg syndrome and is experiencing significant sleep disturbances. Which of the following may be a first-line treatment?
   A. Iron supplements
   B. Beta-blocker
   C. Calcium channel blocker
   D. Muscle relaxant

9. Sleep disorders have many risks and complications. Strokes are found to be a higher risk in which of the following sleep disorders?
   A. Restless leg syndrome
   B. Insomnia
   C. Obstructive sleep apnea
   D. Narcolepsy

10. Migraines with an aura can increase the risk of strokes. Which of the following is NOT considered a physiological cause for the strokes?
    A. Embolic event
    B. Hypercoaguable state
    C. Hypertensive crisis
    D. Hyperviscosity

11. Which of the following would be considered a red flag for an increased risk of a stroke in patients with aura-producing migraines?
    A. Aura of visual hallucinations
    B. Duration of the aura greater than 1 hour

C. Aura accompanied with severe headache
  D. Aura with normal EEG waveforms

12. A resting tremor presents more commonly with which of the following characteristics?
    A. It usually presents unilaterally.
    B. It occurs with fast oscillations.
    C. Head and voice are commonly affected.
    D. Distractions improve the tremor.

13. A patient presents with dystonic tremor. Which of the following is considered a characteristic sign of dystonic tremors?
    A. Fast tremor improves during sleep
    B. Very regular tremor
    C. Only presents with a vertical head shake
    D. Affects head greater than hands and arms

14. Which of the following is the most accurate differentiation between benign essential tremor (BET) and Parkinson's disease (PD)?
    A. PD is an action tremor and improves with rest.
    B. BET experiences a more rapid frequency than PD.
    C. Both BET and PD present with greater unilateral symptoms.
    D. PD has a greater familiar association than BET.

15. Mr. J is admitted with a history of Parkinson's disease. He is demonstrating signs of Lewy body subcortical dementia. Which of the following is a more commonly associated sign of subcortical dementia?
    A. Short-term memory loss
    B. Language abnormality
    C. Difficulty with complex tasks
    D. Word-finding problems

16. A 60-year-old patient presents with behavioral and personality changes, decline in language, and bilateral frontal lobe neuronal loss. Which of the following types of dementia is the most likely cause?
    A. Alzheimer's dementia
    B. Lewy body dementia
    C. Frontotemporal dementia
    D. Vascular dementia

17. A patient with peripheral neuropathy, such as Guillain–Barré, presents with which of the following?
    A. Hyperactive reflexes
    B. Disappearing or absent reflexes
    C. Unilateral loss of reflexes
    D. Neuropathic pain syndromes

18. An injury to the median ulnar nerve with paresthesia to the wrist and fingers may be a result of which of the following?
    A. Radial nerve palsy
    B. Cubital tunnel syndrome
    C. Carpal tunnel syndrome
    D. Brachial plexus injury

19. Which of the following is the most common age group for the onset of symptoms for multiple sclerosis?
    A. Over age of 65 years
    B. Adolescent to 35 years of age
    C. Middle age
    D. Pediatrics

20. Which of the following is NOT a known risk for development of multiple sclerosis?
    A. Single genetic abnormality
    B. Living north of the equator
    C. Vitamin D deficiency
    D. Viral infection

21. A young woman presents with weakness and neuropathies. She is being worked up for multiple sclerosis (MS) and undergoes a lumbar puncture with cerebrospinal fluid (CSF) analysis. Which of the following CSF lab results would most likely be found in MS?
    A. Elevated CSF protein levels
    B. Elevated lymphocytes in CSF
    C. Decrease in immunoglobulin G (IgG) synthesis
    D. Increased oligoclonal bands

22. Which of the following changes seen on MRI is most diagnostic of multiple sclerosis?
    A. Cortical atrophy
    B. Corpus thinning
    C. Periventricular white matter lesions
    D. Obstructive hydrocephalus

23. Cerebrospinal fluid abnormalities are commonly found in multiple sclerosis (MS) patients. Which of the following is the most characteristic finding in MS patients?
    A. Normal opening pressures
    B. Slight elevation of white blood cell count
    C. Normal protein level
    D. Presence of oligoclonal bands

24. Which of the following is the LEAST likely potential side effect of deep brain stimulation?
    A. Rigidity
    B. Abnormal gaze
    C. Vertigo
    D. Disinhibition

25. Which of the following is the MOST common reason for a patient with early undiagnosed Parkinson's disease to seek medical care?

    A. Resting tremor
    B. Muscle rigidity
    C. Unstable gait with bradykinesia
    D. Dizziness and episodes vertigo

26. One test that clinicians use to identify onset of dementia is which of the following?

    A. Mini–Mental State Exam
    B. Geriatric evaluation for dementia
    C. Glasgow Outcome Scale
    D. Framingham profile

27. A 50-year-old man presents to the neurological clinic with a history of gradual choreic movements of face and arms, experiencing frequent falls, changes in speech, and weight loss. Upon assessment of his family history, it was noted his father died when he was a child with similar issues. Which of the following is the MOST likely diagnosis?

    A. Parkinson's disease
    B. Benign essential tremors
    C. Huntington's disease
    D. Tourette's syndrome

28. In the terminal stages of Huntington's disease, which of the following would the nurse expect the patient to see?

    A. Ambulatory but unsteady gait
    B. Cachetic, incontinent, and lethargic
    C. Flaccid paralysis
    D. Comatose state

29. Which of the following neurological disease processes commonly presents with "wing beating" tremors, dysarthria, and unsteady gait?

    A. Amyotrophic lateral sclerosis
    B. Huntington's disease
    C. Wilson's disease
    D. Tourette's syndrome

## CHAPTER 2: CEREBROVASCULAR DISORDERS

1. Which of the following is the most accurate statement regarding the medical management of paroxysmal atrial fibrillation (PAF) with anticoagulation therapy?

    A. If episodes occur more than two times a month and last for greater than 5 minutes, then anticoagulate.
    B. Monitor PAF with a loop recorder and anticoagulate if atrial fibrillation becomes continuous.

C. PAF has significantly lower risk for embolic stroke and can be managed with aspirin (acetylsalicylic acid).
D. PAF should be anticoagulated unless contraindicated.

2. A patient hospitalized following an acute stroke was found to have a patent foramen ovale (PFO). An ultrasound of the lower extremities identified deep venous thrombosis. Which of the following would be the initial recommended treatment?
   A. Dual antiplatelet therapy
   B. Ablation treatment
   C. Anticoagulation therapy
   D. PFO closure

3. When determining the outcome of a stroke patient, which of the following assessment tools is most commonly utilized?
   A. Glasgow Outcome Scale
   B. Modified Rankin Scale
   C. Thrombolysis in Cerebral Infarction Scale
   D. CHADS2 score

4. Which of the following is recommended for preventing complications of patients with hemorrhagic strokes in the acute setting?
   A. Intravenous heparin infusion
   B. Elastic compression stockings
   C. Clear liquid diet
   D. Intermittent pneumatic compression

5. Which of the following techniques is suggested to improve continence in stroke patients?
   A. Prompted scheduled voiding
   B. Placing an indwelling urinary catheter
   C. Scheduled intermittent catheterization
   D. Assessing prior voiding schedules

6. Which of the following is a common complication of stroke?
   A. Chronic headache
   B. Trigeminal neuralgia
   C. Shoulder pain and subluxation
   D. Hip fractures

7. Central pain after a stroke is best managed with which of the following regimens?
   A. Toradol and Dilaudid
   B. Lamotrigine (Lamictal) and amitriptyline
   C. Nonpharmacological management with transcutaneous electrical stimulation
   D. Alternating heat and cold compresses

8. After a stroke with hemiparesis of the upper extremity, joint contractures can commonly occur on the affected limb. Which of the following interventions is considered the best for preventing the contractures?

A. Immobilizing the extremity
   B. Applying hand splints
   C. Daily stretching of the hemiparetic limb
   D. Surgical release of tendons and muscle

9. Which of the following is NOT a common complication of dysphagia in a stroke patient?

   A. Pneumonia
   B. Malnutrition
   C. Failure to thrive
   D. Weight loss

10. Which of the following requires patients to seek care in a timely fashion with a stroke?

    A. Early recognition of signs of a stroke
    B. Living close to a hospital
    C. Being knowledgeable in the option of thrombolytics for treating a stroke
    D. Knowing where their closest comprehensive stroke center is located

11. Which of the following is NOT a recommendation for emergency medical services when responding to a patient with signs of a stroke?

    A. Prioritize the potential stroke patient.
    B. Minimize time spent at the scene prior to transport.
    C. Perform a full National Institutes of Health Stroke Scale (NIHSS) assessment to improve communication with the ED staff.
    D. Transport quickly to the most appropriate hospital.

12. Which of the following statements best describes the purpose of emergency medical services using an assessment tool to recognize large vessel obstructions?

    A. To facilitate transfer to endovascular centers
    B. To identify a stroke and prealert the hospital for shorter response times
    C. To identify intravenous thrombolytic patients
    D. To recognize signs of a stroke

13. Which of the following patients would NOT be a candidate for intravenous alteplase?

    A. Patient with recent diagnosis of infective endocarditis
    B. Patient on aspirin and Plavix
    C. Patient with renal disease on dialysis
    D. 96-year-old woman

14. A patient presents within 1 hour of left-sided weakness and aphasia. During the admission history, it is noted the patient is on Eliquis for atrial fibrillation. Which of the following is a true statement?

    A. Patient is a candidate for intravenous (IV) alteplase due to the time window.
    B. A prothrombin time with international normalized ratio should be obtained before IV alteplase is considered.
    C. Patient is not a candidate for IV alteplase but may be a candidate for endovascular therapy.
    D. Administer a reversal agent for Eliquis and then administer the IV alteplase.

15. A stroke patient continues to have difficulty with swallow and has failed the videofluoroscopy test. Which of the following is the most accurate statement?
    A. Allow the patient to eat since this is a quality-of-life issue.
    B. Total parenteral nutrition is the recommended route for nutrition.
    C. Gastric tube is recommended to provide tube feeding.
    D. Clear liquids may be started until the swallow improves for solid food.

16. Which of the following protocols does NOT lower the risk of aspiration pneumonia in stroke patients?
    A. Dysphagia screen prior to oral intake
    B. Oral hygiene protocols
    C. Daily chest radiographics
    D. Speech therapist consult

17. Which of the following would have the highest risk of vasospasms following a subarachnoid hemorrhage?
    A. Large volume of blood in the ventricles
    B. Hunt and Hess grade II score
    C. Glasgow Coma Scale score of 14
    D. Surgical clipping of aneurysm after 14 days

18. Which of the following syndromes associated with subarachnoid hemorrhage following aneurysm rupture may complicate the management of vasospasms?
    A. Hydrocephalus
    B. Delayed ischemic injury
    C. Cerebral salt wasting syndrome
    D. Syndrome of inappropriate antidiuretic hormone

19. A patient is 8 days postsubarachnoid hemorrhage and has been noted to have a decrease in level of consciousness. The following are the patient's vital signs:
    A. Blood pressure (BP) 118/62 mmHg
    B. Heart rate (HR) 82 beats/min
    C. Respiratory rate (RR) 24 breaths/min
    D. 24-hour intake and output demonstrates a positive fluid balance of 2 L

    Based upon the above findings, which of the following would be the most appropriate intervention at this time?
    A. Initiate vasoconstrictor to keep BP >160 mmHg.
    B. Obtain a noncontrast CT scan.
    C. Administer a diuretic.
    D. Administer a 1,000-mL bolus of normal saline.

20. Medical management of vasospasms following subarachnoid hemorrhage is recommended as the initial intervention. If the vasospasms do not resolve, which of the following is NOT a recommended treatment for vasospasms?
    A. Surgical clipping
    B. Angioplasty

C. Intraarterial vasodilator
D. Intraarterial antispasmodic

21. Which of the following is a contraindication to induced hypertension in managing vasospasms?

    A. Coiled basilar tip aneurysm
    B. Clipped anterior communicating artery aneurysm
    C. Presence of more than one coiled aneurysm
    D. Unsecured aneurysm

22. Which of the following is the most common cause of strokes in the pediatric population?

    A. Congenital heart disease with thromboembolism
    B. Central nervous system (CNS) vasculitis
    C. Neurofibromatosis
    D. CNS infections

23. A patient presents with signs of a postural stroke. Upon assessment of the patient's recent history, which of the following would most likely indicate a vertebral dissection?

    A. Recent diagnosis of cerebral aneurysm
    B. Recent fall
    C. Chiropractor neck manipulation
    D. Hypertensive crisis

24. A vertebral dissection can present with ischemic stroke from occlusion of the artery or hemorrhagic stroke. Which of the following is the most common type of hemorrhage from a vertebral dissection?

    A. Intraparenchymal hemorrhage
    B. Epidural hematoma
    C. Subdural hematoma
    D. Subarachnoid hemorrhage

25. Which of the following best describes a cavernous malformation?

    A. Development of bilateral collateral vessels around the intracranial internal carotid artery
    B. Dural thrombosis caused by hypercoagulable state
    C. Tightly packed clusters of vessels displace brain tissue
    D. Inflammation of the cerebral vasculature

26. A patient with a subarachnoid hemorrhage has a ventriculostomy placed and cerebrospinal fluid (CSF) is being drained. What is a potential complication of overdrainage of the CSF?

    A. Effacement of the ventricles
    B. Subdural hemorrhage
    C. Cerebral edema
    D. Increased intracranial pressure

27. Which of the following is NOT considered a complication of surgical clipping of an aneurysm?

    A. Incomplete clipping of aneurysm
    B. Distal embolization

C. Rupture of the aneurysm
D. Inadvertent clipping of surrounding artery

28. An arteriovenous malformation is resected. Postoperatively, the patient has a neurological change. This is most likely due to which of the following etiology?

    A. Increased perfusion pressure resulting in cerebral edema
    B. Subdural hematoma
    C. Metabolic encephalopathy
    D. Postictal following generalized seizure

29. Dislodgment of plaque from the carotid artery can result in an ischemic stroke. Which of the following best describes amaurosis fugax?

    A. Symptoms result of pseudotumor cerebri
    B. Contralateral loss of motor function
    C. Ipsilateral impairment of vision
    D. Results in presentation of Todd's paralysis

30. The ability of the brain to regenerate and restore function after neuronal tissue loss with a stroke is a concept called?

    A. Neuroplasticity
    B. Scarring
    C. Neuronal replication
    D. Regenerative balance

31. Which of the following is the MOST important purpose of rapid and intense rehabilitation within the first month following a stroke?

    A. Improve patient's mentation.
    B. Prevent contractures.
    C. Capitalize on highest period of time for neuroplasticity.
    D. Assist with moving the patient toward self-care.

32. Which of the following is the BEST description of the DASH diet, which is recommended to prevent hypertension?

    A. High protein and low salt and potassium
    B. Low protein and high fat and vegetables
    C. High protein and fats and low carbohydrates
    D. High in vegetables and fruits and low in dairy

33. Which of the following hemoglobin A1C levels are patients with known diabetes recommended to maintain?

    A. 5%
    B. 6%
    C. 7%
    D. 8%

34. Which visual deficit is most commonly involved with internal carotid artery strokes?

    A. Homonymous hemianopia
    B. Bilateral loss of peripheral vision

C. Contralateral visual field loss
D. Scotoma

35. Sudden bilateral hearing loss with dizziness and ataxia are stroke syndromes that can indicate involvement of which of the following arteries?

    A. Vertebral artery
    B. Posterior cerebral artery
    C. Internal carotid artery
    D. External carotid artery

36. A patient presents with ipsilateral third nerve palsy with contralateral hemiplegia. Which of the following is the stroke syndrome?

    A. Wallenberg's syndrome
    B. Weber's syndrome
    C. Horner's syndrome
    D. Locked-in syndrome

37. Which of the following scales is used to measure the risk for surgical intervention of an arteriovenous malformation?

    A. Spetzler–Martin grading system
    B. Hunt and Hess grading system
    C. Fisher grade
    D. Intracerebral Hemorrhage score

38. A patient presents with hemiplegia of arm and facial droop on the right side. A non-contrast CT scan is obtained. Which of the following is an early sign of a large vessel occlusion?

    A. Hyperdense dot
    B. Hyperdense sign
    C. Infarct of the middle cerebral artery territory
    D. Petechial hemorrhages in basal ganglia

39. Following a subarachnoid hemorrhage, the patient is in the ICU and experiencing neurogenic fevers. External cooling for targeted temperature control is initiated. Which of the following is the MOST important nursing assessment at this time?

    A. Hemodynamics monitoring
    B. Cardiac monitoring
    C. Measurement of urine output
    D. Shivering assessment

## CHAPTER 3: TUMORS OF THE BRAIN AND SPINAL CORD

1. Which of the following statements is most accurate regarding the diagnostic differentiation between a low-grade and high-grade glioma?

    A. High-grade tumors are multifocal.
    B. PET scanning is required to make the differentiation.

C. In high-grade glioma, the T2 signal shows an irregular, enhanced rim around the tumor, whereas the low-grade glioma remains homogenous with little enhancement.
D. Low-grade gliomas cannot be recognized on CT scan, but a high-grade glioma will be identified.

2. Which of the following is the initial treatment of brain swelling with onset or worsening of symptoms in patients with brain tumors?

   A. Levetiracetam (Keppra)
   B. Hypertonic saline
   C. Mannitol
   D. Dexamethasone

3. Which of the following can be a complication of long-term management of brain tumors with steroids?

   A. Aspiration pneumonia
   B. Pneumocystic pneumonitis
   C. Adrenal hypersecretion
   D. Dystonia

4. Which of the following would be the LEAST appropriate initial intervention for a patient admitted with altered mentation and diagnosed with a brain tumor?

   A. Deep vein thrombosis prophylaxis with sequential compression devices
   B. Gastrointestinal prohpylaxis
   C. Continuous enteral feeding
   D. Administration of dexamethasone

5. Which of the following treatment regimens is most commonly recommended in patients diagnosed with glioblastoma multiforme (GBM)?

   A. Debulking surgery only
   B. Debulking surgery and radiotherapy
   C. Debulking surgery, radiotherapy, and chemotherapy
   D. Radiotherapy and chemotherapy only

6. Nonfocal signs of a brain tumor are a result of which of the following?

   A. Brainstem lesion
   B. Cerebral edema
   C. Hydrocephalus
   D. Meningitis

7. Which of the following is the typical description of the headache associated with a brain tumor?

   A. Headache worsens in the morning
   B. Headache described as sharp, knifelike pain
   C. Described as worsening by evening and exacerbated in standing position
   D. Present in periorbital area

8. A lumbar puncture can be used to evaluate the patient for which of the following brain lesions?

   A. Pineal tumor
   B. Pituitary adenoma
   C. Glioblastoma
   D. Brain lymphoma

9. Which of the following is NOT the primary diagnostic/treatment for a suspected central nervous system lymphoma?

   A. Complete surgical resection
   B. Chemotherapy
   C. Radiation therapy
   D. Tumor biopsy

10. Which of the following is unique to the central nervous system?

    A. Capillary beds
    B. Lymphatic system
    C. Kupffer cells
    D. Blood–brain barrier

11. Following radiation therapy for a brain tumor, which of the following complications can mimic tumor progression?

    A. Cerebral edema
    B. Tumor necrosis
    C. Demyelination syndrome
    D. Infarction

12. Which of the following is NOT a complication of steroid therapy in treating brain tumors?

    A. Psychosis
    B. Hyperglycemia
    C. Hyperkalemia
    D. Fluid retention

13. Which vertebral column location has the greatest percentage of spinal cord tumors?

    A. Cervical
    B. Thoracic
    C. Lumbar
    D. Sacral

14. Which of the following best describes a tumor located in the extramedullary/intradural area of the spine?

    A. It occurs outside the spinal cord in the epidural space.
    B. It occurs within the spinal dura but outside the spinal cord.
    C. It occurs within the spinal cord.
    D. It occurs with the vertebral bodies.

15. Which of the following is NOT a common presentation of metastatic tumor to the spinal canal?
    A. Bowel and bladder problems
    B. Weakness of extremities
    C. Localized pain at vertebral area
    D. Bilateral ascending paralysis

16. A patient with metastatic cancer to the spinal column is treated with radiation therapy. Following treatment, which is the most common complication of radiation therapy?
    A. Sensory impairment
    B. Complete motor paralysis
    C. Brown–Sequard syndrome
    D. Spinal fusion

17. Which of the following is best described as a benign vascular neoplasm located in the central nervous system?
    A. Fibromatosis
    B. Pilocytic astrocytoma
    C. Craniopharyngioma
    D. Hemangioblastoma

18. A patient is diagnosed with hemangioblastoma. Which of the following is the most common location for a cerebral hemangioblastoma?
    A. Frontal lobe
    B. Posterior fossa
    C. Pineal gland
    D. Sagittal venous sinus

19. Hemangioblastoma is commonly associated with which of the following autosomal–dominant hereditary syndromes?
    A. von Hippel–Lindau disease
    B. Marfan syndrome
    C. TaySachs
    D. Neurofibromatosis

20. A patient with a craniopharyngioma is scheduled for radiation therapy. Which of the following is a potential complication of radiation treatments?
    A. Neglect syndrome
    B. Hemiparesis
    C. Seizures
    D. Visual losses

## CHAPTER 4: IMMUNE INFECTIONS, PART 1

1. Which of the following is the LEAST common site for intracranial abscess?
    A. Epidural space
    B. Subdural space

C. Cerebellum
D. Frontotemporal area

2. Which of the following is NOT considered a complication of brain abscesses?

    A. Hemorrhagic stroke
    B. Cavernous sinus thrombosis
    C. Cerebral edema
    D. Retrograde meningitis

3. Which of the following diagnostic studies would NOT be recommended in patients with brain abscess?

    A. Erythrocyte sedimentation rate
    B. Lumbar puncture with cerebrospinal fluid analysis
    C. Contrast magnetic resonance imaging
    D. Complete blood count with differential

4. Patients with HIV disease are prone to opportunistic infections of the central nervous system (CNS). Among the opportunistic viral infections, which of the following is the most common cause of a CNS infection in patients with HIV disease?

    A. Neurosyphilis
    B. Herpes simplex types I and II
    C. West Nile virus
    D. *Candida albicans*

## CHAPTER 5: IMMUNE INFECTIONS, PART 2

1. Which of the following is NOT a recognized side effect of interferon in treating multiple sclerosis?

    A. Flu-like symptoms
    B. Psychiatric disease
    C. Hypercoagulopathy
    D. Liver disease

2. Natalizumab (Tysabri) is a drug used to treat multiple sclerosis. Which of the following is its most serious side effect?

    A. Acute kidney injury
    B. Depression
    C. Headaches
    D. Progressive multifocal leukoencephalopathy

3. Which of the following is the strongest known risk factor for multiple sclerosis?

    A. Lack of vitamin D
    B. Family history
    C. Heavy smoking
    D. Exposure to Epstein–Barr virus

4. Which of the following is NOT a physiological change that occurs in multiple sclerosis patients?

    A. Cytotoxic cerebral edema
    B. Nerve conduction dysfunction
    C. Nerve inflammation
    D. Central nervous system loss

5. Which of the following states can trigger a response similar to an exacerbation of multiple sclerosis?

    A. Trauma
    B. Hypoxia
    C. Fever
    D. Shivering

6. Which of the following diagnostic tools is used to diagnose multiple sclerosis?

    A. Hunt and Hess
    B. McDonald Criteria
    C. Glasgow Outcome Scale (GOS)
    D. CHADS2 score

7. Which of the following is the most correct definition of *remission* in patients with myasthenia gravis (MG)?

    A. No muscle weakness while on daily cholinesterase inhibitors
    B. No signs of weakness but weakness of eyelids is acceptable
    C. Presence of ocular muscle weakness only
    D. No signs of any muscle weakness or signs of MG

8. A myasthenia gravis patient presents with increased lacrimation, salivation, and urination. It is determined that he doubled his dose of pyridostigmine to improve motor weakness. Which of the following pupillary changes is most likely to accompany signs of cholinergic crisis?

    A. Mydriasis
    B. Miosis
    C. Bilateral dilated nonreactive pupils
    D. Anisocoria

9. Which of the following medications frequently used in myasthenia gravis is NOT an immunosuppressive agent?

    A. Pyridostigmine
    B. Mycophenolate mofetil
    C. Cyclosporine
    D. Azathioprine

10. Which of the following conditions would be a contraindication to intravenous immunoglobulin treatments?

    A. Pregnancy
    B. Autoimmune disorders

C. Liver dysfunction
D. Renal failure

11. A patient receiving intravenous immunoglobulin for acute exacerbation of myasthenia gravis should have which of the following prior to administration?

    A. Intravenous steroids
    B. Diphenhydramine (Benadryl)
    C. Fluid optimization
    D. Acetaminophen (Tylenol)

12. Which of the following statements best differentiates generalized muscle weakness from myasthenia gravis (MG) and Lambert–Eaton MG?

    A. Eyelid weakness (ptosis) is not present in Lambert–Eaton myasthenic syndrome.
    B. Proximal weakness with autonomic nervous system symptoms is more specific to Lambert–Eaton myasthenic syndrome.
    C. Lambert–Eaton myasthenic syndrome does not involve signs of diplopia.
    D. Lambert–Eaton myasthenic syndrome involves more distal than proximal muscle.

13. Miller Fisher syndrome is a variant of which of the following neurological autoimmune disorders?

    A. Myasthenia gravis
    B. Guillain–Barré syndrome
    C. Multiple sclerosis
    D. Amyotrophic lateral sclerosis

14. Which of the following is considered a significant complication of intravenous immunoglobulin treatments for chronic demyelinating polyneuropathy?

    A. Venous thromboembolism
    B. Thrombocytopenia
    C. Leukocytosis
    D. Angioedema

15. Which of the following are early signs of amyotrophic lateral sclerosis?

    A. Postural drop seizures
    B. Hypotonia and muscle flaccidity
    C. Fasciculations in arms, legs, shoulders, and tongue
    D. Bilateral ascending muscle weakness

16. Which of the following statements best describes the physiology of the medication riluzole (Rilutek) in managing amyotrophic lateral sclerosis?

    A. It prevents the spread to ventilatory muscles, allowing patients to maintain their own spontaneous ventilation.
    B. It has been found to reverse the damage to the motor neurons.
    C. It can stop the progression of the motor neuron damage to produce a remission of the disease process.
    D. It may prolong survival by reducing damage to the motor neurons.

17. A patient with known HIV-positive status presents with history of headache and new-onset seizure. An MRI found a lesion in the brain. Which of the following is the most likely cause of the lesion?
    A. Non-Hodgkin lymphoma
    B. Kaposi sarcoma
    C. Central nervous system lymphoma
    D. Glioblastoma

18. What is the best method used to differentiate Bell's palsy from an ischemic stroke?
    A. Have the patient raise his or her eyebrows.
    B. Ask the patient to open his or her mouth and say, "Ahh."
    C. Assess the nasolabial folds for symmetry.
    D. Assess sensory changes along the trigeminal nerve.

19. Which of the following can cause Bell's palsy?
    A. Bacterial meningitis
    B. Rabies infection
    C. Sinus infections
    D. Herpes simplex infection

20. Which of the following statements best describes the term *encephalomyelitis*?
    A. Leptomeningeal irritation around the brain
    B. Bacterial infection of the brain tissue
    C. Inflammation of the brain and spinal cord
    D. Purulent drainage within meninges

21. A patient with trigeminal neuralgia requires posterior fossa surgery to correct the compression of the trigeminal nerve. Which of these complications is NOT associated specifically with posterior fossa surgeries?
    A. Cerebrospinal fluid leak
    B. Bradycardia
    C. Apnea
    D. Subdural hemorrhage

22. Which of the following is the most common demyelinating event for a patient with multiple sclerosis?
    A. Dysphagia
    B. Ataxia
    C. Facial paresthesia
    D. Optic neuritis

23. Which of the following best describes one of the manifestations of neurosyphilis called *tabes dorsalis*?
    A. Degeneration of posterior columns of the spinal cord
    B. Inflammation of the meninges
    C. New-onset mania or paranoia
    D. Shooting pains across the legs

24. Which of the following is NOT a recognized classification of neurosyphilis by the Centers for Disease Control and Prevention?

    A. Inflammatory vascular
    B. Neuropsychiatric
    C. Meningovascular
    D. Myelopathic

## CHAPTER 6: SEIZURES

1. Which of the following is NOT commonly considered a cause of Lennox–Gastaut syndrome?

    A. Brain injury
    B. Cortical dysplasia
    C. Genetic component
    D. Exposure to toxins

2. A patient presents with progression from acute headache to loss of consciousness and is diagnosed with intracranial hemorrhage. He is in the ICU and remains unresponsive for 24 hours. Which of the following diagnostic studies is recommended at this time to evaluate his "unresponsiveness"?

    A. Cerebral blood flow study
    B. Electroencephalogram
    C. Platelet function test
    D. Coagulation studies

3. A patient is admitted for seizure activity. During the evaluation with continuous EEG, the seizure activity was not associated with EEG identification of epileptic activity. What is this called?

    A. Tonic–clonic generalized seizures
    B. Absence seizures
    C. Nonepileptic seizures
    D. Nonconvulsive status epilepticus

4. Which of the following is NOT commonly found in the postictal period following a status epilepticus?

    A. Neutropenia
    B. Cardiac arrhythmias
    C. Elevated creatine phosphokinase (CPK)
    D. Fever

5. A patient has a seizure while on phenytoin. Phenytoin levels are sent for analysis. Which of the following lab tests should also be obtained to determine the effectiveness of the patient's current phenytoin dosing?

    A. Serum creatinine
    B. Albumin
    C. Liver enzymes
    D. Lipid panel

6. Which of the following is NOT commonly associated with the use of vagal nerve stimulators in epilepsy patients?

    A. Buzzing sensations
    B. Hoarseness
    C. Hiccups
    D. Deeper tone of voice

7. When is the most common age of onset of seizures in patients with Dravet's syndrome?

    A. Under the age of 1 year
    B. Between ages 1 and 5 years
    C. Preadolescencet
    D. Adolescence

8. Which of the following is NOT a well-known cause of status epilepticus?

    A. Alcohol withdrawal
    B. Traumatic brain injury
    C. Neurocysticercosis
    D. Hypocalcemia

9. During tonic–clonic generalized seizures, the patient can exhibit which of the following associated symptoms?

    A. Loss of corneal reflexes
    B. Anhydrosis
    C. Bradycardia
    D. Hypotension

10. Which of the following side effects is more common with the anticonvulsant levetiracetam (Keppra)?

    A. Hair loss
    B. Pancreatitis
    C. Neuropsychiatric symptoms
    D. Liver dysfunction

11. A patient presents with fever, blisters, and peeling skin similar to that of burn patients. Upon obtaining history, the patient is noted to be on an anticonvulsant. Which of the following syndromes is the most likely cause of the patient's presentation?

    A. Dravet syndrome
    B. Stevens–Johnson syndrome
    C. Gerstmann syndrome
    D. Tourette syndrome

12. A patient with seizure activity is admitted to the epilepsy-monitoring unit (EMU). Her anticonvulsant medication is being tapered down. Which of the following is NOT a provocative measure used to induce a seizure in the EMU?

    A. Painful stimulation
    B. Photic stimulation

C. Hyperventilation
D. Sleep deprivation

13. A provoked seizure in an epilepsy-monitoring unit can contribute to an increase in which of the following conditions?

    A. Neurogenic pulmonary edema
    B. Change in type of seizure activity
    C. Aspiration pneumonia
    D. Onset of status epilepticus

14. Which of the following statements best describes a potential complication of tonic–clonic seizures called *postictal psychosis*?

    A. It may occur without prior history of psychosis or any psychiatric history.
    B. It is transient, only lasting between 12 and 24 hours.
    C. It is a result of administering excessive benzodiazepines during the ictal phase.
    D. It follows prolonged periods of hypoxia during the seizure.

15. Which of the following is NOT a strategy typically used to protect a patient from falling while in an epilepsy-monitoring unit?

    A. Sponge bathing rather than showering
    B. Movement beyond bed or chair only in the company of a staff member
    C. Ambulation in the hallway with nonslip socks
    D. Family or identified person to remain with the patient 24/7

16. Which of the following would best prevent sudden unexpected death in epilepsy (SUDEP) during the care of a patient with seizures?

    A. Maintain the patient on supplemental oxygen.
    B. Place pads around the bed.
    C. Continue close observation and cardiac monitoring.
    D. Utilize more pillows in the bed around the patient's head.

## CHAPTER 7: PEDIATRIC AND DEVELOPMENTAL DISORDERS

1. A mother of a child with spina bifida asks you whether there is a risk of her having a second child with spina bifida. What would be the best answer?

    A. This is a rare occurrence and is more likely not to happen again.
    B. There is a significant risk for recurrence with subsequent pregnancies.
    C. It could happen again, but maintaining a better diet will prevent it from repeating.
    D. Genetic testing can tell you whether it was an environmental exposure or a genetic trait.

2. A 14-year-old girl presents with unilateral upper-extremity weakness. Upon imaging, she is diagnosed with a Chiari type II malformation. Which of the following is the cause for the unilateral upper extremity weakness?

    A. Fusion C1 to C2
    B. Compression of cranial nerves

C. Hydrocephalus
D. Syringomyelia

3. An infant with a Chiari malformation can present with brainstem dysfunction. Which of the following is NOT a sign of brainstem dysfunction in an infant?

   A. Atonia
   B. Nystagmus
   C. Dysphagia
   D. Stridor

4. Cerebral palsy can be classified according to muscle tone. Spastic cerebral palsy is the most common and affects which of the following?

   A. Extrapyramidal tract
   B. Central spinal cord
   C. Pyramidal tract in cortex
   D. Cerebellum

5. Which of the following is NOT a commonly used classification of cerebral palsy?

   A. Number of extremities involved
   B. Presence of comorbidities
   C. Muscle tone
   D. Severity of functional limitations

6. The initial recognition of cerebral palsy typically occurs because the child does not reach developmental milestones. Which of the following is the most accurate statement regarding milestones of gross motor development?

   A. Children typically develop head control at 1 month.
   B. Children typically are rolling by 3 months of age.
   C. Children typically are sitting at 6 months of age.
   D. Children typically are walking by 6 months of age.

7. Which of the following is the most common gait abnormality found in spastic cerebral palsy?

   A. Scissoring walk
   B. Toe walking
   C. Ataxic
   D. Toe flicking

8. Which of the following does NOT contribute to a worsening of the movement abnormality in cerebral palsy?

   A. Purposeful movement
   B. Stress
   C. Excitement
   D. Sleep

9. Children with cerebral palsy often have pseudobulbar involvement. Which of the following is NOT considered to be pseudobulbar symptom?

   A. Dysphagia
   B. Dysarthria

C. Dysesthesia
D. Dystonia

10. Which of the following medications is NOT considered treatment for abnormal movement of spasticity in cerebral palsy?

    A. Levodopa/carbidopa
    B. Methadone
    C. Baclofen
    D. Botulinum toxin

11. Following surgical repair of the myelomeningocele, which of the following is the most important assessment of the neonate during early postoperative period?

    A. Measuring head circumference
    B. Assessing lower-extremity sensory function
    C. Auscultation of heart sounds
    D. Assessing upper-extremity motor function

## CHAPTER 8: NEUROLOGICAL TRAUMA: TRAUMATIC BRAIN INJURY

1. In rehabilitation, one of the goals is to assist the patient to become as independent with activities of daily living as possible. Which of the following scales is used to evaluate a patient's independence level for such activities as eating, grooming, and bathing?

    A. Glasgow Outcome Scale
    B. Functional Independence Measure
    C. Independence Outcome Score
    D. Hunt and Hess scale

2. Which of the following intracranial pressure (ICP) waveform analyses would indicate a noncompliant brain and may be seen before the ICP elevates?

    A. P1 component is the highest pulse pressure.
    B. P2 component is greater than P1.
    C. P1, P2, and P3 are in descending order of pulse pressures.
    D. Only P1 and P2 components are present in the pulse pressure.

3. Which of the following "waves" is considered to be a normal occurrence when monitoring intracranial pressure?

    A. A (plateau) waves
    B. B waves
    C. C waves
    D. D waves

4. Propofol is a sedative used on traumatic brain-injured patients to lower intracranial pressure. Which of the following is a potentially lethal complication associated with prolonged use of propofol?

    A. Heart failure
    B. Lipidemia

C. Metabolic acidosis
D. Coronary vasoconstriction and acute myocardial infarction

5. A patient in the ICU following a severe traumatic brain injury develops tachycardia, hyperthermia, and dilated pupils. Which of the following is the most likely cause?

   A. Uncal herniation
   B. Sympathetic storm
   C. Hypothalamic crisis
   D. Subdural hematoma

6. Contractures occur frequently in patients with traumatic brain injury. Which of the following is the most widely used technique to prevent contractures?

   A. Botulinum toxin
   B. Casting
   C. Stretching
   D. Tendon release

7. Which of the following injuries most likely would result in a persistent vegetative state?

   A. Diffuse axonal injury
   B. Subdural hematoma
   C. Coup contracoup
   D. Frontal contusion

8. A severe traumatic brain-injured patient requires sedation in the ICU. Which of the following sedative agents does NOT cause respiratory depression?

   A. Propofol
   B. Fentanyl
   C. Dexmedetomidine
   D. Ativan

9. Which of the following would be the most likely indication for acute hyperventilation therapy in a traumatic brain injured patient?

   A. Presence of cerebral edema
   B. Glasgow Coma Scale of less than 9
   C. Signs of cerebral herniation
   D. Intracranial pressure > 20 mmHg

10. Which of the following trauma patients would be considered at high risk for traumatic brain injury and should have a noncontrast computerized tomography scan performed?

    A. Presence of soft-tissue scalp lacerations
    B. A patient experiencing dizziness following a trip and fall
    C. Presence of headache following soccer ball impact to the head
    D. Facial fractures following a trauma

11. Which of the following is the most common mechanism of injury for a severe traumatic brain injury in the pediatric population?

    A. Falls
    B. Motor vehicle collision
    C. Penetrating trauma
    D. Sports injuries

12. Which of the following is NOT commonly a complication of frontal lobe injury in traumatic brain-injured patients?

    A. Short- and long-term memory losses
    B. Impulsiveness and loss of inhibition
    C. Emotional lability
    D. Visual changes

13. Which of the following is a complication of craniectomy?

    A. Facial droop
    B. Cerebral edema
    C. Hygromas
    D. Increased intracranial pressure

14. Which of the following is the LEAST accurate statement regarding the care of a patient with a decompressive craniectomy?

    A. Wearing of protective head gear until replacement of flap is for patient safety.
    B. Bone flap replacement can occur after the swelling of the brain has receded.
    C. The absence of the bone flap can cause anxiety for the families requiring reassurance.
    D. The site of the absent bone flap should not be palpated due to potential injury of brain matter.

15. Which of the following is considered the mechanism in which new learning occurs after 6 months following traumatic brain injury?

    A. Restitution
    B. Substitution
    C. Reintegration
    D. Recovery

16. Which of the following is NOT a frequently used medication to assist with managing spasticity following a traumatic brain injury?

    A. Baclophen
    B. Clonidine
    C. Gabapentin
    D. Steroids

17. Which of the following is NOT a component of the triad of signs seen in patients with diffuse axonal injury?

    A. Glasgow Coma Scale of less than 8
    B. Rotational mechanism of injury

C. Lack of cerebral edema
D. CT scan without focal mass lesions

18. A patient presents with an anterior fossa fracture after a traumatic brain injury. Which of the following is MOST likely associated with the fracture?

    A. Otorrhea
    B. Rhinorrhea
    C. Battle sign
    D. Epidural hematoma

## CHAPTER 9: NEUROLOGICAL TRAUMA: SPINAL CORD INJURY

1. Which of the following complications would most likely require immediate surgery of a patient with traumatic spinal cord injury?

    A. Bilateral locked facets
    B. Intramedullary hematoma
    C. Subluxation without cord compression
    D. Complete cord injury

2. A spinal cord–injured patient is intubated and being mechanically ventilated. The patient is at high risk for a ventilator-associated pneumonia (VAP). Which of the following is the most appropriate intervention to prevent a VAP?

    A. Head of the bed is flat
    B. Oral care every 2 hours
    C. Suction endotracheal tube every 2 hours
    D. Assisted cough

3. Following a motor vehicle collision, a patient presents with paraplegia and cord compression is found on radiographs. Which of the following is considered the best treatment for a cord compression following a trauma?

    A. High-dose intravenous steroids
    B. Decompressive surgery
    C. Permissive hypertension
    D. Therapeutic hypothermia

4. Your patient arrives by emergency medical service following a fall. He has a history of coronary stents, atrial fibrillation and congestive heart failure. He is noted to have diminished motor and sensory function in his lower extremities. Which of the following is the most likely cause for his motor and sensory deficits?

    A. Hangman's fracture with anterior displacement
    B. Atlantooccipital dislocation
    C. Spinal epidural hematoma
    D. Ischemic stroke

5. Which of the following will increase the risk of vertebral fracture with low mechanism of injuries?

    A. Spinal stenosis
    B. Osteoarthritis

C. Thoracic vertebral injury
D. Cauda equina syndrome

6. Which of the following is NOT considered a correct landmark for localizing the level of spinal cord injury?

    A. Clavicles correlate to C4 level.
    B. Nipple line correlates to C6 level.
    C. Umbilicus correlates to T10 level.
    D. Rectal area correlates to S1 level.

7. The spinal cord begins at the foramen magnum and tapers to end at which of the following levels?

    A. Lumbar 2–3
    B. Lumbar 4–5
    C. Thoracic 8–9
    D. Sacrum

8. A pediatric patient presenting with transient neurological motor abnormalities with spinal trauma is most likely experiencing which of the following spinal cord syndromes?

    A. Central cord syndrome
    B. Brown square cord syndrome
    C. Spinal cord injury without radiographic abnormality
    D. Complete cord injury

# 14

# Answers and Rationales for the Bonus Exam Questions

Disclaimer: These questions are intended for extra practice. The questions may include topics that are not covered in the review.

## CHAPTER 1: CHRONIC NEUROLOGICAL DISORDERS

1. **D**

    Rationale: Huntington's disease is classified as a subcortical dementia and is associated with problems in memory, cognition, and motor control. Huntington's disease is a genetic, incurable, progressive, and eventually fatal disorder. Generally, cognitive changes precede the motor control abnormalities; the rate at which the symptoms progress varies.

2. **D**

    Rationale: *Chorea* refers to involuntary, rapid movements of the limbs, torso, and face. Chorea is commonly associated with Huntington's disease. Blepharospasm is abnormal contraction or twitch of eyelid. Athetosis is twisting or torsions of the trunk. Fasciculations are muscle contractions or twitches.

3. **B**

    Rationale: Genetic testing is used as predictive and confirmatory tests. Genetic testing can predict whether a person is likely to develop Huntington's disease. MRI, lumbar puncture with cerebrospinal fluid analysis, and electromyography testing are used to evaluate patients with neurological symptoms, but genetic testing is most important for the confirmative diagnosis.

4. **C**

    Rationale: Dysphagia, aspiration, and pneumonia are common complications of Huntington's disease during its late stages. Patients in late stages of Huntington's disease will commonly lose the ability to speak and walk but will maintain comprehension of language and the ability to recognize friends and family. Urinary retention is not commonly associated with Huntington's disease.

5. **A**

   Rationale: During thearly stages of Huntington's disease the risk for suicide is at its highest because the person still has the cognitive ability to plan and carry out the suicide. This is also the stage commonly associated with depression. During the middle stages patients develop greater difficulty in thinking and reasoning. In the late stage, patients become completely reliant on caregivers. Patients with Huntington's disease, at end of life, may be unable to communicate or move.

6. **B**

   Rationale: People with restless leg syndrome (RLS) have an uncontrollable urge to move their lower extremities, which is accompanied by abnormal sensations. The sensations are described as aching, throbbing, crawling, and creeping. A classic feature is worsening of symptoms at night, but RLS can occur at other times of the day. It may result in pacing. RLS can have remissions and spontaneous improvements, but can become more severe over time.

7. **C**

   Rationale: Restless leg syndrome (RLS) affects the basal ganglia and the dopamine pathways, as does Parkinson's disease. Patients with Parkinson's disease have a high risk of experiencing RLS. The other neurological disorders, Alzheimer's dementia, Huntington's disease, or myasthenia gravis, do not have a higher risk or association with RLS.

8. **A**

   Rationale: Iron deficiency is considered a significant risk for the development of restless leg syndrome (RLS). Iron supplements can be trialed as the first-line treatment for RLS, especially if the ferritin and transferrin saturations levels are low. Beta-blockers and calcium channel blockers are not used to treat RLS. Benzodiazepines can be used to manage RLS but are not considered the first-line treatment. Other pharmacological treatment for RLS may include anticonvulsants, dopaminergic agents, and opioids.

9. **C**

   Rationale: Obstructive sleep apnea is a type of sleep-disordered breathing characterized by periods of 10 seconds or greater without airflow or breath. This has been shown to be a high risk factor for stroke and right-sided heart failure. Insomnia and restless leg syndrome are both sleep disorders but do not carry a higher risk for stroke. Narcolepsy is not a sleep disorder.

10. **C**

    Rationale: Stroke patients with a history of significant migraines with aura are at a higher risk for ischemic stroke. The proposed physiology includes embolic events due to hypercoagulable or hyperviscosity disorders. Hypertension is not considered an added risk factor for stroke in patients with headaches.

# 14. ANSWERS AND RATIONALES FOR THE BONUS EXAM QUESTIONS

**11. B**

Rationale: Red flags for stroke in patients with aura-producing migraines include an aura lasting for greater than an hour, migraine headache greater than 12 hours, and abnormal neurological signs. Headaches can occur before, during, or after the aura and are not a red flag for a stroke. Normal EEG waveform with an aura is not an increased risk but a typical finding.

**12. A**

Rationale: A resting tremor typically presents unilaterally. It presents a slow oscillation with the head and voice not commonly affected. Distraction can worsen the tremor.

**13. D**

Rationale: Dystonic tremors commonly affect the head more than the hands and arms. Dystonic tremor is usually an irregular tremor and can involve both vertical and horizontal head movement. The tremor is not relieved during sleep.

**14. B**

Rationale: Benign essential tremors (BETs) experience more rapid oscillations of the tremor than Parkinson's disease (PD). PD involves a slower, resting tremor typically occurring with greater symptoms on one side of the body. BET has a familial or genetic trait, whereas PD is not usually considered genetic.

**15. C**

Rationale: Lewy body dementia is a type of subcortical dementia related to Parkinson's disease. The signs of Lewy body dementia commonly present with abnormalities in complex attention and executive function. This includes difficulty with complex tasks, errors in routine tasks, and the inability to multitask. It does not affect memory as much as cortical dementia does. Cortical dementia involves memory loss, language difficulties, and word-finding problems.

**16. C**

Rationale: Frontotemporal dementia commonly presents with behavioral and personality changes such as impulsiveness, compulsiveness, and hoarding. Radiographic scans demonstrate bilateral frontal neuronal loss. Lewy body dementia is associated with Parkinson's disease and does not commonly exhibit neuronal loss. Alzheimer's dementia initially presents with memory and language deficits, not typically behavioral changes. Vascular dementia is a result of ischemic insult to the brain followed acutely by memory, language, and judgment abnormalities.

**17. B**

Rationale: Guillain–Barré syndrome is an autoimmune disorder that involves the peripheral nerves. Peripheral nerves are a part of the lower motor neurons and present with hyporeflexia or loss of reflexes. Upper motor neuron injury results in hyperreflexia or spasticity. Peripheral neuropathies, such as Guillain–Barré, are bilateral.

**18. C**

Rationale: Carpal tunnel syndrome affects the medial ulnar nerve. Cubital tunnel syndrome involves the entrapment of the ulnar nerve at the level of the elbow. Brachial plexus injury involves the group of nerves that travel through the axillary area. Radial nerve palsy involves the radial nerve.

**19. B**

Rationale: Adolescence to the age of 35 years is the most common age for the presentation of onset of multiple sclerosis (MS). MS is rare in pediatrics and in those older than the age of 65 years. Middle-age onset of MS is not as common as young-adult onset.

**20. A**

Rationale: Multiple sclerosis may have a genetic component but is related to multiple genes, not one genetic factor. Known correlations or risks include living north of the equator, vitamin D deficiency, and viral infections.

**21. D**

Rationale: Cerebrospinal fluid analysis diagnostic of multiple sclerosis includes elevated oligoclonal bands, normal opening pressures, minimal elevation of white blood cells, normal protein, and elevated immunoglobulin G synthesis rates.

**22. C**

Rationale: Periventricular white matter lesions are the most characteristic change on MRI to identify multiple sclerosis (MS). Patients with MS may also have cortical atrophy and corpus thinning, but there are other causes for these findings as well. Obstructive hydrocephalus is not a normal finding on MRI for MS patients.

**23. D**

Rationale: Presence of oligoclonal bands is high in 90% of the patients with multiple sclerosis (MS). The other findings are correct for MS but are not diagnostic because they are normal findings in cerebrospinal fluid.

**24. C**

Rationale: Potential side effects of deep brain stimulation (DBS) depend on the placement of the wires. More commonly found side effects include muscle rigidity, abnormal gaze, mania/disinhibition, and affective changes. Vertigo is not a commonly known side effect.

**25. A**

Rationale: Resting tremors are usually early signs of the onset of Parkinson's disease (PD). These tremors are the most common reason that people seek medical attention during the early stages of PD. Other signs of PD include muscle rigidity and bradykinesias but are not commonly the earliest sign of PD. Dizziness and vertigo are not commonly associated with signs of PD.

**26. A**

Rationale: The Mini–Mental Status Exam is the most commonly used tool to evaluate cognition and memory in patients with early dementia. Glasgow Outcome Scale (GOS) is used to evaluate patients following traumatic brain injury (TBI). Framingham's profile is used to determine the risk for stroke. Geriatric evaluation for dementia (GED) is not a known scale.

## 14. ANSWERS AND RATIONALES FOR THE BONUS EXAM QUESTIONS

27. C

Rationale: Huntington's disease is hereditary genetic disorder characterized by abnormal motor movement commonly of the face and arms, gait abnormalities with frequent falls, changes in speech, weight loss, memory loss, and depression. Parkinson's disease presents with resting tremors, bradykinesia, and muscle rigidity. Tourette's syndrome is associated with verbal and motor tics and abnormal behaviors.

28. B

Rationale: Patients with terminal stages of Huntington's disease (HD) frequently present with the appearance of failure to thrive. They are cachetic, experience bowel and bladder incontinence, and are lethargic. They are high-risk patients for aspiration pneumonia. Terminal stages of HD are rarely ambulatory but do not usually progress to comatose states. Flaccid paralysis is not a sign of HD.

29. C

Rationale: Wilson's disease is a hereditary neurological disorder that causes an imbalance in the absorption and excretion of copper, resulting in very high levels of copper. Patients present with uncoordinated gaits, dysarthria/dysphasia, and tremors that appear like "wing-beating." Amyotrophic lateral sclerosis involves motor weakness in both upper and lower motor neurons. Huntington's disease involves abnormal motor movement but does not present with "wing-beating" tremors. Tourette's syndrome is associated with tics of voice and motor.

## CHAPTER 2: CEREBROVASCULAR DISORDERS

1. D

Rationale: Paroxysmal atrial fibrillation (PAF) is managed similar to continuous atrial fibrillation (AF) in regard to anticoagulation. There is no evidence regarding the frequency or duration of AF and the risk for embolic strokes. Monitoring for the presence of AF in patients with appearance of embolic strokes and no history of AF, but if PAF is known, anticoagulation therapy should be initiated unless contraindicated. PAF carries a high risk for stroke and should be managed with anticoagulation therapy, not acetylsalicylic acid unless lone AF.

2. C

Rationale: To a stroke patient with a patent foramen ovale (PFO) and venous source of embolism, anticoagulation therapy is recommended. If there is no source of venous embolism, antiplatelet therapy may be initiated. Ablation treatment is for rapid atrial rates with abnormal pathways, not for PFO. The closure of PFO is not typically performed initially.

3. B

Rationale: The Modified Rankin Scale (mRS) is a commonly used scale to measure the degree of disability or independence with activities of daily living following a stroke. Glasgow Outcome Scale is used to determine the outcomes of patients following traumatic brain injuries. Thrombolysis in Cerebral Infarction (TICI) scores are used to measure the success of reperfusion following a thrombectomy. CHADS2 score estimates the risk of stroke in patients with atrial fibrillation (AF).

4. D

   Rationale: Prevention of complications begins in the acute care setting and continues throughout the rehabilitation period. Prevention of venous thromboembolic events (VTEs) is important following a stroke. In patients with hemorrhagic strokes, intermittent pneumatic compression devices are recommended to prevent VTE until it is determined to be safe to add anticoagulation therapy. Elastic compression stocking is not a recommended intervention to prevent VTE. IV heparin infusion is not recommended following an intracerebral hemorrhage. Clear liquids can increase the risk of aspiration.

5. A

   Rationale: Regularly scheduled prompted voiding can assist with preventing urinary incontinence and is recommended. Intermittent catheterizations should be performed for urinary retention after utilizing bladder scanners. Placement of an indwelling foley should only be for urinary retention after couple attempts of intermittent catheterization.

6. C

   Rationale: Shoulder pain is common following a stroke. The development of shoulder pain is commonly associated with subluxation and motor weakness of the extremity. Trigeminal neuralgia is not a common complication of a stroke. Chronic headaches may develop after hemorrhagic strokes but is not as commonly seen as shoulder pain. Hip displacement with improper positioning can occur but not fractures.

7. B

   Rationale: The best regimen to manage neuropathic pain is with anticonvulsants and/or tricyclic antidepressants. This regimen has been found to have the most improvement in pain management. Nonsteroidal medications may be effective with some neuropathy pain, but long-term use of Toradol is not recommended. Opioids are not recommended with neuropathic pain. Transcutaneous electrical stimulation (TENS) may be more effective with peripheral neuropathies than central neuropathic pain. Alternating heat and cold is not recommended.

8. C

   Rationale: Recommendation of daily stretches has been found to be the most effective at preventing the complication of contractures. Hand splints are often applied on hemiparetic arms, but effectiveness is not well established. Immobilization of the extremity is not recommended and may increase the risk of contractures. Surgical release of tendons and/or muscle may be used to treat contractures but not to prevent them. Another recommended management is control of spasticity.

9. C

   Rationale: Dysphagia following a stroke frequently leads to aspiration pneumonia, weight loss, and malnutrition. Failure to thrive is weight loss, poor appetite, and nutrition and physical inactivity associated with depression. It is not related to dysphagia.

# 14. ANSWERS AND RATIONALES FOR THE BONUS EXAM QUESTIONS

**10. A**

Rationale: Early stroke treatment can only occur if there is early recognition of the signs of a stroke by the patient, family, EMS, and healthcare providers. Living close to a hospital may decrease the time to treatment, but the person will still have to recognize the signs. People should become knowledgeable in both the recognition and treatment options of a stroke, but the essential component for early treatment is early recognition.

**11. C**

Rationale: It is not recommended for the prehospital providers to perform a complete National Institutes of Health Stroke Scale (NIHSS). There are several tools to recognize signs of stroke and signs of large vessel obstruction that take less time to perform. Prioritizing potential stroke patients and minimizing time on-scene will improve time of symptom onset to treatment. Transporting quickly to the most appropriate hospital that can care for the stroke patient will prevent delays of transferring the patient from one hospital to another, thus improving times to treatment.

**12. A**

Rationale: Patients with large vessel obstruction (LVO) strokes are candidates for endovascular therapy and should be transported to a center with endovascular capability. Recognition in the field with specific stroke severity scales for LVO can facilitate transfer to the appropriate facility. Other stroke recognition scales are used to identify signs of a stroke and then prealerting the receiving hospital. LVO recognition is not used to identify IV thrombolytic patients.

**13. A**

Rationale: A patient with the diagnosis of infective endocarditis would have an increased risk for intracranial hemorrhage with thrombolytic therapy. Antiplatelet medications are not contraindicated for intravenous (IV) alteplase. There is not determined age limit for the administration of IV alteplase and can be administered to patient in renal failure on dialysis as long as the INR is below 1.7.

**14. C**

Rationale: A patient on the novel anticoagulants are not candidates for intravenous (IV) alteplase but are candidates for endovascular therapy (mechanical thrombectomy). An international normalized ratio (INR) will not accurately identify the degree of anticoagulation in novel anticoagulants like in vitamin K antagonists. Reversal agents are not recommended to administer unless the patient presents with an intracerebral hemorrhage (ICH).

**15. C**

Rationale: For patients with dysphagia, it is recommended to provide enteral feeding either initially by nasogastric tube or eventually with percutaneous gastric tube (PEG). Enteral feeding should be initiated within 7 days of admission. Total parenteral nutrition (TPN) is not the recommended route in stroke patients. Stroke patients entering hospice care may be allowed to eat for quality of life, but this was not the scenario provided. Clear liquids have higher aspirations risks than solid food and should not be administered to patients with swallow deficits.

16. C

    Rationale: Dysphagia screens and speech therapist consults are to directly evaluate the patient's ability to swallow and risk for aspiration pneumonia. The results can determine the consistency of liquid intake recommended. Oral hygiene protocols include frequent oral care, and use of antimicrobial mouthwash has been found to lower risks of aspiration pneumonia. Chest x-rays can be used to diagnose aspiration pneumonia but not prevent it.

17. A

    Rationale: Risk factors for vasospasms and delayed cerebral ischemia include the volume of blood in the ventricles, poor clinical grades on Hunt and Hess (grades IV and V), hypoglycemia, and early surgery. Hunt and Hess score of II is a low score with a better prognosis and lower risk of vasospasms. Glasgow Coma Scale (GCS) of 14 is a good prognosis and indicates patient's neurological status is a lower risk for vasospasm. Surgical clipping of aneurysm at 14 days postbleed is considered a "late surgery" and decreases risk of vasospasm. Early surgery during vasospasms can increase the risk and severity of vasospasms.

18. C

    Rationale: Cerebral salt wasting syndrome (CSWS) and syndrome of inappropriate antidiuretic hormone (SIADH) both result in hyponatremia but through two different mechanisms. In CSWS, the kidneys lose sodium resulting in diuresis and blood volume loss. This can complicate the management of vasospasm, which requires fluids and vascular volume augmentation. SIADH lowers the sodium by dilutional effects due to volume overload. This does not work against the management strategies of vasospasms. Delayed ischemic injury is a result of vasospasms and is not a factor affecting the management of vasospasms. Hydrocephalus is a complication of subarachnoid hemorrhage (SAH) but is not a concern with fluid augmentation to manage vasospasms.

19. A

    Rationale: This patient is 8 days following a subarachnoid hemorrhage (SAH) and is symptomatic with the most likely reason being vasospasm. Euvolemic or augmentation of hemodynamics and hypertension are recommended to manage vasospasms following an SAH. This patient already appears to be volume augmented with a positive fluid balance of 2 L. Hypertension, typically greater than 160 mmHg, is recommended to improve profusion and prevent delayed ischemic injury. Vasoconstrictors may be utilized with euvolemia. Diuretic would not be indicated during vasospasms. Obtaining a noncontrast CT scan is not an intervention to manage vasospasms.

20. A

    Rationale: Medical management (augmentation hemodynamics and hypertension) is the recommended initial management of vasospasms but if unable to improve cerebral perfusion, interventional techniques are recommended (angioplasty, intraarterial antihypertensives, antisplasmodics). Surgical clipping is a technique used to secure an aneurysm, not to treat vasospasms.

21. D

    Rationale: An "unsecured" aneurysm has not been coiled or surgically clipped. Induced hypertension to manage vasospasm will increase the risk of rebleeds or rupture in the

# 14. ANSWERS AND RATIONALES FOR THE BONUS EXAM QUESTIONS

unsecured aneurysm. Aneurysms that have been surgically clipped or coiled in intervention are considered secured and are less likely to bleed with induced hypertension. The location or the number of secured aneurysms does not make a difference in the use of induced hypertension.

22. A

Rationale: All of the above can cause a stroke in pediatric patients, but congenital heart disease with cerebral thromboembolism events is the most common cause.

23. C

Rationale: Chiropractor manipulation of the neck has caused vertebral and carotid dissection and symptoms of stroke. Recent falls more commonly cause subdural hematomas. Cerebral aneurysms result in subarachnoid hemorrhages when ruptures. Hypertensive crisis results in hemorrhagic strokes and are not related to dissections.

24. D

Rationale: Spontaneous vertebral dissection is divided between ischemic and hemorrhagic. The hemorrhagic type presents as subarachnoid hemorrhage (SAH) caused by the rupture of an intradural vertebral dissecting aneurysm.

25. C

Rationale: Cerebral cavernous malformations are vascular lesions compromised of tightly packed, thin-walled vessels that displace normal neurological tissue. Cavernous malformations can be located in the brain and spinal cord. Internal carotid artery (ICA) narrowing with the development of collateral vessels is called Moyamoya disease. Dural thrombosis is called central venous thrombosis. Central nervous system (CNS) vasculitis is the inflammation of the cerebral vasculature and can cause ischemic or hemorrhagic strokes.

26. B

Rationale: Too rapid or overdrainage of the cerebrospinal fluid (CSF) can lead to bleeding in the subdural space. This may occur unilateral or bilateral. Close monitoring of CSF drainage is important to prevent subdural hematoma (SDH) complications. Overdrainage can eventually produce effacement of ventricles but would be a late complication and is not the primary concern. SDH is more likely the complication of overdrainage. Cerebral edema and increased ICP are not complications of overdrainage of CSF.

27. B

Rationale: Distal embolization is a complication if interventional coiling of the aneurysm, not typically due to surgical clipping of the aneurysm. Incomplete clipping of the aneurysm leading to the development of another aneurysm is a potential complication. Inadvertent clipping of surrounding vessels leading to ischemia and rupture of the aneurysm during surgery are complications of surgical intervention with aneurysms.

28. A

Rationale: Prior to surgical removal of the arteriovenous malformation (AVM), the patient lived with a "steal phenomenon" in which blood flow was routed to the AVM and away from the rest of the brain. Once the AVM is removed, blood flow is redistributed to chronically hypoperfused areas of the brain, resulting in hyperfusion injuries. Intracerebral hemorrhage can occur following an AVM resection, but subdural hematoma (SDH) is not a common complication. Patients with AVM resection can experience seizures, but the scenario does not suggest seizure activity has occurred. There are no labs in the scenario to indicate a metabolic encephalopathy.

**29. C**

Rationale: Amaurosis fugax is the ipsilateral impairment of vision due to retinal occlusion and ischemia. The initial branch of the intracranial internal carotid is the ophthalmic artery, and plaque dislodged from the carotid artery can travel to the ophthalmic artery, resulting in an embolic stroke. Pseudotumor cerebri can present with visual changes but is a result of increased intracranial pressure, not ischemic stroke.

**30. A**

Rationale: Neuroplasticity is a concept that the brain has both restorative and regeneration capabilities. Damage to central nervous system (CNS) cells and neurons is no longer considered to be irreversible injury. Areas of tissue damage can cause scarring but is not providing any regeneration of restoration of function. Neuronal replication and regenerative balance are not concepts used with neuronal healing.

**31. C**

Rationale: Neuroplasticity involves axonal sprouting and reorganizing to improve neuronal pathways. Neuronal sprouting has been found to activate as early as 7 days after a stroke. New connections and pathways are seen within 30 days of a stroke. Rapid, early, and intense rehabilitation can improve neurological outcomes with capitalizing on the time of the highest neuroplasticity. It can also improve patient's mentation and assist with moving the patient toward self-care but is not the most important reason for early rehabilitation.

**32. D**

Rationale: DASH (Dietary Approaches to Stop Hypertension) is a commonly recommended diet to prevent hypertension. It is a diet high in vegetables/fruit and low in dairy products with less saturated and total fat. Low sodium (salt) is recommended but a diet high in potassium, not low. High fat is not recommended.

**33. C**

Rationale: Lowering the HgbA1C levels below 7% in diabetic patients appears to lower the risk of stroke and myocardial infarction (MI). Nondiabetics are recommended to maintain below 6%.

**34. C**

Rationale: Internal carotid artery (ICA) stroke can result in visual deficits, the most common being a contralateral visual field loss. Bilateral losses of peripheral vision occurs when the injury is at the optic chiasm. Homonymous hemianopia occurs in strokes involving the occipital lobe. Scotomas are small areas of visual loss within the fields of vision.

## 14. ANSWERS AND RATIONALES FOR THE BONUS EXAM QUESTIONS

**35. A**

Rationale: Posterior strokes resulting from vertebral or basilar artery involvement can result in bilateral hearing losses, ataxia, dizziness, dysarthria, nystagmus, and vertigo. Posterior cerebral artery (PCA) results more in visual deficits. Internal carotid artery (ICA) can cause contralateral hemiplegia. External carotid artery (ECA) is not a commonly involved artery for a stroke.

**36. B**

Rationale: Weber's syndrome is a posterior stroke of the vertebral–basilar arteries and commonly presents with the ipsilateral ptosis, nonreactive pupil, and contralateral hemiplegia. Wallenberg's syndrome and locked-in syndrome are also syndromes associated with posterior strokes but do not result in the ipsilateral third nerve palsy. Horner's syndrome can be associated with posterior strokes and is the ipsilateral loss of sympathetic inner action to the face.

**37. A**

Rationale: Spetzler–Martin grading system is used to calculate the surgical risk of arteriovenous malformation (AVM). The scale is based upon the size of the AVM, the eloquence of the brain tissue, and the pattern of venous drainage. The Hunt and Hess grading system measures the severity of the subarachnoid hemorrhage (SAH). Intracerebral hemorrhage (ICH) score is used to predict 0-day mortality. Fisher grade is designed to predict vasospasms after SAH.

**38. B**

Rationale: Increased density within the occluded middle cerebral artery (MCA) is called a hyperdense sign and is an early finding of large vessel obstruction (LVO). Hyperdense dot is a more distal occlusion of the MCA and is not considered an LVO. Presence of an infarct indicates a late not early sign of an infarct. Petechial hemorrhages fund in the basal ganglia does not indicate an LVO.

**39. D**

Rationale: Shivering is a physiological consequence of lowering a body temperature. Shivering can increase metabolism, intracranial pressure (ICP), and prevent effective cooling. Monitoring for presence and severity of shivering is very important during the initiation and maintenance of targeted temperature control. Hemodynamics and cardiac monitoring should also be included, but shivering assessment is most important at this time. Measurement of urine output is important, but shivering assessment is a priority.

## CHAPTER 3: TUMORS OF THE BRAIN AND SPINAL CORD

**1. C**

Rationale: In glioblastoma multiforme and anaplastic astrocytoma (high-grade gliomas), the T2 signal in MRI will show an irregular, enhancing rim of the tumor. This is a result of necrosis and loss of blood–brain barrier allowing uptake of the contrast. In low-grade gliomas, the tumor is homogeneously hyperintense on T2 with little enhancement. Multifocal lesions are more likely associated with metastasis to the brain. PET scanning is used to assist with diagnosing brain tumor with increased metabolism but is not required to assist with the differentiation. Low-grade glioma can appear isodense on a noncontrast CT scan, but lesion can usually be identified.

2. D

Dexamethasone is the initial treatment for cerebral edema or new onset symptoms in brain tumors. In many patients, the early use of dexamethasone can show improvement in symptoms within hours and can prevent further brain tissue shifting. Hypertonic saline and mannitol infusions are second-line therapy for managing cerebral edema. Keppra, an anticonvulsant, may be used to manage seizures but is controversial in prophylactic prevention of seizures in brain tumors.

3. B

Pneumocystic pneumonitis is a potential complication of long-term use of steroids (dexamethasone) in managing brain tumors and edema. Some oncology neurologists prescribe trimethoprim–sulfamethoxazole (Baytril) to prevent the complication. Aspiration pneumonia is a potential complication if patients are unable to swallow or protect airway with a brain tumor but is not a result of the steroid therapy. Adrenal suppression (not hypersecretion) can occur if the steroid is suddenly withdrawn. Dystonia is not a complication of steroid therapy.

4. C

Rationale: Tube feeding in a patient with altered mentation unable to swallow may be indicated early within the hospital stay to provide adequate nutrition but is not considered the "initial" intervention on admission. Deep venous thrombosis (DVT) prophylaxis with sequential compression devices (SCDs), gastrointestinal (GI) prophylaxis, and administration of dexamethasone are all three initial managements of a brain tumor patient with altered mentation to prevent complications and begin to manage the cerebral edema.

5. C

Rationale: Treatment of glioblastoma multiforme (GBM) is aimed at multiple levels and different pathways to improve efficacy. Surgical debulking is usually recommended unless in an eloquent area such as the motor strip. This can be followed by radiotherapy and chemotherapy.

6. B

Rationale: Cerebral edema results in presentation with nonfocal neurological symptoms such as altered level of consciousness. Cerebral edema can affect broader area of the brain, resulting in the nonfocal deficits. Brainstem lesion is more in a focal area of the brain and can present with cranial nerve deficits. Hydrocephalus presents with headache, nausea and vomiting, and commonly vertigo or dizziness. Meningitis presents with headache, fever, and nuchal rigidity.

7. A

Rationale: Headache is a common symptom of brain tumors. It is commonly described as a dull, vague headache that worsens in the morning or in a recumbent position. If the headache is associated with vomiting, the symptom is associated with increased intracranial pressure (ICP).

# 14. ANSWERS AND RATIONALES FOR THE BONUS EXAM QUESTIONS

8. **D**

   Rationale: A lumbar puncture and cerebrospinal fluid (CSF) analysis may be used to assist with the diagnosis of brain lymphoma or medulloblastoma. Pituitary tumors can be diagnosed with abnormal endocrine functions. Glioblastoma and pineal tumors are identified with radiographic scans.

9. **A**

   Rationale: The standard treatment of a CNS lymphoma is a tumor biopsy followed by chemotherapy and/or radiation therapy. The tumor can be very radiation sensitive. A total tumor resection is not recommended with suspected CNS lymphomas.

10. **D**

    Rationale: The blood–brain barrier (BBB) is unique to the CNS. This is a tight cellular junction that prevents most drugs from crossing into the brain cells. Many chemotherapy drugs used to treat other cancers cannot cross the BBB to treat a CNS tumor. The brain itself does not have a lymphatic system like other areas of the body. Kupffer cells are macrophages that line the liver to filter bacteria from the blood and are not present in the CNS. Capillary beds are not unique to the CNS.

11. **B**

    Rationale: Tumor necrosis following radiation therapy can cause edema and increased enhancement. This results in a difficulty to distinguish radiation necrosis from progression of the disease process. Radiation necrosis can be treated with steroid treatment. Cerebral edema is a potential complication of radiation therapy but does not mimic tumor progression on radiographic studies. Infarction and demyelination does not mimic tumor progression on the diagnostic radiographic studies.

12. **C**

    Rationale: Prescription of steroid therapy is common in treating cerebral edema and neurological changes in patients with brain tumors. Complications of steroid therapy include mood swings, including psychosis, fluid retention, hyperglycemia, and hypokalemia (not hyperkalemia).

13. **B**

    Rationale: The distribution of spinal tumor per vertebral column locations correlates with the amount of cord tissue in each area. The thoracic area has the largest spinal cord diameter so accounts to approximately 50% of the location for spinal tumors.

14. **B**

    Rationale: The term "extradural" indicates that the spinal tumor is outside the epidural space. Intradural, the tumor is within the dura and extramedullary indicates the tumor is outside the spinal cord itself. "Intramedullary" indicates that it is located within the tissue of the spinal cord. Extradural tumors can be invasive of bone and vertebral bodies.

15. **D**

    Rationale: Metastatic lesions in the spinal canal commonly cause bowel and bladder problems, weakness of extremities, and localized pain with percussion of the vertebral column. Bilateral ascending paralysis may actually indicate a neuromuscular weakness called Guillain–Barré.

16. A

Rationale: Radiation therapy of the spine can result in complications. The most common complication can be sensory deficits. These sensory changes include chronic progressive sensory changes or loss of sensation at the level of radiation. Motor losses and paralysis can occur but are not common. Brown-Sequard syndrome is a combination of sensory and motor and can occur with some spinal tumors but not commonly associated with radiation therapy. Spinal fusion is not considered a complication of radiation therapy.

17. D

Rationale: Hemangioblastoma is a benign vascular neoplasm arises almost exclusively from the CNS. This tumor has a dense vascular component and sometimes called Lindau tumors. Pilocytic astrocytoma is a low-grade astrocytoma and is not considered a vascular tumor. Craniopharyngioma is a nonglial tumor but is not a vascular lesion. Fibromatosis is a group of soft tissue tumors.

18. B

Rationale: Hemangioblastomas are most commonly located in the posterior fossa as an intraaxial tumor in adult patients. Frontal lobe is more commonly associated with gliomas. Pineal tumors are located on the pineal gland but are not classified as hemangioblastoma. Hemangioblastoma is rarely located in the sagittal venous sinus area.

19. A

Rationale: Approximately 25% of the hemangioblastomas are associated with von Hipple–Lindau syndrome. It is an autosomal-dominant hereditary syndrome and may be involving CNS hemangioblastoma, retinal angiomatosis, and visceral tumors. Marfan syndrome and neurofibromatosis are autosomal-dominant hereditary syndromes but are not associated with hemangioblastomas. Tay-Sachs is a recessive autosomal hereditary syndrome and is not associated with hemangioblastoma.

20. D

Rationale: Craniopharyngiomas are commonly located near the pituitary gland, optic chiasm, and third ventricle. Radiation therapy can cause damage to the optic tract and chiasm, resulting in visual losses. Seizures can occur with any tumor but are not specific to craniopharyngioma. Neglect syndrome and hemiparesis are more common with masses occurring within the lobar portions of the brain.

## CHAPTER 4: IMMUNE INFECTIONS, PART 1

1. C

Rationale: The most common areas for brain abscesses in cerebral tissue include frontotemporal, frontoparietal, and parietal. The epidural and subdural spaces are also common areas for intracranial abscess. The least common include cerebellar and occipital.

2. A

Rationale: An infectious source, such as a brain abscess, in the vicinity of the venous dural sinuses can lead to thrombosis due to the hypercoagulable state. The cavernous sinus is most commonly involved. Inflammation and cerebral edema commonly surrounds the brain abscess. The abscess can cause meningitis.

3. B

Rationale: Brain abscess commonly results in an increased intracranial pressure (ICP) so a lumbar puncture is not recommended due to the risk of transtentorial herniation. The cerebrospinal fluid (CSF) analysis does not yield specific results to assist with the diagnosis. Erythrocyte sedimentation rate (ESR) and complete blood count (CBC) with differential are commonly obtained to identify an infection. MRI is the most diagnostic for a brain abscess.

4. B

Rationale: Among the opportunistic infections of the CNS in patients with HIV disease are the herpes viruses, including herpes simplex types I and II, herpes varicella-zoster, and cytomegalovirus (CMV). Neurosyphilis is a bacterium, and *Candida albicans* is a fungal infection. Both are more commonly found in patients with HIV disease but are not virus infections.

## CHAPTER 5: IMMUNE INFECTIONS, PART 2

1. C

Rationale: Hypercoagulable state is not a recognized side effect of interferon. Flulike symptoms occur in almost 100% of the patients receiving interferon. Psychiatric disorders, including depression, are common side effects. Liver disease is a noted complication of interferon.

2. D

Rationale: Progressive multifocal leukoencephalopathy (PML) is a rare type of brain infection. Patients with weak immune systems, through either immunosuppressive agents or illness such as HIV, are at a greater risk for PML when given natalizumab. Depression and headaches are side effects of natalizumab but are not as serious. Acute kidney injury (AKI) is not a side effect of natalizumab.

3. B

Rationale: Family history is the strongest known risk factor for multiple sclerosis (MS). It is more common among first-degree relatives with a rapid decrease in second-degree relatives. Lack of vitamin D, history of heavy smoking, and exposure to Epstein–Barr virus are identified risk factors but are not considered the strongest risk for MS.

4. A

Rationale: Cytotoxic cerebral edema is a physiological change that occurs in patients with hypoxic/anoxic brain injuries. Multiple sclerosis (MS) patients experience conduction abnormalities of the CNS nerves, inflammation, and CNS loss.

5. **C**

Rationale: Pseudoexacerbations of multiple sclerosis (MS) refers to changes in neurological function triggered by fever, infection, heat, and fatigue. These symptoms occur due to decompensation of existing central nervous system (CNS) scars and not new lesions. Hypoxia, trauma, and shivering are not known causes of pseudoexacerbation of MS symptoms.

6. **B**

Rationale: The McDonald Criteria are created to provide a more reliable diagnosis for multiple sclerosis (MS). Hunt and Hess score is used to measure the severity of subarachnoid hemorrhage (SAH). Glasgow Outcome Scale (GOS) is used in patients with traumatic brain injury to measure the neurological recovery. CHADS2 scores are used to determine the risk for stroke with atrial fibrillation (AF) patients.

7. **B**

Rationale: Remission of myasthenia gravis (MG) indicates no symptoms or signs—weakness of eyelids is acceptable but no other muscle weakness is allowed. Presence of ocular weakness only is called *ocular MG*. It is not considered remission if the asymptomatic MG patient is on cholinesterase inhibitors.

8. **B**

Rationale: Miosis (constricted pupil) is associated with cholinergic crisis (parasympathetic nervous stimulation). Mydriasis is dilated pupil and can be found with sympathetic nervous system stimulation. Bilateral dilated nonreactive pupils indicate an increase in intracranial pressure (ICP). Anisocoria is a condition in which one pupil is larger than the other.

9. **A**

Rationale: Pyridostigmine is an acetylcholinesterase inhibitor. It is not a nonsteroidal immunosuppressant. Mycophenolate mofetil, cyclosporine, and azathioprine are nonsteroidal immunosuppressants commonly used with myasthenia gravis (MG) patients.

10. **D**

Rationale: Intravenous immunoglobulin (IVIG) is contraindicated in patients with renal failure or insufficiency. Acute renal injury is not a common adverse reaction to IVIG but can result in irreversible injury. It is not contraindicated in pregnancy and liver dysfunction. IVIG is actually indicated and primarily used to manage autoimmune disorders.

11. **C**

Rationale: Administering fluids prior to administration of intravenous immunoglobulin (IVIG) may lower the risk of thromboembolic events and acute kidney injury. Acetaminophen and benadryl are used prior to IV contrast to lower the risk of anaphylactic reaction, but it is not routinely recommended when administering IVIG. IV steroids are not required prior to initiation of IVIG treatments.

## 14. ANSWERS AND RATIONALES FOR THE BONUS EXAM QUESTIONS

**12. B**

Rationale: Myasthenia gravis (MG) involves proximal muscle weakness but does not involve the autonomic nervous system (ANS). Lambert–Eaton myasthenic syndrome presents similar to MG but includes ANS symptoms. Lambert–Eaton myasthenic syndrome does include distal muscle weakness, diplopia, and ptosis similar to MG.

**13. B**

Rationale: Guillain–Barré syndrome (GBS) typically presents with bilateral ascending weakness. Miller Fisher syndrome is the variant of GBS and is characterized by abnormal muscle coordination, eyelid weakness, and absence of deep tendon reflexes.

**14. A**

Rationale: Intravenous immunoglobulin (IVIG) treatments can cause hypercoagulable state leading to venous thromboembolic events (VTEs), such as deep venous thrombosis (DVT) and pulmonary embolism (PE). Neutropenia is a potential side effect, not leukocytosis. Anaphylactic reactions can occur with IVIG therapy but is not angioedema specifically. Thrombocytopenia is not a complication of IVIG.

**15. C**

Rationale: Muscle fasciculations of arms, legs, shoulders, and tongue are subtle early signs of amyotrophic lateral sclerosis (ALS) and are commonly missed initially. Other signs include muscle cramping, slurred and nasal speech, and difficulty chewing and swallowing. Muscle tightness (spasticity) is more commonly found early than hypotonia and muscle flaccidity. ALS typically has asymmetrical muscle weakness. Bilateral ascending muscle weakness is more likely Guillain–Barré. Postural drop seizure is not a sign of ALS.

**16. D**

Rationale: Riluzole (Rilutek) prolongs survival by several months by decreasing glutamate levels and reducing damage to the motor neurons. It does not reverse the damage or cause a remission of the disease process. It does not affect the ventilatory muscles specifically.

**17. C**

Rationale: Central nervous system (CNS) lymphoma is a fairly common cause of a brain lesion in a patient with HIV disease. Non-Hodgkin lymphoma is more commonly found in the spinal region in HIV patients spread through the leptomeninges. It is rarely found as a brain lesion. Kaposi sarcoma is the most common systemic tumor in HIV patients but is rarely spread to the CNS. HIV patients are not at a greater risk for glioblastoma.

**18. A**

Rationale: Having the patient raise their eyebrows allows for the assessment of the forehead movement. A stroke patient will still be able to wrinkle the forehead even with facial drooping. Bell's palsy will never spare the forehead. It will be flaccid. Asking the patient to say "ahh" assesses for soft palate and swallow. Assessing nasolabial folds is used to determine facial drop but cannot differentiate between stroke and Bell's palsy.

19. **D**

    Rationale: The most common reason for Bell's palsy is viral infection such as herpes simplex and viral meningitis. The infection causes swelling and inflammation of the facial nerve resulting sudden weakness or paralysis of the face. It is not commonly associated with bacterial infections such as bacterial meningitis and sinus infections. Rabies infection is not associated with Bell's palsy.

20. **C**

    Rationale: Encephalomyelitis is the inflammation of brain and spinal cord tissue, usually a result of viral infection. Encephalitis is the inflammation of brain tissue. It can be a result of bacterial infection but includes both brain and spine. Purulent drainage within the meninges is a result of bacterial meningitis.

21. **D**

    Rationale: Posterior fossa surgeries are commonly associated with cerebrospinal fluid (CSF) leaks, bradycardia, central nervous system (CNS) infections, and apnea. Subdural hemorrhage is not considered a common complication of posterior fossa surgeries.

22. **D**

    Rationale: Optic neuritis is commonly the first sign and demyelinating event of multiple sclerosis (MS). It involves visual losses and eye pain. Ataxia, dysphagia, and facial paresthesia are not common demyelinating events experienced by MS patients.

23. **A**

    Rationale: Tabes dorsalis is one of the manifestations of neurosyphilis. Tabes dorsalis is a slowly progressive degeneration of the posterior columns and posterior nerve roots of the spinal cord. It commonly presents with ataxia and paralysis. All the other signs, inflammation, paranoia, and shooting pains are common manifestation of neurosyphilis but does not describe tabes dorsalis.

24. **A**

    Rationale: The Centers for Disease Control and Prevention classifies neurosyphilis into three patient groups: neuropsychiatric, meningovascular, and myelopathic. These classifications are based upon the predominant presentation of the patient. Inflammatory vascular neurosyphilis is not a classification.

## CHAPTER 6: SEIZURES

1. **D**

    Rationale: Exposure to toxins is not considered a risk factor for development of Lennox–Gastaut. Brain injury during delivery or at an early age and cortical dysplasia are identified risk factors. The disorder has a genetic component with mutations of several genes.

2. **B**

    Rationale: Nonconvulsive status epilepticus (NCSE) may be the cause for unresponsiveness in patients following intracerebral hemorrhage (ICH). An EEG is recommended

## 14. ANSWERS AND RATIONALES FOR THE BONUS EXAM QUESTIONS

to identify NCSE before end-of-life discussions, and brain death testing is performed. Platelet function tests and coagulation studies may be performed but are not used to evaluate a patient's unresponsiveness.

3. C

Rationale: Nonepileptic seizure (NES) may resemble epileptic seizure activity but frequently demonstrate atypical features of epileptic seizures. The diagnosis is made during continuous EEG by observing the seizure activity noting no epileptic seizure activity on EEG. This is commonly a result of conversion syndrome and has been called "pseudoseizures." Tonic–clonic and absence seizures are both forms of generalized seizures with epileptic activity on EEG. Nonconvulsive status epilepticus (NCSE) is epileptic activity on EEG without the clinical signs of seizures.

4. A

Rationale: Generalized seizures and status epilepticus (SE) cause an acute elevation of catecholamines. Fever and cardiac arrhythmias are commonly found with the elevated catecholamines and prolonged seizures. Prolonged muscle activity can cause the breakdown of muscle cells and release of creatine protein kinase (CPK) and potassium. Leukocytosis, not neutropenia, can commonly occur following SE.

5. B

Rationale: When obtaining total phenytoin levels, the results will include both phenytoin bound and unbound to albumin. Only the unbound or free phenytoin is active. The phenytoin bound to albumin does not cross the blood–brain barrier. Some hospitals have the capability to send "free phenytoin drug levels, which are more accurate. If using a total phenytoin level, it must be corrected to the patient's albumin level.

6. D

Rationale: Vagal nerve stimulation (VNS) does not typically result in the patient developing hiccups. When bursts of stimulation are applied, the patient can experience buzzing sensations, hoarseness, and deeper tone of voice.

7. A

Rationale: Generally, seizures begin within the first year of life with Dravet's syndrome. This is a genetic disorder with identified gene mutations. Seizures may be of different classifications and types such as tonic–clonic, absence, myoclonic, and atonic seizures.

8. D

Rationale: Alcohol withdrawal, traumatic brain injury, and neurocysticercosis are commonly associated neurological disease processes that can result in status epilepticus (SE). Hypocalcemia is a known cause of a seizure but is not as well known for SE as other answers.

9. A

Rationale: Loss of corneal reflexes and pupillary light reflexes commonly occur in generalized seizures. Generalized tonic–clonic seizures can be associated with sympathetic discharge. Associated symptoms due to the sympathetic discharge include tachycardia, hypertension, diaphoresis (not anhydrosis), and increased bronchial secretions.

10. C

Rationale: Neuropsychiatric symptoms are known complications of Keppra use. These can range from mild (agitation, hostility, depression) to serious psychiatric reactions (psychosis, hallucinations, and suicidal thoughts). Hair loss is not a known side effect of Keppra. Pancreatitis and liver dysfunction are not commonly experienced side effects of Keppra.

11. B

Rationale: Steven–Johnson's syndrome is a toxic epidermal necrolysis of skin caused by drug complications. Symptoms include fever, blisters, peeling of skin, and necrosis. Several of the anticonvulsants have shown rare complications of Stevens–Johnson's syndrome. Dravet's syndrome is severe myoclonic activity present within the first year of life. Gerstmann syndrome is a neuropsychiatric disorder characterized by a group of symptoms related to the parietal lobe. Tourette's syndrome is a neurodevelopmental disorder characterized by repeated involuntary movements and uncontrollable sounds.

12. A

Rationale: The goal of an epilepsy-monitoring unit is to observe the seizure activity on video and EEG to localize or determine the seizure classification. Anticonvulsants are frequently tapered or discontinued to initiate a seizure. Other techniques used to induce a seizure include photic stimulation, hyperventilation, sleep deprivation, and exercise. Painful stimulation is not a technique used to induce a seizure.

13. D

Rationale: The use of seizure-activating measures (provocation) may cause patients to experience seizures of greater frequency and/or severity than their normal seizure pattern, thus increasing the risk of an adverse event such as status epilepticus. Neurogenic pulmonary edema and aspiration pneumonia are complications of seizures but are not necessarily increased with provoked seizures. Provoking the patient's seizure does not trigger a change in the type of seizure the patient experiences.

14. A

Rationale: Symptoms of postictal psychosis vary from mood disturbance, confusion, visual, auditory, tactile and olfactory hallucinations, and paranoid ideation with or without delirium to more severe and serious disturbances in behavior including, physical aggression and self-harm. It manifests as an episode of psychosis occurring within a week of a seizure or (more commonly) cluster of generalized tonic–clonic seizures. It may occur without prior history of postictal psychosis or any psychiatric history. Postictal psychosis may last from several days to months. It is not a result of the benzodiazepines or periods of hypoxia.

15. C

Rationale: Ambulating in the hallway can be an increased risk for falls if the patient has a seizure. The issue is not slipping but having a seizure while standing or walking

# 14. ANSWERS AND RATIONALES FOR THE BONUS EXAM QUESTIONS

that can result in a fall. Sponge bathing rather than showering can prevent patients in epilepsy-monitoring unit (EMU) from having a seizure while showering and falling. Anytime the patient is up and moving about in the room, he or she should be accompanied by a staff member to prevent the patient from falling if a seizure occurs during that time. Family or an identified person is encouraged to remain with the patient at all times for safety purposes.

16. **C**

    Rationale: Sudden unexpected death in epilepsy (SUDEP) is a complication of seizures and can be a result of the catecholamine response. Patients have died from cardiac arrhythmias and respiratory arrest. Continuous close observation and cardiac monitoring can quickly identify a seizure and any rhythm abnormalities. Supplemental oxygen is not required unless saturations are low. A pulse oximetry is recommended to identify the patient's oxygenation levels continuously. Placing pads around the bed is a safety issue to decrease risk of injury if the patient falls out of bed but is not the best prevention of SUDEP compared to the close observation and monitoring. Utilization of more pillows around the head may actually increase the risk of suffocation during a seizure.

## CHAPTER 7: PEDIATRIC AND DEVELOPMENTAL DISORDERS

1. **B**

    Rationale: There is almost a 50-fold increased risk of having a second child born with spina bifida (SB) in subsequent pregnancies. Genetic counseling is recommended, but genetic testing is not always able to accurately identify the traits. Diets fortified with vitamin B can lower the risk but may not prevent the occurrence completely.

2. **D**

    Rationale: Syringomyelia is the forcing of cerebrospinal fluid (CSF) into the spinal cord, resulting in central cord syndrome. Typically, symptoms are unilateral because the fluid tends to collect on one side of the cord. Central cord syndrome presents with upper-extremity weakness and abnormal sensory. Fusion of C1 to C2 results in neck pain and limited movement. Compression of cranial nerves from the medulla may cause dysarthria and dysphagia. Hydrocephalus results in dizziness, nausea and vomiting, and headache.

3. **A**

    Rationale: Atonia is not a symptom of brainstem dysfunction in infants with Chiari malformation. Brainstem dysfunction in infants present primarily with apnea, nystagmus, and dysphagia.

4. **C**

    Rationale: Spastic cerebral palsy (CP) is due to pyramidal tract lesions in the cortex. This type of CP is characterized by spasticity, hyperreflexia, and clonus activity. Extrapyramidal tract lesions (basal ganglia), also called dyskinetic CP, are characterized by abnormal motor movement. CP is caused by lesions in the brain only, not in the spinal cord.

5. **B**

   Rationale: Patients with cerebral palsy (CP) are commonly classified by the number of extremities involved (monoplegia, diplegia, triplegia, quadriplegia), muscle tone (spasticity, hypotonia, dyskinetic), and the severity of their functional limitations (mild, moderate, severe). CP typically has comorbidities, but their presence is not utilized for classification.

6. **C**

   Rationale: Children are typically sitting at the age of 6 months. Head control usually occurs at 2 months, rolling at 4 months and walking by 1 year of age.

7. **A**

   Rationale: Scissoring walk is the most common gait for a spastic cerebral palsy (CP). This involves the crossing of the feet while walking. Toe walking, toe flicking and ataxic gaits are also found in CP but are not the most common.

8. **D**

   Rationale: The abnormal movement of CP does not increase during sleep. The movement is usually normal or decreased during sleep. Stress, excitement, and purposeful movement can increase the abnormal movements.

9. **C**

   Rationale: Dysesthesia is an unpleasant abnormal sense of touch and is not considered a pseudobulbar symptom. Dysarthria, dysphagia, and dystonia are considered bulbar sigs.

10. **B**

    Rationale: Methadone is an opioid analgesic and is not used to manage abnormal motor movements. Antiparkinson's drugs, such as levodopa/carbidopa, have been used to manage some of the abnormal movements of cerebral palsy (CP). Baclofen is an antispasmodic and used for treating spasticity. Botulinum toxin may be used primarily for lower limb spasticity. Benzodiazepines and anticonvulsants have also been used in managing abnormal motor movements in CP.

11. **A**

    Rationale: An early postoperative complication following closure of myelomeningocele is ventriculomegaly due to the alteration in flow of cerebrospinal fluid (CSF). Cranial ultrasound and measuring head circumference in the neonate postoperatively can be used to recognize ventriculomegaly. Sensory and motor of the lower extremities are assessed but are not as high of priority as head circumference in early postoperative period. Auscultation of heart sounds is a normal assessment routine and not higher priority.

## CHAPTER 8: NEUROLOGICAL TRAUMA: TRAUMATIC BRAIN INJURY

1. **B**

   Rationale: The Functional Independence Measure (FIM) tool is an 18-item assessment scale that is commonly used in rehabilitation to evaluate the patient's degree of

# 14. ANSWERS AND RATIONALES FOR THE BONUS EXAM QUESTIONS

independence for activities of daily living, including transfers. Glasgow Coma Outcome Scale (GCOS) is an evaluation of the patient's neurological outcome, not necessarily to determine the level of independence. Independence outcome score is not a real tool. Hunt and Hess score is used to determine the severity of subarachnoid hemorrhage (SAH).

2. **B**

   Rationale: The pressure waveform is a triple wave pressure reading with each wave labeled P1, P2, and P3. P1 is the highest pulse pressure wave, with P2 and P3 in descending order. When the P2 component is greater than the P1, it indicates that the brain is noncompliant and the intracranial pressure (ICP) is increasing.

3. **C**

   Rationale: C waves are periodic, self-limited elevations of intracranial pressure (ICP) greater than 20 mmHg occurring for less than 5 minutes. This is considered a normal reaction. B waves are periodic and self-limiting but can elevate to higher pressures (up to 50 mmHg) for longer periods of time. A (plateau) wave is associated with poor compliance and prognosis. The ICP is sustained at high pressures for long period of times. There are no D waves.

4. **C**

   Rationale: Propofol infusion syndrome can be life-threatening complication of prolonged use of propofol and includes refractory metabolic acidosis, rhabdomyolysis, and acute renal failure. Serum creatinine kinase (CK) and pH need to be monitored while the patient is on the infusion. Heart failure and coronary vasoconstriction are not common complication of propofol infusion. Propofol's mixture is high in lipids and can lead to elevated lipids and triglycerides but is not considered a lethal complication.

5. **B**

   Rationale: Sympathetic storm can occur after 24 hours following a severe traumatic brain injury (TBI) up to several weeks postinjury. Symptoms include posturing, tachycardia, hypertension, dilated pupils, sweating, and hyperthermia. Uncal herniation would result in unilateral pupil dilation and loss of consciousness. The hypothalamus controls homeostasis but does not produce the symptoms above in the scenario. Subdural hematoma (SDH) can result in unilateral neurological symptoms and signs of uncal herniation.

6. **C**

   Rationale: Stretching is the most widely used technique to prevent contractures in traumatic brain injury (TBI) patients. It is effective if performed regularly. Botulinum toxin injections can be used in patients with spasticity but is not as common or considered first-line treatment. Casting and surgical tendon releases are late techniques and are not as common.

7. **A**

   Rationale: Diffuse axonal injury (DAI) is the shearing of the axons and injuries can result in severe neurological deficits, including persistent vegetative state, especially in the brainstem. Subdural hematoma (SDH) is a common injury with traumatic brain injury (TBI) and causes neurological deficits but does not commonly result in vegetative states. Coup contracoup is a mechanism of injury associated with TBI. It does not commonly result in vegetative states. Frontal contusions in TBI patients frequently result in altered cognition and behavior.

8. **C**

Rationale: Dexmedetomidine (Precedex) is an alpha-2-adrenergic used for sedation and control of agitation. It does not cause respiratory depression and permits intermittent neurological assessment. Propofol is also a good sedative for intermittent neurological assessment because of the short half-life but can cause respiratory depression. Fentanyl is an opioid and is used for pain management as well as sedation. Ativan is a benzodiazepine used for agitation and sedation. Both of these classifications of medications can cause respiratory depression.

9. **C**

Rationale: Only patients demonstrating signs of herniation should be candidates for temporary hyperventilation to a $PaCO_2$ level of 30 to 35 mmHg and is considered a last resort. Presence of cerebral edema or Glasgow Coma Scale (GCS) of less than 9 is not an indication for hyperventilation. Intracranial pressure (ICP) > 20 mmHg is considered elevated, but hyperventilation is not a first-line management of increased ICP.

10. **D**

Rationale: The presence of facial fractures in a trauma patient increases the likelihood of traumatic brain injury (TBI). Soft tissue lacerations, dizziness, and headaches are not commonly signs of severe TBI or indications for routine CT scans. Other indications for CT scan include vomiting, altered mentation, loss of consciousness, intoxication, and signs of basilar skull fractures.

11. **B**

Rationale: Motor vehicle collision (MVC) is the leading mechanism of neurological injury, disability, and death in the pediatric population. Falls are not as common but are found more often in children younger than 10 years of age. Sports injuries with traumatic brain injury (TBI) are also not as common as injury from MVC and occur more often in the preadolescent and adolescent age groups. Penetrating trauma to the head is less common than blunt.

12. **D**

Rationale: Frontal lobe injury is common in patients with traumatic brain injury (TBI). This area of the brain is responsible for the executive functions of the brain. Complications of injury to the frontal lobes include loss of inhibition, attention deficits, short- and long-term memory problems, motor deficits, and emotional lability. Visual changes are not as commonly experienced in TBI patients.

13. **C**

Rationale: Hygromas, hydrocephalus, and infections are well-known complications of craniectomies. A craniectomy is typically performed to manage cerebral edema and

## 14. ANSWERS AND RATIONALES FOR THE BONUS EXAM QUESTIONS

increased intracranial pressure (ICP). Facial droop is not a common complication of craniectomy.

14. **D**

Rationale: The site of the absent bone flap should be lightly palpated for fluctuations in fluid level and distention. Wearing protective head gear when out of bed can protect the open skull area from trauma and is considered a patient safety intervention. Bone flaps can either be replaced or alternative material can be used to build the skull. This commonly occurs after the brain swelling has subsided and the patient is stable for surgery. The absence of the bone flap can cause anxiety for the patient and family, and reassurance may be needed for them regarding the procedure and process for reconstruction of the skull.

15. **B**

Rationale: Restitution reflects the early healing and recovery following TBI and is the reactivation neural pathways. Substitution reflects transmission of neural function from injured to noninjured brain tissue, compensation of the losses. Substitution is thought to occur predominantly after 6 months when new learning is occurring. Reintegration is the initiation of preinjury routines following rehabilitation. Recovery is the result of restitution.

16. **D**

Rationale: Steroids are not used to manage spasticity. They are used as anti-inflammatory agents to manage edema and swelling. Baclophen is an antispasmodic used to manage spasticity. Clonidine, alpha-agonist, and gabepentin, an anticonvulsant medication, are used to manage spasticity following traumatic brain injury (TBI).

17. **C**

Rationale: Traumatic brain injuries with diffuse axonal injury (DAI) commonly experience an acceleration/decelerational rotational injury causing the neuronal axons to shear. The patient usually presents with Glasgow Coma Scale (GCS) of less than 8. CT scans will not demonstrate mass lesions such as hematomas. Diffuse cerebral edema can be present with DAI. MRI is a more sensitive imaging modality than CT for petechial hemorrhages at the gray/white junction.

18. **B**

Rationale: Basilar skull fracture through the anterior fossa presents with otorrhea and raccoon eyes. A fracture through the medial fossa results in rhinorrhea and battle sign (bruising on the mastoid process).
Epidural hematoma (EDH) is complication of depressed skull fractures but not a complication of basilar skull fracture.

## CHAPTER 9: NEUROLOGICAL TRAUMA: SPINAL CORD INJURY

1. **A**

Rationale: Bilateral locked facets will prevent the realignment of the spine with traction and may require immediate surgery to decompress the spinal cord. Intramedullay hematoma is blood within the central portion of the spinal cord and does not require surgery. Subluxation without cord compression can be managed initially with traction to realign the spine. In a complete cord injury, the damage is done, and immediate surgical intervention is not going to improve outcomes.

2. **B**

Rationale: Frequent oral care has been found to decontaminate the mouth of pathogens, decreasing aspiration of bacteria and ventilator-associated pneumonia (VAP). Head of the bed should be elevated, not flat, to prevent aspiration. Endotracheal (ET) tube suctioning is only recommended when needed and should not be performed every 2 hours routinely. Assisted cough is a maneuver used with spinal cord–injured patients who are unable to generate an effective cough. It is not related to preventing VAP.

3. **B**

Rationale: Rapid surgical decompression of the spinal cord can limit injury to the cord. High-dose steroids are no longer recommended following spinal cord trauma. Maintaining perfusion to the spinal cord with permissive hypertension is recommended in most patients but is not used instead of surgical decompression. Therapeutic hypothermia is not a recommended treatment for spinal cord trauma.

4. **C**

Rationale: The hint in this scenario is that the patient has a history of atrial fibrillation (AF) and is more likely being anticoagulated. Hangman's fracture and altantooccipital dislocation with cord involvement will produce quadriplegia, not just lower-extremity (LE) weakness. This scenario is not a high suspicion for an ischemic stroke.

5. **B**

Rationale: Osteoporosis and osteoarthritis can cause loss of bone and impaired joint mobility in the spine. Low mechanisms of injury can result in vertebral fractures, most commonly in the cervical area due to the mobility of these joints. Thoracic vertebrae are least likely to be injured because of the lack of mobility. Spinal stenosis and cauda equina syndrome can cause neurological deficits but are not considered high risk for spinal cord injury with low mechanism of injury.

6. **B**

Rationale: Nipple line correlates to T4 level, not the C6 level. Clavicles do correlate to the level of C4, responsible for innervations to the diaphragm. Umbilicus is at T10 level, and the rectal area correlates to S1 level.

7. **A**

Rationale: The spinal cord terminates at the level of the lumbar 2–3 vertebrae. Below that level, it becomes strands of nerves called conus medullaris.

8. **C**

Rationale: Spinal cord injury without radiographic abnormality (SCIWORA) can be found in pediatric patients following a spine trauma. They commonly present with

## 14. ANSWERS AND RATIONALES FOR THE BONUS EXAM QUESTIONS

symptoms of cord injury (motor abnormalities) but without any radiographic signs of vertebral fractures. This usually results in temporary motor deficits. Central cord syndrome results in greater upper-extremity than lower-extremity weaknesses. Brown-Sequard cord syndrome is a hemisection compression of the cord, commonly a result of herniated disc. Complete cord injury would not result in transient or temporary signs of motor weakness.

# Index

abdominal binders, 169, 221, 243–244
abdominal compartment syndrome (ACS), 150
abscess. *See* brain abscess
ACA. *See* anterior cerebral artery
acceleration injury, 141–142, 223
acetylcholine, 20, 227, 233
   in myasthenia gravis, 86, 244
   in Parkinson's disease, 8, 14
acetylcholinesterase
   agents, 227
   inhibitors, 20, 241, 300
acoustic neuroma, 54, 57, Q*175*, 214, 248
ACS. *See* abdominal compartment syndrome
acupuncture, 18–19, 238
acute kidney injury (AKI), 60, 105, 117, 217, 236, 254, 299, 300
AD. *See* Alzheimer's disease
ADHD. *See* attention deficit hyperactivity disorder
AEDs. *See* antiepileptic drugs
AF. *See* atrial fibrillation
AH. *See* autonomic hyperreflexia
AKI. *See* acute kidney injury
allodyne, 11
allodynia, 131, Q*161*, 246
ALS. *See* amyotrophic lateral sclerosis
alteplase, 40, 41, 42, 44, Q*153*, 214, 228, 245, 291
altered mental status (AMS), 58, 76, 94, 98, 235
Alzheimer's disease (AD), 4, 7–8, 214
   cognitive impairments of, 12
   diagnosis, 16–17
   drugs for, 20
   pathological changes in, 8
   risk factors for, 4
   rummaging and pillaging, 13
   stages (I–IV), 12–13
   symptoms, 12, 13
   word substitution, 12

amnesia
   antegrade, 149
   posttraumatic, 147, 148, 149
   retrograde, 102, 109, 149
AMS. *See* altered mental status
amyloid plaques/amyloid deposits, 8, 17, 73
amyotrophic lateral sclerosis (ALS), Q*15*, Q*16*, Q*199*, 252
   classification, 84
   corticospinal tract degeneration, 89
   diagnosis, 97
   management, 100
   medication for, 99–100
   presentation and symptoms, 88–89, 239
   risk factors for, 89
   signs and symptoms, 93–94, 216, 301
analgesics, 19, 80, 153–154, 251, 306
aneurysm, 32, Q*57*, Q*62*. *See also* subarachnoid hemorrhage
   cerebral, 31, 35, Q*71*, 233, 235, 293
   Charcot–Bouchard, 228, 232, 239
   fusiform, 33, Q*113*, 231, 239
   giant, 231, 232, 239
   intracerebral, 33, 35
   locations, 35
   mycotic, 33, 231, 232
   rupture, 31, 33, 34, 35, 38, 44–45, Q*65*, 228, 232
   saccular/berry, 33, 231
   unsecured, 292–293
angioedema, 44, 214, 234, 301
anterior cerebral artery (ACA), 36, 37, 214, 220, 225, 226, 233, 250
anterior cord syndrome, 165, 220, 235
anticholinergics, 20, 133, Q*158*, 246
anticholinesterase medications, Q*29*, Q*43*, 97, 98–99, 101, 227, 229
anticoagulation therapy, Q*1*, 31, 32, 43, 225, 241, 289, 290

*Note: Numbers that appear in boldface italic denote Practice Exam question numbers and numbers that appear in italic denote Bonus Exam question numbers, the answers and rationales for which appear in Chapter 12 and Chapter 14, respectively.*

anticonvulsants
  for cerebral palsy, 306
  complications with use of, 304
  for neuropathic pain, 18, 98, 252, 290
  for restless leg syndrome, 286
  for seizures, 105, 106, 110, 223, 245, 296, 304
  side effects, Q10
  and spina bifida, 127
antiemetics, 19, 20
antiepileptic drugs (AEDs), 112, 117, 118, 154, 233
  phenytoin, Q5, 113, 242, 244
  side effects of, 115–116, 240
antihistamines, 20, 44
antispasmodics, 100, 133–134
antiplatelet therapy, 31, 157, 289
antithrombotic agents, 31, 247
aphasia, 11, Q14, 37, 64–65, 213, 214, 227, 234, 236
Aquaduct of Sylvius, 5
arachnoid villi, 5, 6, 9, 81, 213, 250
arrhythmias, 118, 224, 303, 305
arteriovenous malformation (AVM), Q28, 31, 33, Q37, 40, 228, 235, 243, 293–294, 295
aspirin, 31, 42, Q169, 225, 228
astrocytes, 50, 52
astrocytoma, Q23, 50, 52, 53, Q159, Q208, 223, 226, 233, 246, 253, 295, 298
atlantoaxial instability, 164
ataxia, 56, 76, 94, 129, 215, 216, 217, 227, 229, 233, 295, 302
atrial fibrillation (AF), Q13, 30, 31, 224, 225, 248, 255, 289, 290, 300, 310
attention deficit hyperactivity disorder (ADHD), Q172, 248
aura, 11, Q19, Q55, 108, 226, 228, 231, 239, 286–287
aural fullness, 12, Q41, 229
automatisms, 109, 114, Q176, 248–249, 253
autonomic hyperreflexia (AH), 169–170, 171, 221, 240, 242–243
autopsy, 8, 16, 17, 73
AVM. See arteriovenous malformation

barbiturate coma, 154
basilar artery, 37, 225, 226, 233, 241, 242, 295
basilar skull fracture, Q17, 144, 146, 147, 154, 155, 156, 225, 308, 309
BBB. See blood–brain barrier
Bell's palsy, Q7, Q18, Q19, 245, 301–302

benign headaches
  abortive management techniques for, 19
  characteristics of, 11
  diagnosis by exclusion, 16
  indications for preventive management, 20
  management, Q210, 254
  populations affected by, 3
  types, 3. See also cluster headaches; migraines
Beta-2 transferrin, 146
bladder dysfunction, 55, 59, 66, 221
blood–brain barrier (BBB), 50, 52, 62, 297
blunt trauma, 141, 166, 221
bone flap, 153, 309
bone spurs. See osteophytes
bradycardia, 168, 171, 221, 225, 234, 243, 246, 302
bradykinesia, 4, 14–15
brain abscess, Q2, Q3, 72, 75, 78, 79, 81, 298–299
brain biopsy, 61, 79, 80, 215, 244
brain pacemaker. See deep brain stimulation
brain tumors, 49–66, Q72. See also individual tumors
  anaplastic, 53
  benign, 53, 54, 65, 231, 246
  brain injury mechanisms, 53
  complications, 64–66
  diagnoses, 59–61, Q86, 235
  genetic syndromes and, 50
  grading of, 51–52, 53, 65
  headache in, Q7, 54, 56, 58, 296–297
  hydrocephalus and, 50, 53, 54, 58, 65
  locations, 49, 51, 52, 54, 56, 58, 65, Q205, 240
  medical management, Q2–4, 61–63
  metastatic/secondary, 49, 52
  pathophysiology, 52–54, Q56
  in pediatric population, Q1, 50, 54
  primary, 49, 52, 215, 240
  prognosis, Q14, Q56
  risk factors for, Q39, Q49, 229
  surgical management, 63–64
  surgical resection, 60, 63, 64–65, Q103, Q116, 234, 238, 239–240
  symptoms/assessment, 54–59
Brown-Sequard syndrome, Q101, 165, 220, 235, 237, 298
Brudzinski's sign, 74, 230, 236
burning pain. See neuropathic pain
burst fractures, Q85, 161–162, 163, 168

carotid endarterectomy (CE), Q53, 231, 237
cauda equina syndrome (CES), 165, 310

*Note: Numbers that appear in boldface italic denote Practice Exam question numbers and numbers that appear in italic denote Bonus Exam question numbers, the answers and rationales for which appear in Chapter 12 and Chapter 14, respectively.*

cavernous malformations, Q25, Q145, 244, 293
CBF. *See* cerebral blood flow
CE. *See* carotid endarterectomy
central cord syndrome, 164–165, 235, 237, 305, 311
central pontine myelinolysis (CPM), 152
central venous thrombosis (CVT), Q118, Q123, Q124, Q127, 240, 241
cerebral angiogram, 40, 214, 244, 245
cerebral blood flow (CBF), 29, 143, 151, 152–153, Q182, 214, 217, 250, 251
cerebral edema, 42, 46, 216, 232, 238, 241, 251, 252, 293, 299
　cytotoxic, 72, 143, 229, 236, 299
　infections and, 65–66, 78, 81, 85
　management, 296, 297, 308–309
　mannitol for, 152, 226, 250
　presentation, 296
　steroids for, 61, Q187, 250, 297
　in traumatic brain injuries, 143, 144, 148, 151, 152, 154
　vasogenic, 72, Q93, 143, 224, 229, 236
cerebral palsy (CP), Q4–10, Q35, Q104, Q161, Q192, 251
　diagnosis, 130–131, 132
　etiology, 126, 238, 242
　maternal infections and risk of, 127, 254
　medications for, 133–134
　motor abnormalities of, 130
　newborn's risk for development of, 126–127
　presentation and effects, Q10, 124, 224
　preventive intervention for, Q213
　sensory abnormalities, 131
　spastic, Q4, Q7, 305
　and strabismus, 135–136
　surgical management for, 134–135
　symptoms, 130–131, 135–136
cerebral perfusion, 43, 85, 151, 228, 292
cerebral perfusion pressure (CPP), 151, Q204, 253
cerebral salt wasting syndrome (CSWS), 46, 224, 237, 249, 292
cerebrospinal fluid (CSF), 9, 23
　in encephalitis, analysis of, 79
　glucose levels in meningitis, 77–78
　in Guillain-Barré, analysis of, 97
　hydrocephalus, imbalance in, 5–6, 15, 17, 53
　leak, Q22, 23, 64, 71, 144, 155, 226, 241, 249, 302
　leptomeningeal tumor spread, 54, 61
　in multiple sclerosis, characteristics of, 96
　in neurocysticercosis, analysis of, 79
　obstruction, 5
　production, 5, 9
　reabsorption, 5, 6, 9
　removal/drainage, Q5, 17, 23, 146
cerebrovascular disorders, 29–46
　complications, 44–46
　diagnoses, 38–40
　medical management, 40–43
　pathophysiology, 33–36
　surgical management, 43–44
　symptoms/assessment, 36–38
CES. *See* cauda equina syndrome
chemotherapy, 2, 59, 62, 240, 243, 244, 246, 252, 296, 297
Chiari malformations
　classification, Q26, 123, Q211
　diagnosis, 132
　headaches in, 128–129
　hydrocephalus in, Q60, 131–132, 135, 218
　location, 123
　spine deformities in, 129
　surgical management for, 134, 135
　symptoms, 128–130, 131
　type I, 123, 125, 128, 129
　type II, Q2, 123, 125, 128, 129, 136, 227, 243
　type III, 123, 125–126
　type IV, 123, 126, 254
chronic inflammatory demyelinating polyneuropathy (CIDP), Q14, 88, 102
chronic traumatic encephalopathy (CTE), 143, 157
CIDP. *See* chronic inflammatory demyelinating polyneuropathy
Circle of Willis, 34, 35
CJD. *See* Creutzfeldt–Jakob disease
cluster headaches
　populations affected by, 3
　symptoms, 11, Q219, 255
CN. *See* cranial nerves
complex regional pain syndrome (CRPS), 10
concussion, Q25, 147, 157, 162, 221, 227
contrecoup injury, 142, 223
contusion, 144–145, 148, 149, 161, 245, 250, 255, 308
corpus callosotomy, 116–117
coup–contrecoup injury, 142
coup injury, Q3, 142, 223
CP. *See* cerebral palsy
CPM. *See* central pontine myelinolysis
CPP. *See* cerebral perfusion pressure
cranial nerves (CN), 214, 224, 247, 254
　in acoustic neuroma, 54, 57, Q175
　in amyotrophic lateral sclerosis, 93
　in basilar skull fractures, 156
　in brainstem lesions, 55
　in Chiari malformations, 129

cranial nerves (*cont.*)
  in epidural hematoma, 149
  in Guillain–Barré, 93
  in meningitis, 74, Q75
  in multiple sclerosis, 90
craniectomy, Q13, Q14, 134, 153, **Q156**, 218, 245–246, 308–309
craniopharyngioma, 54, 57, 298
craniotomy, 81, 153
  awake, 63
  decompressive, 154, 241, 245
Creutzfeldt–Jakob disease (CJD), *Q138*
  diagnosis, 80
  neuronal tissue loss, 73
  occurrence, 70
  symptoms, 76–77
  transmission, 73, 254
  variant, 70, 73, 77
CRPS. *See* complex regional pain syndrome
CSF. *See* cerebrospinal fluid
CSWS. *See* cerebral salt wasting syndrome
CTE. *See* chronic traumatic encephalopathy
Cushing's triad, 148, 249
CVT. *See* central venous thrombosis

DAI. *See* diffuse axonal injury
DBS. *See* deep brain stimulation
deceleration injury, 141–142, 223
deep brain stimulation (DBS), 22, 23, Q24, 213, 288
deep tendon reflexes (DTRs), 240, 248, 301
degenerative spine disorders, 6
dementia, 14, 16, 143
  cortical, 4, 157. *See also* Alzheimer's disease
  encephalopathy and, 84, 94
  Lewy body, 287
  risks of, 4
  subcortical, 4, Q15, 213. *See also* Parkinson's disease
  test for, Q26, 288–289
depressed skull fracture, 144, 255
  complications, 156, 310
  surgical debridement post, 150
DHE. *See* dihydroergotamine mesylate
DI. *See* diabetes insipidus
diabetes insipidus (DI), 56, 66, **Q164**, 247
diffuse axonal injury (DAI), 142, 144, 149, *Q281*, 307–308, 309
dihydroergotamine mesylate (DHE), 19
direct injury, 142

disc(s)
  herniation, 9, **Q58**, 161, 165, 227, 231
  protrusion/propulsion, 6, 9, **Q58**, 231
distraction injury, 162
dopamine
  agents, 20–21. *See also* levodopa
  agonists, 21, 63
  in Parkinson's disease, 8, 14, 17
dorsal horn, 7
DTRs. *See* deep tendon reflexes

ecchymosis, 146
EDH. *See* epidural hematoma
EEG. *See* electroencephalogram
Ehlers–Danlos disease, **Q142**, 232, 243, 245
electroencephalogram (EEG), 79, 80, 110, 112, 154, 217, 223, 224, 226, 239, 245, 246, 287, 302–303, 304
electromyogram (EMG), 96–97, 226, 285
embolic stroke, 252, 289, 294
  cardioembolic, 30, 31
  causes, **Q6**, 30, 224
  occurrence, 30
  presentation, 30, 34, 223
  prevention, Q13, 31, 225
  timing, 30
embolization, 63, 224, 293
EMG. *See* electromyogram
EMU. *See* epilepsy monitoring unit
encephalitis, 6, 238
  diagnosis, 79
  etiology, 69–70
  herpes simplex/HSE, 70, 80–81
  medications for, 80–81
  symptoms, 76, 216
  viral, 70, 76, 80–81, 239
encephalomyelitis, *Q20*, 302
encephalopathy, **Q108**, 238
  bovine spongiform/BSE, 70
  causes, 85
  classification/grading, 95–96
  complications, 102
  cysticercosis, 81
  definition, 84–85
  diagnosis, 97–98
  etiology, 90
  hepatic/HE, 95–96, 98, 100, 238
  hypertensive/reversible, 85, 97–98
  ischemic–hypoxic, 89
  management, 100

---

*Note: Numbers that appear in boldface italic denote Practice Exam question numbers and numbers that appear in italic denote Bonus Exam question numbers, the answers and rationales for which appear in Chapter 12 and Chapter 14, respectively.*

posterior reversible encephalopathy
  syndrome (PRES), 85
 symptoms, 94–95
 transmissible spongiform (TSE), 70
 Wernicke's, 85, 94–95, 100, 102, 216
ependymoma, 50, 52, 53, 65, 233
epidural hematoma (EDH), 145, 149–150, 165,
  220, 226, 227, 232, 249, 250, 309
epilepsy, Q4, 76, 105, 106, 115. See also
  seizure/seizures
 childhood, 110
 complications, 115, 117–119
 diagnostic studies for, 112
 nursing admission assessment, 111
 pacemaker-like devices for, 117
 sleep deprivation and, 107
 sudden death in patients, 115,
  117–118, 305
 surgical procedure for, 116
epilepsy monitoring unit (EMU), Q12, Q13,
  Q15, 107, 112, 304, 305
extrapyramidal tracts, 8, 306

facetectomy, 23
facial pain, 2, 16, 22
FFP. See fresh frozen plasma
FIM. See Functional Independence Measure
flaccidity, 94, 130, 224, 301
fMRI. See functional magnetic resonance
  imaging
forced vital capacity (FVC), 99, 168–169, 221
fresh frozen plasma (FFP), 43, 157
Functional Independence Measure (FIM), 167,
  225, 306–307
functional magnetic resonance imaging (fMRI),
  60, 63, 64, 217
FVC. See forced vital capacity

GABA. See gamma-aminobutyric acid
gabapentin, 18, 233, 252
gamma-aminobutyric acid (GABA), 106,
  233, 242
GB. See Guillain–Barré
GBM. See glioblastoma multiform
GCS. See Glasgow Coma Scale
generalized seizure, 107–110, 226, 234,
  239, 246, 303, 304
 absence, 109
 atonic (drop), 109, 236
 febrile, 110
 nursing assessment and observation, 114
 nursing care post, 114–115
 surgical procedure for, 116–117
 types, 110

Glasgow Coma Scale (GCS), 34, 147, 148, 151,
  219, 252, 292, 308, 309
glioblastoma multiform (GBM), Q5, 53, Q139,
  Q196, 218, 230, 296
gliomas, 50–53, 62, 233, 244, 295–296, 298
glutamate, 106, 301
Guillain–Barré (GB), Q48, 228, 243, 287, 298
 chronic form of, 88, 102
 diagnosis, 97
 multiple sclerosis, comparison with, 87–88
 paralysis in, 91–92, 230
 peripheral nerves involved in, 87–88
 presentation, Q17, Q20, 87, 239, 301
 symptoms, 91–93
 triggers for, 88, Q100, 237

hallucinations, 21, 77, 94, 108, 115, 226, 253, 304
halo test, 146, 223–224, 243–244
Hangman's fracture, 163, 310
HD. See Huntington's disease
head of the bed (HOB), 155, 219, 226, 234, 242
headaches. See also benign headaches; cluster
  headaches; migraines
 in brain tumors, Q7, 54, 56, 58, 296–297
 in cerebrovascular disorders, 32, 35, 36, 38
 in Chiari malformations, 128–129
 in encephalitis, 216
 in hydrocephalus, 15, 58
 in meningitis, 74
 posttraumatic, 157
 in subarachnoid hemorrhage, 229, 234
hemangioblastoma, Q18, Q19, 298
hemorrhagic stroke, 230–231
 classification, 31. See also intracerebral
  hemorrhage; subarachnoid hemorrhage
 occurrence, 29
 risk factors for, 30, 32. See also hypertension
heparin, Q166, 225, 247, 290
herniation
 cerebellar, 123, 125, 218, 249
 in Chiari malformations, 125, 129, 133, 134
 disc, 9, Q58, 161, 165, 227, 231
 syndrome, 35, 78
 tonsillar, 125, 218
 uncal, 149
hippocampus, 7, 8
HOB. See head of the bed
Horner's syndrome, 37, 229, 242, 295
Hunt and Hess score, 36, 220, 235, 292, 295,
  300, 307
Huntington's disease (HD), Q1–5, Q28,
  285–286, 289
hydrocephalus, 5–6, 131–132, 135, 308
 acute, 15

hydrocephalus (*cont.*)
  assessment in children, 15
  brain tumors and, 50, 53, 54, 58, 65
  in Chiari malformations, **Q60**, 131–132, 135, 218
  communicating, 6, 213, 232
  CSF imbalance in, 5–6, 15, 17, 53
  decompensated congenital, 15
  diagnosis, 17
  etiology, 6
  in hemorrhagic strokes, 40, 46
  in infections, 72, 76, 81
  noncommunicating/obstructive, 5, 50, 53, 65, 125, 213, 232, 255
  normal pressure/NPH, 15, 17, **Q110**, **Q119**, **Q188**, **Q203**, 213, 229, 239, 250
  surgical management, 23, **Q203**
  symptoms, 15
  ventriculoperitoneal shunt for, 135, 238, 240, 253
hydromyelia, 124, 135
hyperalgesia, 10–11, 131
hyperglycemia, 42, 61, 77, 105, 153, 219, 228, 246, 252, 297
hyperextension, 161, 164, 168, 235
hyperflexion, 161, **Q81**, 234–235
hypernatremia, 66, 100, 152
hypertension, 232, 239, 304, 307, 310
  autonomic hyperreflexia and, 170, 171, 221, 242–243
  DASH diet for prevention of, *Q32*, 294
  and encephalopathy, 85, 97–98, 216
  in spinal cord injury, 169–170, 171, 222, 240
  as stroke risk factor, 30, 32, 34, 246, 253
  in traumatic brain injury, 224
  in vasospasm treatment, 45, 236, 292–293
hyperventilation, **Q63**, 112, 219, 250
hyponatremia, 46, 105, 153, 223, 224, 228, 237, 249, 292
hypotension, 41, **Q91**, 116, 168, 171, 219
  orthostatic, 24, **Q144**, 169, 221, 243
  postural, 92, 169
  in traumatic brain injuries, 145, 150–151, 153–154, 228, 249
hypovolemia, 152, 225, 249
hypoxia, 89, 126, 143, 145, 150–151, 154, 161, 219, 228, 299, 304

ICH. *See* intracerebral hemorrhage
ICP. *See* intracranial pressure

indirect injury, 142
infections, 69–102. *See also individual infections*
  complications, 81–82, 101–102
  diagnoses, 77–80, 96–98
  medical management, 80–81, 98–100
  pathophysiology, 71–73, 86–90
  signs and symptoms, 90–96
  surgical management, 81, 100
  symptoms/assessment, 74–77
INR. *See* international normalized ratio
international normalized ratio (INR), 40, 41, 43, 44, 247, 248, 291
intracerebral hemorrhage (ICH), 31–33, **Q52**, 228
  causes, 32–33, **Q34**, 232
  clinical presentation, 38
  lobar, **Q40**, 229
  pathophysiology, 34–35
  sites, 32
  management/treatment, 42–43
  medications for, 43
intracranial pressure (ICP), Q2–4, 218, 226, 232, 234, 236
  in brain tumors, 58–59
  increased, 54, 58, 148, **Q173**, 247, 248, 293, 296, 308
  indicator of, 148
  lowering of, **Q76**, 155
  in meningitis, 72, 78
  potential treatments for increased, 154
  in subarachnoid hemorrhage, 46
  in traumatic brain injuries, 143, 150–155, **Q165**, 219, 247
intravenous immunoglobulin (IVIG), 99, 300
intraventricular extension, 40
intraventricular hemorrhage (IVH), 35, 40, 228
ischemic injury/ischemia, 1, 29, 45, 126, 162, 163, 224, 231, 236, 292, 293, 294
ischemic stroke, **Q157**
  hemorrhagic transformation in, 34
  injury zones, **Q11**, 33–34, 38
  medications for, 42, **Q169**
  noncontrast CT for diagnosis, 38
  nursing care for patients, **Q160**, **Q163**, 246–247
  occurrence, 29
  risk factors for, 30, 32. *See also* hypertension
  sleep apnea in, **Q78**, 234, 286
  treatment, 33, 40–41, **Q78**
IVH. *See* intraventricular hemorrhage
IVIG. *See* intravenous immunoglobulin

---

*Note: Numbers that appear in boldface italic denote Practice Exam question numbers and numbers that appear in italic denote Bonus Exam question numbers, the answers and rationales for which appear in Chapter 12 and Chapter 14, respectively.*

Kernig's sign, 74, 230, 236
Korsakoff's syndrome, 85, 102

lactulose, 100
laminectomy, 23, 134
large vessel obstruction (LVO), 43–44, 291, 295
last known normal (LKN), 39, 41, 44
Lennox–Gastaut syndrome, Q*1*, 110, Q*193*, 216, 251, Q*275*, 302
leptomeningeal tumors, 54, 58, 61, 62, Q*143*, 243, 244
levodopa, 20–21, 213, 306
Lewy bodies, 17, 287
Lhermitte's sign, 90, Q*120*, 240
LKN. *See* last known normal
LMNs. *See* lower motor neurons
lobectomy, temporal, 116
LOC. *See* loss of consciousness
locked-in syndrome, Q*24*, 37, 224, 225, 226, 242, 252, 295
loss of consciousness (LOC), 38, 42, 45, 54, 109, 148, 149, 227, 229
Lou Gehrig's disease. *See* amyotrophic lateral sclerosis
lower motor neurons (LMNs), 83, 87, 165, 248
LP. *See* lumbar puncture
lumbar puncture (LP), Q*8*, 17, 78, Q*90*, 97, 236, 240, 285, 297, 299
LVO. *See* large vessel obstruction

magnetic resonance angiography (MRA), 166, 235
mannitol, Q*69*, 143, 152, Q*178*, 226, 236, 247, 248, 249, 250, 296
MAP. *See* mean arterial pressure
maternal serum alpha-fetoprotein (MSAFP), 133, 239, 241
MBI. *See* Modified Barthel Index
MCA. *See* middle cerebral artery
mean arterial pressure (MAP), 151, 168, 221, 253
medulloblastoma, 58, 215, 223, 297
memory
  long-term, 7, 13, 309
  loss, 12, 13, 20, 37, 55, 100, 102, 149, 227. *See also* amnesia
  short-term, 7, 13, 91, 148, 309
  types, 8
Ménière's disease
  endolymphatic hydrops, 7
  occurrence, 3
  microsurgical intervention for, 23
  symptoms, 7, 12, Q*41*, Q*146*, 244. *See also* vertigo
  treatment, 20, 246

meningioma, 51, 65, 239
meningitis, 6, Q*51*, 156
  antibiotic therapy for, 80
  bacterial, 69, 71, 74, 77–78, 80, 81, Q*96*, Q*220*, 237
  in children, 74, 80
  complications, 81
  diagnosis, 77–78
  effect on cranial nerves, 74
  in infants, 75
  meningococcal, 71, 75, 232
  pathophysiology, 71–72
  routes of entry, 71
  signs and symptoms, 71, 74–75
  steroids for treatment, 74, 80
  vaccine for, Q*66*
  viral, 69, 72, 77–78, 80, 237, 302
meningocele, 125, 136–137, 233, 243
MG. *See* myasthenia gravis
microglial cells, 51, 52
microvascular decompression (MVD), 22–23
middle cerebral artery (MCA), 34, 36, 43, 214, 220, 225, 233, 252, 295
migraines, 213, 231, 286–287
  characteristics of, 11
  medications for, 19–20
  populations affected by, 3
  symptoms, 11
Modified Barthel Index (MBI), 167
Moyamoya disease, Q*37*, 228, 245, 293
MRA. *See* magnetic resonance angiography
MS. *See* multiple sclerosis
MSAFP. *See* maternal serum alpha-fetoprotein
multiple sclerosis (MS), Q*1–6*, Q*114*, 232, 241. *See also* trigeminal neuralgia
  clinical presentations, 2, 83, 288
  demyelination of nerve fibers, Q*22*, 86, 302
  diagnosis, Q*22*, 96, 288, 299
  Guillain–Barré, comparison with, 87–88
  management, Q*128*
  medications for, 98
  remissions and relapses, 83, 239
  risk factors for, Q*20*, 288, 299–300
  symptoms, 90–91
  types, 84
  viral infections as trigger for, 84
muscle tone
  in cerebral palsy (CP) patients, 306
  increase of, 8, 14
  inhibition of, 8. *See also* Parkinson's disease
  loss of, 109, 248
  low, 129, 130
MVD. *See* microvascular decompression

myasthenia gravis (MG), Q*7–12*, 301
    associated autoimmune disorders, 84, Q*141*, 243
    cholinergic crisis, 101, 216, 300
    cholinergic drug testing for, Q*29*, Q*43*, 97
    complications, 101
    diagnosis, 96–97
    diurnal pattern of strength in patients, 87
    factors that worsen, 87
    medications for, 98–99
    myasthenia crisis, 101, 215
    pathophysiology, 86
    presentation, Q*149*, 239, 244
    refractory, 215–216
    signs, ocular, 91, 300
    surgical management, 100
myelogram/myelography, 17–18, 215, 230
myelomeningocele, 124–125, 218, 233, 235, 243, 306
    complications, 136–137
    in neonates, 131–132, 218
    nursing care for neonates, 134
    surgical management, Q*11*, 135
myelopathy, 6, 225

nasogastric tube (NG), 154, 225, 291
National Institutes of Health Stroke Scale (NIHSS), 39–40, Q*186*, 220, 227, 228, 250, 291
NCSE. *See* nonconvulsive status epilepticus
negative inspiratory force (NIF), 168–169, 221
neurocysticercosis, 72–73, 237, 303
    cause, 69, 255
    complications, 81–82
    cysticidal medications for, 80
    diagnosis, 78–79
    occurrence, 69
    seizures in, 76
    symptoms, 76
neurofibromatosis, 50, 214, 230, 245, 253, 298
neurogenic claudication, 15–16
neurogenic shock, 168, 171, 221, 225, 242
neuroleptic agents, 5, Q*79*, 234
neurological deterioration, 34, 38, 148
neurological trauma, chronic, 1–25
    assessment/symptoms, 10–16
    complications, 23–25
    diagnoses, 16–18
    medical management, 18–21
    pathophysiology, 7–9
    surgical management, 21–23
neuroma, 52–53. *See also* acoustic neuroma
neuropathic pain, 1, 10, 59, 90, 232
    causes, 2, 7
    deafferentation of, 7
    depression and anxiety in, 23–24
    management, 18–19, 21–22, Q*73*, 98, Q*198*, 233, 252, 290
neuroplasticity, 158, 294
neurosyphilis, Q*23*, Q*24*, 299, 302
NG. *See* nasogastric tube
NIF. *See* negative inspiratory force
NIHSS. *See* National Institutes of Health Stroke Scale
nimodipine, 45, 214
noncontrast CT, 31, 38, 42, 148, 214, 244, 292, 296
nonconvulsive status epilepticus (NCSE), 110, 217, 302–303
nonsteroid anti-inflammatory drugs (NSAIDs), 18, 98, 233
NSAIDs. *See* nonsteroid anti-inflammatory drugs

odontoid fracture, 163, 164, 166, 168
OGT. *See* orogastric tube
oligodendroglioma, 50, 233
oligodendrocytes, 50, 52, 86
opioids, 21, 22, 233, 252, 286
orogastric tube (OGT), 154–155, 251–252
osmotic diuretics, 152, 219–220, 233, 236. *See also* mannitol
osteoarthritis, 6, 164, 225, 310
osteophytes, 6, 9, Q*28*, 227

Parkinson's disease (PD), 4–5, Q*14*, Q*15*, 213–214, 233, 235, 288–289
    acetylcholine and, 8, 14
    autonomic dysfunction, 24
    causes, 5
    diagnosis, 17
    dopamine and, 8, 14, 24
    drugs for, 20–21, 24
    dyskinesias, 20–21
    parkinsonism, 4, 5, 21
    postural instability, 24
    retropulsion, 24
    symptoms, 8, 14–15, 24. *See also* bradykinesia; rigidity; tremors
PCA. *See* posterior cerebral artery
PCC. *See* prothrombin complex concentrate

---

*Note: Numbers that appear in boldface italic denote Practice Exam question numbers and numbers that appear in italic denote Bonus Exam question numbers, the answers and rationales for which appear in Chapter 12 and Chapter 14, respectively.*

PD. *See* Parkinson's disease
pediatric and developmental disorders, 123–137. *See also individual disorders*
  complications, 135–137
  diagnoses, 132–133
  medical management, 133–134
  pathophysiology, 125–128
  surgical management, 134–135
  symptoms/assessment, 128–132
penetrating injury, 142, 165, 221
penumbra, Q*11*, 33–34, 224
perforating injury, 142
peripheral neuropathy pain. *See* polyneuropathy
periventricular leukomalacia (PVL), 127, 132
PET. *See* positive emission tomography
phantom limb pain/phantom leg pain, 10
pig tapeworm, 69, 72, 80, Q*102*, 237–238
pineal tumors, Q*217*, 255, 297, 298
pituitary adenoma, 56–57, Q*80*, 233, 244, 297
  laboratory tests for, 60–61
  prolactinoma, 63, 234
  secreting, 57
  signs of, 56, Q*194*, 251
  surgical management, 63–64
  transphenoidal approach for resection, 63–64, 66, Q*180*, 249
pituitary tumor. *See* pituitary adenoma
plasmapheresis, Q*36*, 99, 228
poikilothermia, 170, 246
polyneuropathy, 1, 2, 87
positive emission tomography (PET), 17, 60, 112, 214, 215, 243, 296
posterior cerebral artery (PCA), 214, 225, 295
posterior reversible encephalopathy syndrome (PRES), 85, 216
postictal psychosis, Q*14*, 115, 304
PRES. *See* posterior reversible encephalopathy syndrome
prion diseases, 70, 73, Q*88*, 236, 243
proprioception, 165, 167, 220, 235
prothrombin complex concentrate (PCC), 43, 157
pseudotumor cerebri, Q*129*, 239, 241, 294
PVL. *See* periventricular leukomalacia

radiation therapy, Q*16*, Q*20*, 49, 62, Q*134*, 242, 297, 298
radiculalagia, 1
radiculopathy, 6, Q*15*, 16, 59, 76, 82, 225
Ranchos Los Amigos, 150, 220
rebleed, 43, 44–45, 230–231, 292
repetitive injuries, 143, 155, 157. *See also* chronic traumatic encephalopathy

residual limb pain. *See* phantom limb pain/phantom leg pain
restless leg syndrome (RLS), Q*6–9*, 286
rhabdomyolysis, 105, 117, 118, 217, 249, 307
rhinorrhea, 11, 64, 144, 146, 155, 309
rigidity
  cogwheel, 4, 14, 15
  "lead pipe," 14
  nuchal, 36, 71, 74, 75, 77, 296
RLS. *See* restless leg syndrome
rotational injury, 142, 162, 309

SAH. *See* subarachnoid hemorrhage
SB. *See* spina bifida
SBS. *See* shaken baby syndrome
schwannoma, 50, 53, 214
SCI. *See* spinal cord injury
SCIWORA. *See* spinal cord injury without radiographic abnormality
scoliosis, 129, 130, 135, 136
SDH. *See* subdural hematoma
SDR. *See* selective dorsal rhizotomy
SE. *See* status epilepticus
secondary injuries, 228, 230
  brain, Q*32*, 143, 145–146, 150, 153, 154
  spinal cord, 162–163
seizure/seizures, 105–119, 304–305
  anticonvulsants for management, 105, 106, 110, 223, 245, 296, 304
  autonomic, Q*206*, 236, 253
  benzodiazepines in stopping, Q*131*, 242
  brain damage during, 105
  in brain tumors, 65, 240
  causes, 107
  in children, Q*193*
  classification, Q*77*, 108, 218
  complex partial, 108, 109, 226, 234, 253
  complications, Q*109*, 115, 117–119
  diagnoses, 111–113
  epileptic, 105. *See also* epilepsy
  generalized. *See* generalized seizure
  idiopathic, 106
  Jacksonian march, 108
  medical management, 113–116
  medications for, 116
  in neurocysticercosis, 76
  neurotransmitters to inhibit, Q*67*
  nonepileptic/psychogenic, 110, 223, 234, 303
  nursing assessment during, Q*50*, 111, 114
  nursing care during, 113–114
  pathophysiology, 106–107
  precautions, 113
  prophylaxis post traumatic brain injury, 154
  refractory, 223, 242

seizure/seizures (cont.)
  signs of impending, Q*31*, 227–228
  simple partial, 108, 111, 226, 234, 236, 239, 253
  somatosensory, 108
  stages, 111
  surgical management, 116–117
  symptoms/assessment, Q*31*, 107–111
  thresholds, 107
  tonic–clonic, Q*9*, Q*42*, 115, 117, Q*147*, 250, 303–304
selective dorsal rhizotomy (SDR), 134–135
shaken baby syndrome (SBS), 144
shooting pain. See neuropathic pain
SIADH. See syndrome of inappropriate antidiuretic hormone
spasticity, 130, 133, 135, 224, 240, 248, 287, 290, 301, 306, 308, 309
spina bifida (SB), 126. See also meningocele; myelomeningocele
  causes, 124, 127, 245
  complications, Q*82*, 136
  diagnosis, Q*111*, Q*125*, 132–133, 239
  forms of, Q*70*, 124–125
  occulta, 124, 125, 131, 233, 243
  prevention, Q*154*, 245
  risks for development of, Q*1*, Q*97*, 127–128, 237
  symptoms, 131
spinal cord injury (SCI), Q*1–8*, Q*47*, 161–172, 310–311. See also individual injuries
  assessment/diagnoses, Q*30*, 165–167, 227
  classification/grading, 220
  complete, 164
  complications, Q*106*, Q*137*, 170–171
  incomplete, 164, 167
  mechanisms of injury, Q*21*, 161–163, 226
  medical/surgical management, Q*133*, 167–168
  nursing interventions, 168–170
  rehabilitation, 171–172, 230
  traumatic injuries, Q*87*, 163–165
spinal cord injury without radiographic abnormality (SCIWORA), Q*8*, 310–311
spinal shock, Q*121*, 170–171, 222, 240, 242, 243
spinal tumors, Q*13–15*, 298
  complications, 66
  diagnosis, 215
  location, 52, 297
  signs and symptoms, 59
  surgical resection of, 64

spondylosis, 6, 225
statins, 31, 42, Q*177*, 237, 241, 249
status epilepticus (SE), 105, 111, 116, 217, 303
stenosis, 6–7, 15–16
  central, 6, 7, 23, 225
  cervical, 16
  foraminal, 7, 227
  lateral recess, 7, 18
  spinal, 15, 23, 310
steroids, 241, 250, 301, 309, 310
  for angioedema, 44
  for cerebral edema, 61–62, 296
  corticosteroids, 98, 216, 236
  for meningitis, 74, 80
  for traumatic brain injury, Q*191*, 251
stroke, Q*6–11*, Q*16*, Q*22–24*, 29–31, 301
  assessment, Q*3*, Q*18*, 39–40. See also National Institutes of Health Stroke Scale
  cause, Q*22*, Q*130*
  definition, Q*218*, 255
  education for patients, Q*181*, 249–250, 251
  embolic. See embolic stroke
  FAST recognition, Q*185*, Q*197*, 250, 252
  hemorrhagic. See hemorrhagic stroke
  ischemic. See ischemic stroke
  large vessel obstruction (LVO), Q*12*, 39, 43, 44, 291, 295
  left hemispheric, 34
  mimics, 39, 40
  neuroplasticity after, 294
  occurrence, 29
  patent foramen ovale and, Q*2*, 30, 289
  posterior, 40, 250, 252, 295
  prevention, 31
  rehabilitation, Q*31*
  risk factors for, Q*11*, 30, 32, Q*202*
  syndromes, 36–37
  thrombotic. See thrombotic stroke
  treatment/management, Q*2*, 40–42, 291
  types, Q*2*, 29
  in women, 36
stump pain. See phantom limb pain/phantom leg pain
subarachnoid hemorrhage (SAH), 6, Q*92*, Q*94*, 223, 250
  causes, 31–32, 35, 145. See also aneurysm
  complications, 44–46, Q*90*, Q*107*, 238
  diagnosis, 40, Q*83*
  grades, 235
  intervention, Q*19*

---

Note: Numbers that appear in boldface italic denote Practice Exam question numbers and numbers that appear in italic denote Bonus Exam question numbers, the answers and rationales for which appear in Chapter 12 and Chapter 14, respectively.

presentation, Q74, 229, 234, 235
severity, 36
subarachnoid precautions, 45
symptoms, 38, 234
subdural hematoma (SDH), Q54, 143, 144, 145, 149, 219, 231, 232, 250, 293, 294, 307–308
subluxation, 161, 163, 164, 168, 229, 290
sudden unexplained death epilepsy patients (SUDEP), Q16, 115, 117–118, 305
SUDEP. *See* sudden unexplained death epilepsy patients
sympathectomy, 21
syndrome of inappropriate antidiuretic hormone (SIADH), 46, 56, 237, 249, 292
syringomyelia, 124, 128, 135, 305
syrinx, 132, 135, 233

*Taenia solium*. *See* pig tapeworm
TBI. *See* traumatic brain injury
TCD. *See* transcranial Doppler
tethered cord syndrome, 136–137
thalamic pain syndrome, 1
thiamine (vitamin B1), 85, 100
thrombectomy, 39, 43–44, 290, 291
thrombolytic therapy/thrombolytics, Q33, 39, 40, 41, 42, 43, 227, 253, 291
thrombotic stroke
  occurrence, 29
  presentation, 30, 223
  prevention, 31
  timing, 30
thymectomy, 100, 216, 243
TIAs. *See* transient ischemic attacks
tic douloureux. *See* trigeminal neuralgia
TN. *See* trigeminal neuralgia
Todd's paralysis, 111, 238–239
tonsils, 123, 125, 128, 132, 227. *See also* Chiari malformations
Tourette's syndrome (TS), Q79, 248, 289, 304
transcranial Doppler (TCD), 45, 214, 244
transient ischemic attacks (TIAs), 29, 34, Q99, 214, 223, 227, 237
transmissible spongiform encephalopathy (TSE), 70
traumatic brain injury (TBI), Q4–6, Q8–12, 141–158, 219, 307–310. *See also individual injuries*
  anoxic, Q44
  assessment/diagnoses, Q5, Q9, 146–150
  in children, 143–144
  classifications based on GCS, 147
  complications, 156–158, 307
  cranial nerve injuries in, Q214
  gunshot injuries/wounds, 142, 162, 220

hypotension in, 145, 150–151, 153–154, 228, 249
intracranial pressure in, 143, 150–155, Q165, 247
mechanisms of injury, Q12, 141–144
medical/surgical intervention, 150–154
mild/MTBI, 143, 147, 155, 157–158
by motor vehicle collision (MVC), 141, 143, Q136, 308
noncontrast CT scan indications of, 148
nursing interventions, Q17, 154–156, Q190
rehabilitation, 158
steroids for, Q191
traumatic injuries, 144–146
tremors, 56, Q68, 233, 234
  benign essential/BET, Q14, Q84, Q95, 235, 236–237, 287
  dystonic, Q13, 287
  head, 237
  in Parkinson's disease, 4, 14
  "pill rolling," 14
  resting, Q12, 287, 288, 289
  "wing-beating," 289
tricyclic antidepressants, 18, 19, 98, 233, 252
trigeminal neuralgia (TN), 19, Q132, 242, 247. *See also* multiple sclerosis
  autoimmune disorders and, Q61
  etiology, 2
  location of pain, 11
  pain history for diagnosis, 16
  pain syndrome in, Q64, 232, 245
  posterior fossa surgery for, Q21, 302
  treatment, Q105, 238
triptans, 19, 157
TS. *See* Tourette's syndrome
TSE. *See* transmissible spongiform encephalopathy
tumors. *See* brain tumors; spinal tumors

UMNs. *See* upper motor neurons
upper motor neurons (UMNs), 83, 88–89, Q170, 248

vagal nerve stimulator (VNS), Q6, 117, 217, 303
VAP. *See* ventilator-associated pneumonia
vasospasms (VSs), Q17, Q18, Q20, Q21, 45, 145, 214, 223, 236, 238, 244, 292, 295
venous thromboembolism (VTE), 221, 241, 290, 301
ventilator-associated pneumonia (VAP), Q2, Q195, 251–252, 310
ventriculoperitoneal (VP) shunt, 17, 23, 213
  complications, 24–25, 135

ventriculoperitoneal (VP) shunt (*cont.*)
   for hydrocephalus management, 135, 238, 240, 253
vertigo, 3, 12, 244, 288, 295, 296. *See also* Ménière's disease
   in acoustic neuroma, 57
   medication for, 20
   surgical technique for treatment of, 23

vitamin K antagonist (VKA), 31, 40, 291
VKA. *See* vitamin K antagonist
VNS. *See* vagal nerve stimulator
VP shunt. *See* ventriculoperitoneal shunt
VSs. *See* vasospasms
VTE. *See* venous thromboembolism

Wada test, 112, 217
wafers, 62

---

*Note: Numbers that appear in boldface italic denote Practice Exam question numbers and numbers that appear in italic denote Bonus Exam question numbers, the answers and rationales for which appear in Chapter 12 and Chapter 14, respectively.*

www.ingramcontent.com/pod-product-compliance
Ingram Content Group UK Ltd.
Pitfield, Milton Keynes, MK11 3LW, UK
UKHW051849210426
5322IPUK00024B/622